COMMUNICATING SOCIAL CHANGE

Communicating Social Change: Structure, Culture, and Agency explores the use of communication to transform global, national, and local structures of power that create and sustain oppressive conditions. Author Mohan J. Dutta describes the social challenges that exist in current globalization politics, and examines the communicative processes, strategies, and tactics through which social change interventions are constituted in response to the challenges. Using empirical evidence and case studies, he documents the ways through which those in power create conditions at the margins, and he provides a theoretical base for discussing the ways in which these positions of power are resisted through communication processes, strategies, and tactics. The interplay of power and control with resistance is woven through each of the chapters in the book.

This exceptional volume highlights the points of intersection between the theory and praxis of social change communication, creating theoretical entry points for the praxis of social change. It is intended for communication scholars and students studying activism, social movements, and communication for social change, and it will also resonate in such disciplines as development, sociology, and social work, and with those who are studying social transformations.

Mohan J. Dutta is Professor of Communication and Associate Dean for Research and Graduate Education in Liberal Arts at Purdue University, where he teaches and conducts research in international health communication, critical cultural theory, poverty in healthcare, politics of resistance, and public policy and social change. In recognition of his scholarly productivity, Professor Dutta has been recognized as the Lewis Donohew Outstanding Scholar in Health Communication, and as the Lim Chong Yah Professor of Communication and New Media at the National University of Singapore. Currently, he serves as senior editor of the journal *Health Communication*.

COMMUNICATION SERIES
Jennings Bryant / Dolf Zillmann, General Editors

COMMUNICATING SOCIAL CHANGE

Structure, Culture, and Agency

Mohan J. Dutta

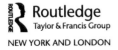

Routledge
Taylor & Francis Group

NEW YORK AND LONDON

First published 2011
by Routledge
711 Third Avenue, New York, NY 10017

Simultaneously published in the UK
by Routledge
2 Park Square, Milton Park, Abingdon, Oxon OX14 4RN

Routledge is an imprint of the Taylor & Francis Group, an informa business

© 2011 Taylor & Francis

Typeset in Bembo by
Keystroke, Station Road, Codsall, Wolverhampton

The right of Mohan J. Dutta to be identified as author of this work has been asserted by him in accordance with sections 77 and 78 of the Copyright, Designs and Patents Act 1988.

Trademark Notice: Product or corporate names may be trademarks or registered trademarks, and are used only for identification and explanation without intent to infringe.

Library of Congress Cataloging-in-Publication Data
Dutta, Mohan J.
Communicating social change: structure, culture, and agency / Mohan J. Dutta.
p. cm.
1. Social change. 2. Communication–Social aspects. I. Title.
HM831.D88 2011
302.2–dc22
2010036231

ISBN: 978–0–415–87873–9 (hbk)
ISBN: 978–0–415–87874–6 (pbk)
ISBN: 978–0–203–83434–3 (ebk)

To Debalina for dreaming a better world together
To Ma for the lessons in dreaming
To Nana for nurturing the seeds of every dream

And for Shloke
So that you may dream!

CONTENTS

PREFACE

Communicating Social Change: Structure, Culture, and Agency describes not only the social challenges constituted in the realm of current globalization politics, but also the communicative processes, strategies, and tactics through which social change interventions are constituted in response to these social challenges. In doing so, the goal of the book is to theorize about the communicative possibilities for transforming global, national, and local structures of power that create and sustain oppressive conditions in various sectors of the globe. Communication is theorized in terms of its transformative capacities in bringing about changes in oppressive political, economic, and social configurations. Based on empirical evidence, each part documents the various ways through which positions of power create conditions at the margins, offering a theoretical base for discussing the ways in which these positions of power are resisted through communication processes, strategies, and tactics in global spaces and in local sites of articulation. The interplay of power and control with resistance is weaved in through each of the chapters in the book.

Communication is situated at the intersections of structure, culture, and agency; these intersections are articulated through examples and case studies presented in each chapter. With the goal of discussing key social challenges and the communication processes, strategies, and tactics mobilized to deal with these challenges, the book is divided into two parts. Part I discusses the key social challenges in the various sectors, focusing on the ways in which marginalization is constituted amidst contemporary globalization politics. Part II builds on the discussions of the social challenges in Part I to articulate the ways in which communication serves as an entry point for transforming the social structures that sustain the inequities reviewed in Part I. Discussions of dialogue, performance, organizing, participation, and mediated processes of social change draw attention to the role of communication in articulating entry points for change. Parts I and II of the book are set up to create points of dialogue with each other, demonstrating the constitutive role of structures and the transformative role of communication. The chapters in Parts I and II are wrapped up by discussions about the pragmatic implications of social change theories in communication. Ultimately, the book points the reader toward various ways in which communication comes to bring about transformations in unequal global structures.

ACKNOWLEDGEMENTS

This book embodies the values that my joint family, Dutta Bari, taught me. I was born in a house of communist teachers, who believed in the value of change, gave their lives to it, and continue to dedicate their passion and energy to the politics of change so that the world may be a better place for those in the margins of society. As I pen this book, joint families in the Indian context are continuing to disappear in the face of the politics of modernization, fragmentation, and development. It is in the face of this onslaught of the images and material interventions of development and modernity that I cherish and will always cherish the life that I grew up amidst, surrounded by the loving care of my mothers and aunts, the politically engaged guidance of my uncles, and the friendships of my brothers and sisters.

It is almost a decade now since my grandmother Nana passed away, but her values of compassion, courage, and political involvement inspire me. Godaikaka and Boro pishi, your teachings and lessons through a life lived in sacrifice continue to model many of the values that found their way into the pages of this book. Pishimoni, your tireless work with Rittwick inspired me to take up the politics and performance of social change. Thank you Baba for the lessons in Marxist theory. You guided me through the works of Marx, Lenin, Engels, Trotsky, and later in life, Howard Zinn and Noam Chomsky. Ma, your love is a pillar of strength and your unshakeable faith an inspiration to always do better than the last time. We are lucky to have your presence in our lives; your endless support, love, and faith saw through the wrapping up of the book. Munna, Tuku, Tattu, Babai, thanks for the arguments, for the many moments of play, and for being my younger siblings. Bordi, Chordi, and Didibhai, thanks for your love. Ria, Rua, and Gulli, each of you are wonderful sources of joy and promises of the future. Thanks also to my maternal uncles and aunts, the Biswas family, for their unfettered love, kindness, and generosity of spirit.

The Banerjee household (my other joint family of thakuma, uncles, aunts, and siblings) adopted me as a son, giving me a loving home in Gauhati, and embracing me amidst their laughter, happiness, and struggles. Thank you Ma (my mother from Gauhati) for your honesty and love, and for always checking on the progress of the book. Baba, your quiet support is an inspiration for us all. Thank you Tito, Bonnie, Shreyoshi, and Amod for loving me as an elder brother.

I am grateful to the Department of Communication at Purdue University and the many faculty and students that have and continue to make Purdue an intellectually stimulating place to be in. I owe my journey to my colleagues and students here at Purdue who continue to inspire through their very high standards of scholarship. The very different ways of looking at the world and engaging with it at Purdue create intellectually enriching experiences, pushing the boundaries of knowledge through debates and conversations.

I would especially like to express my gratitude to my colleague and mentor Patrice Buzzanell for the many conversations, the great food, the love, and the continued support through the many transformations that I have gone through. That change is what makes life worth living, this I have learned from you. I remember that one day Patrice when you told me in your caring way "I see you as an activist." These words continue to inspire me and make me think about the possibilities of my own activism as I engage in my research and writing. I am grateful to Heather Zoller for her critical thoughts and activist politics, Teri Thompson for her continued inspiration, Barbara Sharf for her generous support, and Beverly Sypher for her encouragement. Vicki Biggs has played a pivotal role in the writing of this book by supporting me in my other job as the Director of Graduate Studies at Purdue. Her competent and involved participation in the management of the graduate program ensured that I had enough time to focus on writing the book. Graduate students enrolled in my courses at Purdue have engaged with the ideas presented here, and offered very important feedback through their questions, discussions, and analyses.

I am also grateful to the Communication and New Media program and the Asia Research Institute at the National University of Singapore where I started this project. Special thanks to my friend and colleague Milagros Rivera for her love, kindness, and generosity of spirit.

As a native, the brown man whose agency has at once been historically stripped, whose language has been forever stolen, whose dreams have been forever contaminated with the desire for the colonizer and his way of life, whose imaginations have been forever disrupted violently by the interventions of altruism carried out by the missionaries and later by the modernizers who promised development, and whose voice has been (cons)trained in the phonetics and dictions of the Anglophone world, I have struggled with finding my own agency and situating it amidst the various cultural tropes and criticisms of structures. These struggles have played out through my writings, through my advising, and through my teaching. I thank my sojourners-cum-advisees Debalina Mookerjee, Rebecca DeSouza,

Ambar Basu, Mahuya Pal, Induk Kim, Iccha Basnyat, Chuck Morris, Raven Pfister, Nadine Yehya, Lalatendu Acharya, Raihan Jamil, Shaunak Sastry, Zhuo Ban, Christine Spinetta, Sydney Dillard, Uttaran Dutta, Rahul Rastogi, Rati Kumar, Christina Jones, Min Jiang, Wonjun Chung, Agaptus Anaele, and Soumitro Sen for their courage in treading the difficult terrains of contingent identities, fragmented knowledge claims, and interrupted narratives. Each one of you have taught me in different ways the value of critically interrogating our own privileges as we imagine a socially just world, and struggle to make relevant our own work to this politics of social change. Thanks to my editor Linda Bathgate at Routledge for believing in the project and for working with me on it. Thanks also to Katherine Ghezzi at Routledge for all the assistance with the nuts and bolts of the project.

I thank my wife Debalina for her critical questions that have forced me to rethink many of my own positions, for her courage and persistence, for her strength as a partner, for so many of her sacrifices, and for her faith in me. You have given me the legitimacy through which I speak, write, teach, and learn to dream a better world with you. Thank you for the humor, patience, understanding, friendship, and love that have nurtured this project to fruition. And finally, a heartfelt thanks to Shloke for your patience as the many hours I spent with the computer also meant that you had to sacrifice the many hours of playtime with baba. Your smiles sustained the process of writing this book. Your unconditional love reaffirms in me the faith that alternative rationalities of love, sustenance, and nurturing have much to offer to this world!

Mohan J. Dutta
West Lafayette, IN

INTRODUCTION

Contemporary processes and practices of social change across the globe are situated on the landscape of globalization (Guidry, Kennedy, & Zald, 2000; Pal & Dutta, 2008a, 2008b; Robertson, 1992). Globalization is constituted in the increasing flow of goods, capital, labor and services across national borders; economically, it is defined and marked by *neoliberalism*[1] as the primary political and economic organizing framework for social relations, institutional frameworks, policy-making, and implementation of policies across various sectors of the globe (Dutta, 2009; Ganesh, Zoller, & Cheney, 2005; Harvey, 2005; Pal & Dutta, 2008a, 2008b). As a social, cultural, economic, and political process, it has been marked by the hegemony of the neoliberal logic as the primary organizing framework for constituting relationships among nation states, key political actors in these nation states, non-governmental organizations (NGOs), transnational corporations (TNCs), global policy-making bodies, activist groups, and wider publics in the various sectors of the globe (England & Ward, 2007). The neoliberal logic is fundamentally an economic logic that operates on the basis of the idea that opening up markets to competitions among global corporations accompanied by minimum interventions of the state would ensure the most efficient and effective political economic system. Therefore, proponents of the neoliberal logic argue that the public sectors around the globe ought to be privatized so that these sectors could operate most efficiently and effectively. The advent of the neoliberal logic on the global stage has been marked by the power and control of global organizations such as the international financial institutions (IFIs): World Bank and International Monetary Fund (IMF), as well as the Global Agreement on Trade and Tariffs (GATT), which later evolved into the World Trade Organization (WTO), created with the goals of minimizing the barriers to global trade, and maximizing trading opportunities for transnational corporations (TNCs) across national borders (World Bank 2000a, 2000b, 2000c,

2001). The neoliberal logic of power and control has been and continues to be carried out through the linkages among TNCs, IFIs, the WTO, national governments, and local elites, also referred to as neoliberal hegemony, with a critical role played by the debts doled out by the IFIs as mechanisms for setting up structural adjustment programs in nation states across the globe.

Examining the role of globalization processes dictated by the neoliberal logic across the various sectors of the globe, scholars have observed the increasing inequalities in society, both within nation states as well as across nation states (Millen & Holtz, 2000; Millen, Irwin, & Kim, 2000). Simultaneously, the distribution of communicative spaces and the opportunities to participate in these spaces are unequally distributed, with increasing gaps in access to communicative infrastructures between the rich and the poor (Dutta, 2008c, 2009; Dutta & Pal, 2010; Kim, 2008; Pal & Dutta, 2008a, 2008b). These disparities have been observed within local spaces, within nation states, as well as across the various sectors of the globe. Of particular interest here is the increasing marginalization of the poorer sectors of the globe with limited access to material resources as well as to platforms for articulating their voices (Dutta, 2008c, 2009; Dutta-Bergman, 2004a, 2004b; Pal & Dutta, 2008a, 2008b). Marginalization here refers to the continued construction of a group, class, sector at the bottom of a social system, with no access or limited access to the basic resources for living. The markers of marginalization vary widely, including categories such as class, caste, race, gender, nationality of origin, and sexual orientation, although almost all forms of marginalization carry an economic logic with them with the emphasis on the lack of access to basic resources. The question of the margins has become of increasing interest to contemporary scholars as globalization processes have participated in creating these margins and sustaining them, often operating on the basis of violence to delegitimize the rights of the communities at the margins (Dutta, 2009; Dutta & Pal, 2010; Farmer, 2003; Millen et al., 2000). For instance, under the name of structural adjustment programs and development initiatives, collective lands belonging to indigenous people worldwide are being usurped for the purposes of developing mining projects, hydroelectric projects, manufacturing plants and so on. In the state of Orissa in India, the state-sponsored Operation Greenhunt is utilizing police and military violence to thwart tribal resistance to projects of mining and industrialization in the region (Padhi, Pradhan, & Manjit, 2010). Similar stories of state-enacted violence against local resistance are also evident in the Andean-region countries of Ecuador, Peru, Bolivia, Colombia, and Venezuela (Burt & Mauceri, 2004).

Of interest to communication scholars are opportunities for engaging with these margins with the goal of creating spaces for listening to the margins, as well as for creating possibilities for transforming the globalization processes that continually participate in the creation of the margins, and in the enactment of violence on the margins (Dutta, 2008c, 2009; Dutta & Pal, 2010; Kim & Dutta, 2009). For the purposes of this book, we will engage with those margins of contemporary societies that are systematically erased from dominant discursive spaces of knowledge production. Even as the increasing power and control in the hands of neoliberal hegemony are carrying out the exploitation of the subaltern sectors,[2] communicative processes and practices of change are being articulated among the subaltern spaces in the midst of these very structures. These spaces across the globe demonstrate the ways in which communicative practices of social change are enacted in combination with material practices to disrupt the oppressive and exploitative structures of neoliberalism (Pal & Dutta, 2008b). The overall purpose of this book is to understand these practices of social change at the margins that seek to disrupt dominant structures and bring about transformations in these structures. The culture-centered approach reviewed in the book as an organizing framework for understanding social change communication departs from the dominant approaches to communication for social change by fundamentally noting the capacity of marginalized communities to consciously and strategically participate in processes of change that are meaningful to them (Basu & Dutta, 2008a, 2008b; Desmarais, 2007; Dutta, 2008c; Reed, 2005; Stolle-McAllister, 2005). The resistive possibilities of social change communication presented here will be situated in the backdrop of and in conversation with the dominant articulations of social change communication that are evident in the mainstream literature on development communication (Lerner, 1967, 1968; Melkote & Steeves, 2001; Rogers, 1962, 1973, 1974, 1983).

The definition of communicating social change advocated here is built upon the primary idea that social change reflects some form of change in the traditional forms of organizing and conceptualizing organizational processes, commitments, and philosophies (Dutta & Pal, 2010; Kim, 2008; Pal, 2008; Reed, 2005). Essential to the idea of social change therefore is the construction of departures from the accepted configuration in society, as a process that departs from the mainstream, and furthermore, as a process that challenges the hegemony of the mainstream. The mainstream or dominant configuration is the status quo that reflects the interests of the dominant actors in society, maintaining and propagating the goals of these dominant actors. In the contemporary global scenario, communicative processes in the mainstream are constituted with the goals of maintaining the interests of the power elite, and continuing to reinforce the increasing class differentials within the neoliberal framework (Dutta, 2009; Dutta & Pal, 2010). These existing processes, commitments, and philosophies of dominant actors are situated within the rules, roles, and goals of structures. Structures here refer to ways of organizing institutional processes and resources that enable or constrain access to resources. Social change, therefore, is conceptualized in the context of the goals of communicative process, strategies and tactics directed at changing these structures in contemporary globalization that are primarily driven by the neoliberal logic. It is on the basis of the principle of transformation in social structures that the culture-centered approach is proposed as an organizing principle for engaging with the communicative processes, strategies and tactics that lie at the heart of contemporary efforts of social change (Basu & Dutta, 2008a, 2008b; Dutta, 2008c, 2009; Dutta & Pal, 2010; Kim & Dutta, 2009). For example, the World Social Forums (WSF) have emerged as popular sites of resistive politics against neoliberalism, bringing together over 5,000 activists from 117 countries at the first WSF meeting in Porto Alegre, Brazil in 2001, and increasing that number to 155,000 activists from 135 countries by the 2005 meeting (Moghadam, 2009). The WSF are an exemplar of participatory consciousness of local collectives, communities and networks as they articulate alternate values and principles of organizing in their dialogic engagement at global sites. The ultimate goal of this book is to offer a framework for understanding communicative principles of resistance set on the canvas of the articulations of local, national, and global structures that continue to perpetuate inequities, injustices, and silences across the globe. Attending to the ways in which marginalized communities across the globe participate in processes of structural transformation, the book documents various instances of culture-centered processes of social change communication against the backdrop of globalization that are directed at creating points of access and justice for the poor, underserved, and marginalized sectors of the globe.

Theoretical Trajectory

Situated on the foundations of postcolonial and subaltern studies theories, the culture-centered approach to communication is committed to the goals of transformative politics through the enunciation of the marginalizing processes in global hegemonic structures and through the creation of dialogic possibilities for engaging with the voices at the margins that stand in resistance to the neo-liberal policies that perpetuate inequalities and the marginalization of the poor (Cousineau, 2009). The culture-centered approach proposes a paradigm shift in the theorizing of communication for social change by recognizing and foregrounding the agency of the subaltern sectors in participating in processes of social change and structural transformation (Dutta, 2006, 2007, 2008a, 2008b, 2008c; Dutta-Bergman, 2004a, 2004b). Dialogues with the margins create entry points for multiple counter-hegemonies that simultaneously seek to transform the hegemony of the neoliberal logic through a wide range of communicative practices and processes, and narrate the stories of resistance in the subaltern sectors that are directed toward disrupting the dominant structures of exploitation and oppression (Blaser, Feit, & McRae, 2004; Bradshaw & Linneker, 2001; Brecher, Costello, & Smith, 2000). The culture-centered approach engages with the questions of structures and the ways in which these structures constitute the margins, and simultaneously seeks to challenge the structures through a wide range of communicative practices. On one hand, the culture-centered approach enters into the discursive spaces of transformative politics by deconstructing the marginalizing processes and practices of neoliberal hegemony; on the other hand, it participates in co-constructive possibilities for listening to the voices of the groups at the margins and narrates the stories of subaltern resistance that are directed toward transforming structures. The communicative lens adopted in this book articulates the goals of the culture-centered approach to communication for social change in participating in transformative politics for challenging global structures of inequity.

Postcolonial Theory

With its emphasis on interrogating the structures of colonialism and neocolonialism that continue to circulate through dominant discursive spaces, postcolonial theory explores the intersections of discursive representations, economic interests and forms of control in global spaces (Dutta, 2009; Shome & Hegde, 2002). Postcolonial studies, as a field of inquiry, not only seeks to understand the processes underlying colonization, but also is committed to an emancipatory politics that attempts to undo these processes of colonization; it is fundamentally transformative in seeking to alter those knowledge structures that erase the stories of violence inherent in global neocolonial configurations and create spaces for listening to the voices of the subaltern sectors of the globe. Connecting the histories and geographies of colonialism with the project of modernity and modern knowledge structures, postcolonial scholarship attempts to "redo such epistemic structures by writing against them, over them, and from below them by inviting reconnections to obliterated presents that never made their way into the history of knowledge" (Shome & Hegde, 2002, p. 250). The deconstructive move in the postcolonial approach creates openings for disciplinary transformations through the interrogation of the taken-for-granted assumptions in West-centric productions of knowledge (Broadfoot & Munshi, 2007; Dutta-Bergman, 2005a, 2005b; Mosse, 2001; Munshi & Kurian, 2007; Pal & Dutta, 2008a, 2008b). One of the key threads of the postcolonial approach to communicative processes is in its examination of colonial discourses that circulate and reify the material inequities across the globe (Dutta, 2009).

This transformative impulse of postcolonial studies is reflected in Gayatri Spivak's (1999) interrogation of the colonial histories and geographies of disciplinary structures and institutional knowledge that constitute the Anglo-European academy. Her work helps locate communication theory in the realm of the neocolonial politics of globalization processes, the formations of the new world order, dialogic opportunities with marginalized communities that are erased by the dominant economic logics of globalization, and the possibilities of transformative politics in the context of globalization processes (Spivak, 1999). Furthermore, her scholarship has charted an intellectual trajectory that covers feminist deconstruction, Marxist critiques of international divisions of labor and the global flow of capital, critiques of imperial and colonial discourses, and critiques of race in the context of the intersections among nationality, ethnicity, and the politics of representation in a neocolonial world (Landry & MacLean, 1996). Applying the postcolonial lens to the project of social change calls for a deconstructive turn in theorizing that attends to the mobilization of knowledge for the purposes of serving the material inequities of neocolonialism. For instance, in his deconstruction of the democracy promotion, civil society, and nation-building initiatives sponsored by the United States, Dutta-Bergman (2005a, 2005b) demonstrates the ways in which the language of democracy is utilized in order to co-opt participatory spaces, erase subaltern voices of resistance, and enact control over Third World spaces in opening them up to foreign capital and as markets for TNCs.[3] Similarly, Dutta and Pal (2010) note the ways in which the language of public diplomacy and dialogue are utilized in order to hide the agendas of power and control enacted by TNCs in conjunction with powerful nation states at the center.

In situating the scholarship of communication for social change in the realm of postcolonial studies, this book responds to the call issued by Raka Shome and Radha Hegde (2002), who suggest the imminent need for communication theorizing that locates communication processes in the realm of the historical and geographical contexts of postcolonial politics, and explores the intersections between communication and postcoloniality in the realm of the relationships among nation states in the geopolitical landscape. It demonstrates that communication scholars are particularly well suited to interrogate the communicative practices that connect transnational corporations, nation states, and global structures, and offer strategies and concepts for engaging postcolonial studies in communication theorizing and practice. Dutta (2009) notes that the application of postcolonial theory to projects of social change move beyond the discursive turn in postcolonial theory that foregrounds identity politics in the realm of the subjective to investigating and interrupting the discourses of neocolonialism that continue to operate across the globe in economic and material terms, continuing to enact and deepen class differentials within geospatial configurations. Although global corporations emerge as centers of power in the global landscape, they continue to exert their influence through the geographical dominance of the nation states at the center that continue to serve as the sites of operation and influence of these corporations. For instance, the environmental policies that regulate the operation of transnational petrochemicals play out within the landscape of the nation state, being subjected to national policies and specific policy-based stances of nation states such as the United States at sites of global policy-making. Even as postcolonial scholars draw attention to concepts such as hybrid identities and fragmented sites of power, Dutta (2009) notes the importance of returning to the concept of the nation state as a vital entry point for the enactment of hegemonic discourses and practices of material exploitation and oppression that operate on the foundations of geographic differentials in positions of access to power. Ultimately, then, our adoption of postcolonial theory for the purposes of understanding and engaging in communicative processes of social change is contingent upon the exploration of the linkages between postcolonial theorizing and the materialities of global oppression and exploitation.

Subaltern Studies Theory

Subaltern studies theory emphasizes writing history from below, seeking to invert the dominant epistemic structures that write the narratives of history from the vantage points of dominant social actors and erase the narratives of those sectors that are constituted at the margins of the margins (Guha, 2001; Spivak, 1988). Guha (1981) depicts subalternity in the realm of subordination in terms of "class, caste, age, gender and office or in any other way," attending to the violent erasures that are constituted at the complex intersections of the fragmented and intersecting identifiers. Situating itself amidst a complex critique of modernity, the subaltern studies project attends to the erasure of the subaltern participant, as she gets constituted within discourse and within its legal–political structures. The project is interested in exploring the roots of material and discursive erasure, and therefore, is particularly relevant for theorizing of communication for social change as it offers insights into the ways in which the margins are created and erased, and simultaneously offers an entry point for listening to the voices at the margins. It is on the framework of these margins that cultural communities enact their ability to challenge their marginalization and envision possibilities of social change by imaging alternative worlds (Dutta, 2009). The foundations of subaltern studies theorizing are guided by the desire to rewrite the narratives that constitute the discursive spaces of history by listening to locally situated voices that have been systematically erased (Dutta, 2007, 2008a, 2008b, 2008c, 2009). Interrogating the absences and erasures in dominant epistemic structures, the subaltern studies project deconstructs the narrativizing of history, asking questions such as: Whose stories are circulated in the dominant epistemic structures? What are the agendas and desires that get constituted in these stories? And in the telling of the stories from certain classed, raced, gendered standpoints, what are the narratives that get erased from the discursive spaces of knowledge construction?

Therefore, the subaltern studies project seeks to create alternative discursive spaces that challenge the hegemony of the mainstream (Guha, 1981). The very essence of writing history from below is to challenge the dominant constructions of knowledge, with specific focus on that which is left out of such dominant constructions. It is in asking this question of what is left out that the project engages with questions of agendas, motives, and interests, interrogating the overarching goals of dominant epistemic and ontological structures. Subaltern studies is concerned with the condition of being erased from the dominant discursive spaces and from the dominant narratives of knowledge (Guha, 1981, 1983). The project introduced questions of voice and access in contesting the dominant constructions of knowledge and the political economic functions of such knowledge in maintaining the status quo. Situating the mainstream knowledge as subject of inquiry, it demonstrated how such knowledge continues to serve positions of power and maintain social structures that sustain the conditions of marginality enacted in the realms of race, class, gender, caste, nationality, occupation, and position within the social structure. The interrogation of erasures in dominant discourses then creates spaces for dialogues with subaltern communities. The objective of the subaltern studies project is to document the historiography of the people by documenting their agency and politics, which had always been left out of dominant discursive spaces of knowledge. The appeal of the subaltern studies project is captured by Said (1988) in the foreword of the book *Selected subaltern studies*, co-edited by Guha and Spivak:

> As an alternative discourse then, the work of the Subaltern scholars can be seen as an analogue of all those recent attempts in the West and throughout the rest of the world to articulate the hidden or suppressed accounts of numerous groups—women, minorities, disadvantaged or disposed groups, refugees, exiles, etc. . . . This is another way of underlining the concern with politics and power.

Its interjection with issues of power makes subaltern studies a paradigm that radically challenges modernist epistemologies and monolithic notions of modernity. Evident is the influence of postcolonial thinking in subaltern studies (Prakash, 1994; Beverley, 2001).

Because the effort of the subaltern scholars is to recover the history of the marginalized "other" against the institutionalized system of knowledge constructed by the West and the national elite in postcolonial states, it becomes a critique of the dominant system of knowledge production itself, legitimized by the West. At the same time it is postmodern as it endeavors to bring about "epistemological rupture" (Beverley, 2001, p. 15) or what Lyotard regards as interrupting grand metanarratives. Dynamic in its multidisciplinarity, subaltern studies allows for studies in different colonial situations. Though it relies on postcolonialism, it is distinct in its scholarly inquiry as it is not only invested in documenting the record of colonial domination, but in tracking the "[subaltern] positions that could not be properly recognized and named" (Prakash, 1994, p. 1486). Hence, it is a study to "displace the question of power" (Prakash, 1994, p. xvi) from the elitist agenda by drawing attention to the "other." The project of communicating for social change offered in this book envisions communicative processes that interrupt the erasures in mainstream discourses of development, and engage with subaltern voices in seeking spaces for transformative politics and redistributive justice.

Culture-Centered Approach

The culture-centered approach concerns itself with the voices of marginalized groups and explores the interaction between culture and structure that create conditions of marginality (Dutta, 2008a, 2008b, 2008c, 2009; Dutta-Bergman, 2004a, 2004b). Structures are the institutional frameworks, ways of organizing, rules and roles in mainstream society that constrain and enable access to resources. Culture is defined in terms of the local contexts, frameworks of meaning making and interpretation, and spaces of shared meanings, values, and interactions (Dutta, 2008c). The interactions between the continuous and dynamic elements of culture provide the context for cultural meanings that are in flux (Dutta, 2008c). It is through the expression, interpretation, and reinterpretation of culturally circulated meanings that individuals and communities enact their agency. Agency here taps into the fundamental human capacity to enact choices in negotiating structures (Basu & Dutta, 2008a, 2008b; Dutta, 2008a, 2008b, 2008c; Dutta & Basu, 2008). The culture-centered approach, at its heart, recognizes the agency of subaltern communities in negotiating structures and in seeking spaces of change (Dutta-Bergman, 2004a, 2004b). The philosophy here is writing theory from below, and defining praxis through the engagement with subaltern classes who have traditionally been marginalized and absent in dominant theories and models. The culture-centered approach engages with these silences and absences and generates meanings through a participatory framework.

According to Dutta (2008c), power is differentially distributed and determines the nature and content of the dominant discourses, which, in turn, support the dominant positions of power, a view that is often ignored by the dominant models of communication theorizing. Although power is fragmented and is played out at multiple sites, it is also rooted in material realities (Dutta, 2008c, 2009). Therefore, critiquing the discursive turn in the dominant literature on critical approaches in communication, the culture-centered approach emphasizes the relevance of attending to the material realities of control and resistance. As noted by Cloud (2005), the realm of the symbolic is constrained by and contingent upon the exigencies in the realm of the material. It is therefore in this domain of material inequities that the culture-centered approach proposes the necessity of discursive deconstruction. Discourses are approached in terms of their relationship to the material, attending to the ways in which they perpetuate material inequities. Therefore, the culture-centered approach interrogates the circulation of dominant discourses to serve the agendas of the dominant political and economic actors within social systems, simultaneously perpetuating the exploitation of the poorer classes (Dutta & Pal, 2010). For instance, Chevron (a petrochemical TNC based in the United States) utilizes its material access to dominant sites and spaces of power to delegitimize and downplay the negative health effects of the oil spills caused by the operation of Chevron in Ecuador (Sawyer, 2006). The discursive strategy of delegitimizing the claims of the subaltern sectors in a weaker nation state (Ecuador) is achieved through the claims of scientific expertise, corruption, and fabrication in the Third World, downplaying of Third World subaltern agency and accusations of falsification within the dominant discursive spaces of public relations, crisis management, and legal communications that are traditionally accessible to Chevron. It is against this backdrop of material inequity in the politics of representation in communicative and juridical frameworks that the culture-centered approach explores avenues for organizing in the subaltern sectors such that alternative subaltern discourses can be heard in achieving material transformations (in this case, getting Chevron to pay and clean up the oil spills in Ecuador). The materiality of the practices of TNCs needs to be interrogated in the backdrop of the dominant discourses of "corporate social responsibility" and "sustainability" that are often used by TNCs to hide their agendas of profiteering by the exploitation of the subaltern sectors (Cloud, 2007; Dutta & Pal, 2010; Munshi & Kurian, 2007).

Therefore, the culture-centered approach takes critical thinking to the next level by its emphasis on disenfranchised communities that exist on the peripheries of the dominant system with the goal of disrupting the marginalization of the underserved sectors. What sets apart the culture-centered approach from the discursive approaches to power is its singular interest in understanding those conditions at the margins that have limited access to basic resources. Building upon its roots in subaltern studies (Beverley, 2004a, 2004b; Guha 1981, 2001; Prakash, 1992; Rodríguez, 2001; Said, 1988; Spivak, 1999) and further extending the postmodern thread in subaltern studies to material contexts, the culture-centered approach centralizes listening to subaltern voices that traditionally remain outside the mainstream discursive spaces, arguing that the silencing of the subaltern is deeply intertwined with her oppression in the hands of local, national, and global power structures (Dutta, 2008a, 2008b, 2008c). Therefore, one of the fundamental steps toward resisting the oppression of the subaltern sectors lies in creating points of listening to subaltern voices, where subaltern voices could be heard in meaningful ways that matter to policy-making, implementation of policies, and evaluation of policies (Dutta-Bergman, 2004a, 2004b). For instance, Pal's (2008) ethnography with the farmers of Singur, West Bengal, explored the resistive practices and spaces of agency enacted by farmers who were threatened with eviction by a car manufacturing project. Similarly, Kim's (2008) co-constructive journey with the farmer activists in Korea demonstrated the active ways in which farmers and their families mobilize locally, nationally, and globally to challenge unfair global policies. In doing so, this approach draws attention to the voices on the periphery and aims to disrupt the Eurocentric notion of what constitutes as strategic communicative practices in the mainstream such as corporate social responsibility, crisis management, and public relations that adopt a predominantly managerial perspective.

The emphasis, therefore, is on interrogating the dominant practices of communication for the ways in which they create and sustain conditions at the margins, and on creating spaces of transformation by documenting the ways in which these dominant practices are resisted in marginalized communities. The culture-centered approach necessitates working from within, where cultural members actively participate in defining problems and developing solutions. Therefore, from the standpoint of theorizing communication for social change, the culture-centered approach provides an opening for an epistemic shift in our understanding of what counts as social change communication and what ought to be studied under the purview of communication for social change. Through its discursive engagement with subaltern communities that have hitherto been erased, it resists the dominant discourse of managerial communication (in organizational communication, public relations as well as development communication) by introducing alternative discourses and meaning structures. By bringing forth alternative possibilities that have otherwise been silenced, it creates opportunities for transformative politics, or, more precisely, openings for social change. Central to the participatory process in the culture-centered approach is the interaction between culture, structure, and agency that contributes to the co-construction of meanings by cultural members of a community. These co-constructed meanings offer entry points for transformative politics directed at bringing about shifts in material structures.

Culture

In the culture-centered approach, culture is a complex web of meanings that is always in a state of flux (Dutta, 2007, 2008a, 2008b, 2008c). Dynamic in character, culture is always shifting as it continually interacts with structure, and is constituted through the interactions among cultural participants. The global and local economic and political shifts influence structure, which, in turn, informs culture. Culture gets articulated in the local as the cultural members of the community co-construct meanings of their lives within the local context. Hence, culture can be defined as the communicative process by which shared meanings, beliefs, and practices get produced (Geertz, 1994). It is a shared experience that is central to living and communicating for social groups. Culture is the strongest framework for providing the context of life that shapes knowledge creation, perceptions, sharing of meanings, and behavior changes.

Engaging with culturally situated voices creates a discursive opening for interrogating the ways in which organizational and public relations strategies serving dominant social structures are interpreted, co-constructed and resisted by marginalized publics. In this realm, it is particularly relevant to listen to the discursively constituted spaces in which the local contexts are negotiated by cultural members. Such an outlook on locally situated activist politics is quite distinct from the situational theory of publics in the mainstream communication literature (Grunig & Hunt, 1984, p. 148), which posits that "communication behaviors of publics can best be understood by measuring how members of publics perceive situations in which they are affected by such organizational consequences." Situational theory suggests classifying individuals in relation to the awareness and level of concern about a particular problem. According to Grunig and Hunt (1984), three independent variables—problem recognition, constraint recognition, and level of involvement by the publics—can be used to predict the extent to which publics will seek and process information about that particular situation. Though situational theory turns the lens toward the publics, the theory is driven by the emphasis to benefit the organization, where publics can be predicted and controlled to fulfill the interests of the organization.

But the culture-centered approach departs from a unidirectional flow of communication and raises critical questions. How do the dominant practices of mainstream organizations within social systems become meaningful to cultural members? What are the ways in which these practices are resisted? How do local contexts inform the meanings articulated in the realm of resistive strategies used by marginalized publics? How do these locally enunciated contexts challenge the dominant national and global structures, and the policies that are promoted by these structures? Attending to locally situated discourses and practices through which marginalized community members challenge dominant discourses and structures creates an alternative entry point for communication scholarship.

Structure and Agency

Structures refer to the material reality as defined by policies and institutional networks that privilege certain sections of the population and marginalize others by constraining the availability of resources. Structures define and limit the possibilities that are available to participants as they enact agency to engage in practices that influence their health and well being. At a macro-level, structure refers to resources such as national and international political actors, points of policy formulation, and national and global corporations that work in tandem with the structure at a micro level. The emphasis in the culture-centered approach is to gain a sense of understanding of these structures that limit the possibilities of resources for members of a community. From a communicative standpoint, the emphasis is on understanding the communicative practices that serve the interests of the dominant structures. For instance, a culture-centered examination of public relations theorizing and strategizing in the wake of Hurricane Katrina examines the ways in which the public relations strategies of the Federal Emergency Management Agency (FEMA) maintained the status quo, and simultaneously silenced the voices of the displaced people of New Orleans (see Kim & Dutta, 2009). In post-crisis New Orleans, federal aid to rebuilding and restructuring programs was phrased within the dictates of the neoliberal ideology, turning the city into a neoliberal experiment (Kim & Dutta, 2009). Similarly, critical interrogations of dominant organization practices demonstrate that the organizational emphasis on participatory processes, democratic decision-making, and empowerment emerge as ways of exploiting workers, as more and more work is placed on workers (Cloud, 2007). In her critical analysis of participatory empowerment discourse at the workplace, Cloud (2007, p. 223) regards the "implementation of participatory lean production models as ideological mystifications of class antagonism," thus seeking to blur the lines between the oppositional interests of employers and workers. A culture-centered analysis of the public relations literature addressing crisis response in the aftermath of 9/11, for instance, would interrogate the ways in which the voices of marginalized communities within the United States (such as Muslim minorities) were silenced within the discursive frame.

Similar analysis of dominant messages and campaigns may also be applied to non-profit sectors where efforts are often driven by so-called altruistic reasons (Dutta-Bergman, 2005b). For instance, in the case of the *Santalis*, an indigenous community that resides in multiple pockets in eastern India, Dutta-Bergman (2004a, 2004b) locates poverty as a barrier to this community's search for and articulations of health, thus challenging the campaign strategies of dominant global social actors in the health arena that frame health risks as products of individual behaviors. The author notes: "Marked by the very essence of poverty, hunger is an integral part of Santali life and remains a primary impediment to the achievement of good health" (Dutta-Bergman, 2004a, p. 11). Subsequently, food, or the lack of it, and the overriding need to find food for the family takes precedence over accessing even the marginal health services available to the communities.

Hence, the study among the *Santalis* indicates that not only is it is the structure that determines the meanings for marginalized groups, but also policies mostly disregard the needs of the marginalized, thereby creating structural barriers for them. While structures limit the possibilities of health among *Santalis*, agency is enacted in its interaction with the structures and embodies communicative actions that negotiate these structures. For instance, the structural barriers faced by the *Santalis* informs their culture, where they prioritize accessing food over health. In doing so, *Santalis* enact agency. Agency is explained as the capacity of human beings to engage with structures that encompass their lives, to make meanings through this engagement, and at the same time, creating discursive openings to transform these structures.

Dutta (2008c) locates agency at its interaction with culture and structure. For instance, in the case of Hurricane Katrina, scholarly explorations of agency co-construct narratives with displaced communities that articulate the ways in which the dominant structures were interpreted and the ways in which the communities mobilized to secure resources and to resist the marginalization they faced in the wake of the crisis (Kim & Dutta, 2009). This line of thinking foregrounds the importance of understanding articulations of meanings by engaging participant voices at the local level (Dutta-Bergman, 2004a), which present opportunities for social change by challenging the dominant articulations of social reality and cultural and behavioral norms. It is important to note that structures that frame the lives of marginalized communities operate at multiple levels and that these micro-, meso-, and macro-levels are interdependent and mutually reifying. Foregrounding these structural factors as realities in the lives of marginalized people, the culture-centered approach situates the margin in the realm of the agendas of neoliberal politics, and centers the margin as the site of global processes of social change by listening to the voices of those communities that have historically been erased from platforms of academic enunciation and policy-making.

Margins of the Globe

The key issues around which the margins have been constituted also offer the bases for organizing at the margins; some of these issues are poverty, agriculture, hunger, indigenous rights, health, environmental pollution, and issues of gender. Each of these issues at the margins is defined in the backdrop of the agendas of neoliberal politics and the ways in which these agendas have constructed the margins, determining the political, social, and economic landscapes on which the material experiences of loss and erasure have been constituted. At the heart of the creation and reification of the margins are the ideologies of neoliberal hegemony that operate on the basis of the politics of power and control in contemporary epistemic structures, and the ways in which these politics of power and control disenfranchise certain sectors of society (Dutta, 2008c; Dutta & Pal, 2010; Pal & Dutta, 2008a, 2008b).

The political economy of the neoliberal project plays out in a broad range of discourses around the globe, reiterating itself through academe to policy circuits to the media to popular culture (Dutta, 2009; Dutta & Pal, 2010; Pal & Dutta, 2008a, 2008b). The intersections of the symbolic and the material demonstrate the ways in which discourse constitutes material inequities, justifying the poverty and silences at the margins of contemporary mainstream political economies. The silences of the subaltern sectors in neoliberal policy structures are deeply intertwined with the marginalizing policies that are developed through these structures. We begin by reviewing the core principles of neoliberal politics and the ways in which these principles have been played out in the areas of poverty, hunger, agriculture, indigenous groups, health, and gender. In each of these areas, we explore the intersections of the symbolic and the material, engaging with the politics of dominant structures in global, national, and local pubic spheres that play out the interests of the status quo, simultaneously erasing the questions and concerns of the poor, raced, classed subaltern subject.

Neoliberal Politics

Neoliberalism is fundamentally an economic principle that constitutes the opening up of global markets to corporations that operate across the boundaries of nation states, the minimization of state interventions in the operation of the market, and the increasing privatization of public sectors that are brought under the framework of the free market logic (Harvey, 2005). Markets and privatization are assumed to be the natural order, and this order is accomplished through minimal state intervention (Meur, 2000). Based on the principles of freedom and individual-level liberty, neoliberal theory argues that unregulated markets will optimally regulate social outcomes and will ultimately lead to the most effective use of society's resources (Friedman, 1962). The political-economic idea that lies at the heart of neoliberalism is that human development can be best achieved through the freeing of the human entrepreneurial capacity achieved through private property rights, free market, and free trade (Harvey, 2005; Irwin & Kim, 2000; Dutta & Pal, 2010). Neoliberals place faith in the market, not only as a mechanism for achieving the most productive distribution of resources, but also as a mechanism for regulating social problems (Friedman, 1962; Shakow & Irwin, 2000). Shakow and Irwin (2000) observe:

> To keep price levels stable, neoliberals advocate strict limits on public spending, particularly social spending. Reduced government social spending, they claim, brings many benefits. It checks inflation, promotes private initiative and investment, and creates powerful incentives for poor people to work rather than remain dependent on public resource.
>
> *(p. 54)*

Therefore, inherent in the fundamental tenets of neoliberalism is the reduction in state support for the marginalized sectors of society and the minimization of socially directed programs that are directed at meeting the needs of poor and the underserved. Simultaneously, rather than focusing on the unemployment rates within the state, the emphasis of the state is shifted to minimizing inflation, irrespective of the consequences to unemployment (Harvey, 2005). The privatization of resources and deregulation of the economy are accompanied by the uses of state power to minimize collective capacities of unions and associations to bargain for labor rights and minimum wages, negatively impacting both employment rates as well as minimum wages of workers. The state enacts a wide variety of measures of violence in order to ensure safe and secure spaces for the working of corporations.

The Western ideals of liberty and freedom are drawn out as metaphorical equivalences to guide the moral imperative to free the market under neoliberalism (Friedman, 1962). For example, Shakow and Irwin (2000) note that the languages of freedom and liberty often get played out in the articulations of neoliberalism among economic experts, policy makers, and political leaders. It is precisely this language of freedom and liberty situated amidst Western ideals that takes center-stage in powerful policy circles, academic circles, and think tanks such as the Monte Perlin Society that included the Austrian political philosopher Friedrich von Hayek, the economist Milton Friedman, and the noted philosopher Karl Popper. However, Shakow and Irwin point out that the brand of freedom positioned under neoliberalism is tied to a specific mechanism for controlling and managing the global markets within the interests of TNCs, maintained and negotiated under specific international legislation and commercial agreements that are dictated by the needs of TNCs and are carried out through the participation of nation states in global policy circles. On an international scale, Harvey (2005) delineates the linkage between neoliberalism and neoimperialism, noting that for the US, creating markets abroad for its capital, goods, and services, also often came in the way of exerting direct and indirect forms of control ranging from the support of local coups in the name of democracy promotion (Dutta-Bergman, 2005; Harvey, 2005) to covert violence against popular movements such as in the example of Chile to direct imperial invasion in the form of the most recent invasion of Iraq (Harvey, 2005). The US government in these cases worked hand-in-hand with the local elites in shaping policies that were supportive of US capital and investments, and more broadly, in favor of neoliberal reform abroad. In the example of Chile, the undermining of the populist Allende government worked hand-in-hand with the setting up of a neoliberal agenda by placing US-trained economists in key decision-making positions, accompanied by the support for local business elites in Chile who had tremendous gains to make from the flow of foreign capital into the country. Similarly, the invasion of Iraq was a precursor to the setting up of a neo-liberal state under the leadership of Paul Bremer, head of the Coalition Provisional Authority, carried out through the privatization of public enterprises and resources, the opening up of Iraq's banks to foreign control, the full repatriation of foreign capital, and the elimination of trade barriers, thus turning Iraq into a 'capitalist dream regime' (Harvey, pp. 6-7). The US imperial occupation of Iraq therefore was the precursor to the top-down pushing of neoliberal agendas on Iraq and to the shaping of the Iraqi economic policies to serve the interests of TNCs. Further-more, once wars and invasions have been carried out, large-scale projects of restricting and rebuilding the nation state open up new doors of operation for funding agencies and international aids, further creating domains of profiteering for TNCs and, to a smaller extent, the local elite. For example, a major proportion of the aid for rebuilding Iraq disappeared. In each of these cases, in carrying out the goals of neoliberal restructurings of nation state, the US sponsored large-scale com-munication programs in the name of media restructuring, community relations, civil society building, and nation building (Dutta-Bergman, 2005a, 2005b). Large funds became available to communication researchers and practitioners, for example, to create media relations and community relations activities that were directed at building nation states that would be aligned with the political, geostrate-gic, and most importantly, economic interests of the United States and its TNCs.

Neoliberalism operates through the principles of the market as a govern-ing mechanism on the global scale. Therefore, essential to neoliberalism are the workings and agendas of global corporations that operate across the boundaries of nation states, with the goal of increasing the penetration and reach of global corporations within and across nation states such that the development and industrialization policies of nation states are configured within the dictates and interests of global corporations. These corporations are referred to as transnational corporations (TNCs). The opening up of nation states to foreign capital, and the products and services of TNCs is achieved through the structural adjustment programs and conditional debts issued by international financial institutions such as the World Bank and the International Monetary Fund. The TNCs operate in conjunction with the nation states at the center (United States and UK predominantly) to dictate the policies and scope of the IFIs, and subsequently network with the IFIs to exert various forms of persuasive and coercive tactics (including bribery, sponsoring and supporting coups, and financially supporting pro-free market national elites) on nation states across the globe to force these states to open up to foreign investment and products marketed by TNCs (Griffin, 2009; Payer, 1974). Neoliberalism operates through the interweaving relationships among transnational power brokers and local elites, with the goal of creating and opening up markets for multinational and transnational corporations across nation states, even as the power to shape neoliberal policies is exercised through the political powers of the nation state (for instance, note the historic relationship of the United States with the World Bank and WTO). The nation state on one hand gets situated within the broader political agendas of TNCs that dictate the extent of participation of the nation state in market economics and market reform; on the other hand, it is through the political participation of the nation state in shaping global policies that the neoliberal program is carried out.

As noted by Harvey (2005), neoliberalism operates as a political and economic configuration that achieves its hegemony through the foregrounding of the logic of property rights, free market, and free trade as the universal markers of relationships among global actors. In foregrounding the logic of free trade, neoliberal discourse continually erases the material markers of global inequities perpetuated by the large-scale global adoption of neoliberal policies (Irwin & Kim, 2000). The structural adjustment programs, for instance, impose specific liberalization mandates on nation states and constrain the subsidies and incentives that are often offered to the local industries, thus creating unequal competitions in the global market and resulting in the large-scale consolidation of markets in the hands of TNCs. Even as neoliberal reforms are imposed on developing and underdeveloped nations with minimal resources, the language of such reforms omits the highly protectionist economic strategies used within the powerful imperial configurations (such as the United States) to support local industries, particularly during the developmental phase of these industries (such as the information technology sector in its developmental years). Structural adjustment programs imposed on the Third World in the domain of agriculture have led to increasing consolidation of lands in the hands of TNCs, which then has fostered large-scale inequities and food insecurities by undermining the local agricultural sectors and livelihoods of small-scale local farmers. Trade-related intellectual property rights (TRIPS) imposed by the WTO have consolidated knowledge in the hands of global power structures, often facilitating the exploitation of indigenous resources and knowledge bases in the hands of TNCs on the basis of their inequitable access to juridical structures and legal processes. Indigenous forms of knowledge and resources have been turned into exploitable commodities, thus erasing the access to these resources in indigenous communities and turning these resources into tradable commodities in the marketplace (Dutta & Pal, 2010). Locally grown seeds that have traditionally been retained by farmers at the end of every season to be used in the next season have been replaced by monoculture varieties marketed by TNCs that foster additional markets for fertilizers, pesticides, water, and additional seeds the following year. Similarly, the tax incentives offered to corporations accompanied by the poor implementation of labor laws and the state-based attacks on collective solidarities have resulted in increasing marginalization of the working classes across the globe. The privileging of the interests of the TNCs has become the universal guiding framework for defining global, national, and local policies; local political agendas have become situated within the dictates of global corporate interests, with the continual emphasis on opening up additional markets, privatizing the public sectors, and minimizing the state-based subsidies and infrastructural support for the underserved sectors within nation states.

Increasingly, collective resources such as water and nature (forests) are turned into individually owned private properties to be transacted by TNCs. As the emphasis shifts on privatizing resources and opening up national markets to international investments, attention is shifted away from specific state-based programs that are directed at serving the local needs of individuals and communities at the margins of the neoliberal logic of the marketplace. Furthermore, the state is configured as a mechanism for exerting its power to privatize collective resources and to subject these resources to the principles of the market. As noted by Harvey:

> Enclosure and the assignment of private property rights is considered the best way to protect against the so-called "tragedy of the commons" (the tendency for individuals to super-exploit common property resources such as land and water). Sectors formerly run or regulated by the state must be turned over to the private sphere and be deregulated (freed from any state interference) . . .the ground-rules for market competition must be properly observed, of course. In situations where such rules are not clearly laid out or where property rights are hard to define, the state must use its power to impose or invent market systems (such as trading in pollution rights).
>
> *(p. 65)*

The privatization of collective resources has turned these resources into commodities to be purchased, thus creating additional positions of inaccess at the margins. The marginalization of the poor through economic policies directly affecting agriculture and labor has been exacerbated by the price tags attached to resources such as water.

Although the rhetoric of the free market gets framed as the basic principle of neoliberalism, worth noting in actual practice is the complicit role of the state in serving the interests of corporations by absorbing the risks in markets (as depicted in the recent bailouts) and through the use of state power to create and build markets for corporations. Neoliberal interests are maintained by the state, whose function becomes to ensure a secure and strategic space for the functioning of corporations. The state also plays a key role in privatizing resources such as water, energy, land, education, social security, etc. in order to build new markets for TNCs. Most importantly, the state becomes the mechanism for the enactment of violence in order to silence possibilities of resistance among those groups that are increasingly marginalized by the pro-corporation policies of the state. The military, police, and legal structures are deployed in order to ensure that economic bases are created for the operation of free markets that ultimately serve the political economic needs of private corporations (Mychalejko & Ryan, 2009). In India, for instance, Operation Green Hunt has been launched in the eastern region, deploying military, paramilitary, and police forces to thwart indigenous resistance to projects of privatization, mining, and industrialization that threaten to displace the indigenous communities residing in these regions (Bhattacharya, 2009). Across several regions of India, military, paramilitary, and police forces have been utilized by the state to thwart subaltern resistance to land privatization and enclosure for setting up mining and manufacturing operations by TNCs. Similarly, Shell worked hand in hand with the state, supporting paramilitary interventions in the Niger delta to counter the protests by the Movement for the Survival of the Ogoni People (MOSOP) (Yearley & Forrester, 2000).

Resistance and Transnational Activism

The globalization of neoliberal politics has simultaneously opened up spaces for globally connected networks of solidarity that challenge neoliberal policies and the ways in which such policies are implemented by nation states and global actors to marginalize the subaltern sectors of the globe (Dutta, 2010; Dutta & Pal, 2010; Dutta-Bergman, 2006; Moghadam, 2009; Pal & Dutta, 2008a, 2008b; Reed, 2005). Globally situated and interconnected spaces of communication open up possibilities for grassroots processes of social change that seek to bring about transformations in neoliberal policies. The transformative processes of social change are constituted locally in response to the local ramifications of the structural adjustment programs, and simultaneously are positioned nationally and globally with the goals of challenging neoliberal policies (Dutta & Pal, 2010; Mike, 2009). Local sites of resistance emerge into global processes of social change, creating the entry points for global dialogue about alternatives to neoliberalism (H. Cleaver, 1998; Dellacioppa, 2009).

As Harvey (2005) observes, globalization has a particular bearing on postmodern thinking that necessitates theorizing in new directions, paying attention to "globalization from below" that promises to disrupt the oppressive and exploitative elements of neoliberal politics. The very structures, institutions, and roles that carry out the objectives of TNCs also serve as the sites of enacting global resistance, connecting activist networks across the globe to foreground alternative narratives of progress and development, and to bring about changes in global policies that continue to perpetuate the exploitation of the world's poor (Dellacioppa, 2009; Pal & Dutta, 2008a, 2008b). For instance, the protests against the WTO ministerial meeting in Seattle in 1999, referred to as the "Battle of Seattle," brought together over 40,000 protestors across the globe representing over 700 organizations, and functioned on the capability of activist groups to organize into coalitions and networks across the globe, operating as a network of networks that mobilized through an Internet campaign driven by listservs, bulletin boards, and websites (Reed, 2005). The sites of economic globalization also constitute and coexist with spaces of democratic and participatory globalization that challenge and seek to transform economic globalization policies.

Transnational activism connects the structural and cultural dimensions of global resistance, demonstrating the dialectical tension between the local and the global in enacting resistance to globally distributed power structures (Dellacioppa, 2009; Muñoz Ramírez, 2008; Pal & Dutta, 2008a, 2008b; Papa, Singhal, & Papa, 2006). For example, in response to the implementation of neoliberal policies in Mexico and the marginalization of the indigenous population in the Chiapas region of Mexico, the Zapatista Army of National Liberation (Ejército Zapatista de Liberación Nacional, or EZLN) emerged as an indigenous movement that challenged neoliberal policies of the state and demanded indigenous autonomy, and in doing so, drew upon a transnational solidarity network to articulate a resistive politics against neoliberalism (Dellacioppa, 2009; Muñoz Ramírez, 2008). More specifically, the EZLN was founded in 1983 in the jungles of Chiapas to resist the antidemocratic nature of neoliberal projects sponsored by the Mexican government, the selling of collective indigenous lands to transnational capital, and the historic exploitation of indigenous people. The Zapatista Liberation Army recruited villagers from the local villages of Chiapas, starting conversations in the villages about the problems faced by the communities such as health and access to land, and building health clinics in the villages. As the villages in Chiapas started participating in the EZLN, each village had a representative that would report to the insurgents and meet with each other to discuss the antidemocratic policies of the government and the strategies needed to resist these policies. Of particular concern to the Zapatistas were the continued marginalization of the indigenous population in the face of structural adjustment policies andthe continued erasure of the indigenous population from the state policies that exerted control on indigenous land. In the early 1990s, the revision of article 27 of the Mexican constitution that opened up collective indigenous lands to foreign investment catalyzed the EZLN to take up arms against the government.

Finally, resisting the signing of the North American Free Trade Agreement (NAFTA) in 1994, the Zapatista rebel army took control over five municipalities in Chiapas, demanding work, land, food, housing, health, education, independence, freedom, democracy, justice, and peace in their first communiqué issued from the main balcony in each of the municipalities they had taken over (Dellacioppa, 2009; Muñoz Ramírez, 2008). The Zapatistas functioned on the basis of consensual decision-making that operated at the level of the local communities, and quickly emerged as a global model for organizing against neoliberalism, simultaneously drawing upon global support from transnational actors to resist the neoliberal policies of the Mexican state. The participatory processes of community organizing among the Zapatistas quickly emerged as a model for the development of a transcultural community activist network against neoliberalism (Dellacioppa, 2009). The EZLN rapidly emerged on the global stage as an exemplar of resistive politics against neoliberalism, demonstrating the intersection between the local and the global in the politics of social change. The local cultural politics of the EZLN demonstrates the interplay between structure and agency in challenging global structures of neoliberalism.

As demonstrated with the example of the EZLN, it is in the realm of the control enacted by dominant global actors that resistive strategies are deployed by activist publics and communities dispersed around the globe; just as globalization expands the geographic and material scopes of TNCs, it also opens up new spaces and methods of global organizing directed at social transformation at the global level. Global resistance is at once both modern and postmodern; it explores the material roots of global inequities and simultaneously foregrounds the temporality of discourse that is continuously shifting and open to reinterpretations in complexly layered global structures. The "complex interplay of economic and cultural dynamics" (Papa et al., 2006, p. 201) played out in the realm of transnational activism necessitates an understanding of its implications for communication research (Pal & Dutta, 2008a). For instance, the concept of the "scapes" articulated by Appadurai (1990) demonstrates that public consciousness no longer stretches across national spaces, but "ignites the micro-politics of a nation-state" (Robins, 2000, p. 236). Hence, what are the challenges for communication research in view of these complex global shifts, especially as it enters into conversations about communicative processes of social change (see Pal & Dutta, 2008a)?

In the realm of the materiality of global resistance spaces, there are multiple sites through which activists are organizing in response to global economic restructuring (Dellacioppa, 2009). While working in a community-based setting, grassroots organizers are increasingly networking with transnational activists to effect changes in specific communities, thereby connecting the local and the global (Naples & Desai, 2002). With the growing presence of locally rooted networks structured around global issues, we see complex interaction between local and supranational activism. Though these groups occasionally participate in transnational protest events, their activities remain strongly rooted in the local. Agency is expressed through the continued used of cultural symbols in transformative politics of social change. For example, Zapatismo emerges as a global concept for activist organizing that offers an alternative consensus-based participatory approach to decision-making in communication for social change (Dellacioppa, 2009). Diani (2005) writes that in the North as well as in the South, there has been a reemergence of social movements on a scale unprecedented since the 1960s. These are largely collective actions against neoliberal approaches, promoting a different model of globalization. Several other factors give an impetus to the growing activist interests: growth of voluntary or political organizations mobilizing on transnational issues, the density of interorganizational collaborations between them, participation in major "no global" gatherings such as Genoa in 2001 or Florence in 2002, and the consolidation of a transnational community of professional activists and campaigners. Locally situated cultural articulations and interpretive frames offer avenues for the enactment of agency that challenges local, national and global structures.

Contemporary forms of resistance such as the EZLN open up opportunities to further explore the communicative practices by which local struggles connect with global politics with a potential to contribute to policy formulations. Let's once again consider the transcultural element in the resistive politics of the Zapatistas. In 1996, the Zapatistas issued a call for an "Intercontinental Encounter Against Neoliberalism and for Humanity," holding a global platform for bringing together activists and intellectuals from around the globe to discuss and construct a global alternative to neoliberalization (Dellacioppa, 2009). The issue of transnational activism once again brings up the question that has been raised earlier in this review. Is globalization a process by which collective resistance can help structure a transnational public sphere of contention that would oppose the dominance of the state and transnational corporate interest? This question has become particularly relevant as there is a surge in activist interests in resisting and transforming ideologies, practices, and institutions that support and constitute neoliberalism, that are popularly called "globalization from below" (Ganesh et al., 2005). According to Tarrow (2005), although transnational activism is not a new phenomenon, what is striking about it is its connection to the current wave of globalization and its relation to the changing structure of international politics. It is the latter that provides activists the focal points for collective action, provides them expanded resources and brings them together in transnational coalitions and campaigns.

Tarrow (2005) suggests transnational activists link non-state actors, their states, and international politics with the potential to create a new political arena. Tarrow and della Porta (2005) explain such linkages by suggesting the concept of "complex internationalization" in present times that involves

> expansion of international institutions, international regimes, and the transfer of the resources of local and national actors to the international stage, producing threats, opportunities and resources for international NGOs, transnational social movements and, indirectly, grassroots social movements.
>
> (Tarrow & della Porta, 2005, p. 235)

These actors have varying levels of power. The state is the central actor; international institutions represent both the state interest and their bureaucratic claims; some NGOs gain direct access to both states and institutions, and social movements operate from outside this structure to influence its policies.

Della Porta and Tarrow (2005) have summarized a number of changes that have expanded the scope of the contemporary wave of transnational contention:

- The institutions representing neoliberalism—IMF, World Bank, and the WTO—have become central to targets of resistance.
- These institutions provide a focal point for the global framing of a variety of domestic and international conflicts.
- New electronic technologies enhance the organizing of movements in many venues at once.
- Within transnational contention, tendencies can be seen toward formation of transnational campaigns and coalitions.
- Partial but highly visible successes of campaigns by non-state actors such as the international support for the liberation movement in South Africa, the anti-landmine campaign, the international solidarity movement with the Zapatista rebellion among others.

However, development of conflicts over global issues is not necessarily organized around transnational social movement organizations. Instead, they are rooted at the local and national level, turning simultaneously to various government levels and making linkages between different social and political actors. In addition to active interaction between domestic and international populations of movement organizations, coalitions are formed both at local and global levels. One way local coalition occurs is mobilization by changing the framing of domestic political conflicts. But more interesting is the "global social justice" masterframe of new mobilizations (della Porta & Tarrow, 2005). This, in turn, creates loosely coupled transnational networks that organize around particular campaigns or series of campaigns, using different forms of protests. In other words, the authors argue, the local issues of the struggles remain distinct even though they get connected by sharing a common global agenda. The authors explain:

> Specific concerns with women's rights, labor issues, the defense of the environment, and opposition to war survive, but are bridged together in opposition against "neoliberal globalization." In order to keep different groups together, "tolerant" inclusive identities develop, stressing differences as a positive quality of the movement.
>
> *(della Porta & Tarrow, 2005, p. 12)*

The awareness about local phenomena getting increasingly linked with broader global processes has gained immense importance in the twentieth century (Seidman, 2000). The new global perspective on identities, networks, and communities and the way international processes shape and redefine local ones have prompted social movement theorists to reconsider many of their basic assumptions. Some of the questions, Seidman (2000) summarizes, evoke special interests:

- When does a social process become a global one?
- When does a local social movement become linked enough with the global processes to be considered a global social movement?
- What do global processes mean for the very local processes through which movements create collective identities?
- Who represents movements on the global stage and how are those representations redesigned internationally?
- How do local movements change in response to global resources or audiences?
- What roles do global organizations play in provoking local movements?

Routledge (2000) suggests that it is not Harvey's concept of "militant particularism" of local struggles that becomes globalized, but rather the common ground that is shared between different social movements. Hence, particular social movements are frequently entangled with broader communities of interest that "overlap, intertwine, and coalesce with one another" (Routledge, 2000, p. 27). This community, Routledge (2000) points out, collaborates at particular times and places into a strategic force, such as global days of action. In terms of mobilization of resources, della Porta and Tarrow (2005) have identified two emerging challenges for movements. First, the fragmentation in the social structure has increased social heterogeneity affecting formation of social groups that used to be an important basis for many social movements. Second, increasing individualization of cultures has led to declining solidarity in the society. But della Porta and Tarrow (2005) suggest that to cope with these changes, transnational mobilization has made adaptation to different movement strategies. For instance, flexible networks are formed that allow heterogeneous social forces to become part of one movement.

However, the processes of fragmentation are concomitant to the declining power of the state and the growing importance of private economic actors in global economic policies as a result of an alliance of transnational corporations, financial institutions, and the US government. Alongside the tension of complex heterogeneity, interdependence also contributes to collective action. As mentioned earlier, it also provides the resources for non-state actors to challenge elites and sometimes collaborate with insiders (domestic movements sometime collaborate with political parties) (Tarrow & della Porta, 2005). The international institutions provide new platforms for articulation of claims and development of "new reference public." Also, some of these are amenable to issues such as human rights and sustainable development, thereby making themselves permeable to social movements. In other words, the authors argue, these establishments provide multilevel targets—national, macro-regional, international for social movements. The protests at Seattle, Quebec, and Cancun showed the commonality between these events. Collectively, they drew attention to the increasing inequalities and environmental disasters tied to neoliberal transformations. Thus these protests increased their transnational visibility and demonstrated their linkages and sometimes their power to influence events.

Central to these new-age movements are *networks* of groups and activists. They imbibe an emerging identity, involve in conflictual issues, and follow non-traditional forms of participation. A large majority of the activists who take part in demonstrations against international summits identify themselves with the movements related to globalization. Different names have been proposed for it— no global, Seattle people, globalization from below, global justice, and so on, which indicates that its core goals are yet to be crystallized. Networks, however, are central to globalizing resistance. According to Routledge (2000), solidarity, information sharing, and mutual support contribute to forming networks. He also suggests that the core function of networks is production, exchange, and strategic use of information. There has been a dramatic increase in such international linkages since the late 1980s. Cheaper air travel and new electronic communication technologies have speeded up information flows and enhanced personal contact among activists thus forming a "global electronic fabric of struggle" (see Routledge, 2000, p. 27). Tarrow (2005) suggests these are resources and opportunities particular to our era that transnational activism is building on. Greater access to higher education, emergence of English as the main language of international trade and services, and evidence of formulation of decisions that affect people's lives at international venues play a role in generating activist interest. These resistive sites of change demonstrate the plethora of communicative processes and practices through which agency is enacted through the use of culturally circulated symbols that are situated amidst structures and yet are resistive in their transformative agendas of challenging and changing these structures.

Organization of the Book

It is against the backdrop of this globally situated neoliberal agenda with global, national, and local goals that we start seeing examples of locally situated and globally connected politics of resistance. In other words, resistance gets played out in the domain of the constraining and enabling structures that define the ambit of life experiences at the margins. Reflecting the interplay between structural inequities and the communicative practices of resistance, Chapter 1 examines the theoretical foundations of a social change framework, offering an entry point for studying the interplays between material and symbolic inequities and the practices of resistance in the realm of these inequalities. It will articulate some defining features of social change as well as define the terrain of social change, differentiating between efforts directed at changing marginalizing social structures as opposed to the efforts within the dominant framework that are directed at individual behavior change although they are marketed as such as social change efforts. This distinction is one of the key features of the book, creating an ontological entry point for categorizing the variety of communicative efforts that are typically classified within the broader territory of social change.

The first part of this book is organized by the different contexts that continue to reflect the goals and effects of neoliberal politics. The contexts and issues covered include poverty, hunger, agriculture, indigenous groups, health, and gender. These different contexts offer the backdrop for the clustering of specific issues played out in the realm of neoliberal hegemony. It is also on the landscape of these different contexts of local–global inequities that communicative practices of resistance are constituted with the agendas of bringing about transformations in neoliberal structures. One of the key aspects of globalization has been the increasing disparities between the haves and have-nots, with further marginalization of the poor with limited access to resources. Therefore, Chapter 2 examines the intersections of neoliberal politics, poverty, and hunger. Continuing the thread of economic marginalization even further, Chapter 3 explores the role of neoliberalism in the realm of agriculture, particularly examining the ways in which contemporary neoliberal interventions have placed farmers at the margins. In Chapter 4, we will look at the ways in which neoliberal policies constrain and enable the discursive and material spaces in the broader domain of the health experiences of the subaltern sectors across the globe. Chapter 5 will carry out the theme of experiences at the margins in the realm of neoliberalism by exploring the context of gender as an organizing framework for understanding how neoliberal policies play out in the lives of the women in the marginalized sectors of the globe.

Part II offers ontological and epistemological insights into the ways in which communicative processes of social change are organized. The emphasis of this part of the book is on social change practices that actually seek to bring about transformation in unequal neoliberal structures. Therefore, the emphasis is on examining the inequities and finding spaces where these inequities are consistently challenged. In other words, a transformative politics marks the communicative processes and practices that are outlined in this part, as opposed to the individual behavior change programs in development efforts led by the status quo that are often categorized as social change initiatives. Resistance, therefore, becomes a defining feature of these processes and practices, discursively constituted as efforts that stand in opposition to the organizing framework of the dominant structure that perpetuates the inequities across the globe. In Chapter 6, we engage with the dialogic possibilities of communication, studying the ways in which dialogue brings about possibilities for social change and social transformation, further building upon the ways in which dialogue creates transformative avenues, possibilities for changing unequal structures in neoliberal politics. Chapter 7 looks at performance as a communicative practice, narrating stories of performance-based strategies for social change across the globe. These examples offer the empirical base for looking at the theoretical issues brought about in the performance of stories of marginalization and social change, demonstrating the ways in which performance disrupts the status quo and offers an avenue for reconstituting the organizing principles of neoliberalism. In addition, at the heart of any social change initiative is the organizing of groups, communities, and neighborhoods into cohesive entities that offer the base for challenging the unequal structures. Chapter 8 offers an overview of the communicative processes, strategies, and tactics through which the politics of resistance is organized, brought into its collective existence as a base for challenging the neoliberal structures. Chapter 9 explores the participatory spaces and participatory strategies that are mobilized in subaltern contexts as entry points for social change and transformative politics, bringing to the fore the role of participation in social transformation (see Mosse, 2001). Chapter 10 offers an overview of the mediated practices of social change, looking at the role of mass media across the globe as sites and actors in social changed processes. Beyond the exploration of the role of media as channels of communication, this chapter focuses on the mediated strategies and processes through which social change issues are circulated in discursive spaces, creating alternative entry points to the dominant ideologies of neoliberalism that predominate much of contemporary mass media. The book wraps up with a concluding chapter that connects the threads that flow through the various aspects of communicative practices constituted in the realm of neoliberal hegemony, offering a narrative of counter-globalization, a space for constituting multiple counter-hegemonies that are continually in flux and therefore, continually offering entry points for structural transformation. Theoretically, each of the chapters outlined in Part II offers an overview for understanding the ways in which agency is enacted in the realm of local cultures, drawing upon cultural symbols and markers of resistance to challenge structures of globalization (see Pollack, 2001).

Conclusion

Communicating Social Change: Structure, Culture, and Agency engages with the politics of neoliberalism and the ways in which this politics is resisted through locally situated and globally connected movements of social change. The material and the symbolic work hand in hand to create the positions at the margins; it is also in this realm of the material and the symbolic that the margins offer an entry point for social change, reconstituting the agendas of neoliberal politics and offering alternative epistemological and ontological frameworks for constituting the politics of social change. Ultimately, this book creates a discursive space for engaging with the role of communication in bringing about social transformation.

1

THEORIZING SOCIAL CHANGE COMMUNICATION

The goal of this book is to offer points of intersection between the theory and praxis of social change communication, with the broader agenda of creating theoretical entry points for the praxis of social change. The conceptualization of social change is integral to the ways in which we practice social change initiatives, the strategies developed in these initiatives, the implementation of the initiatives, and the ways in which these initiatives are measured (Dutta, 2008a, 2008b, 2008c; Gumucio-Dagron & Tufte, 2006; Melkote & Steeves, 2001). Social change efforts problematize existing social configurations; these problem configurations offer the primary foundations for developing social change agendas. Essential to a communicative engagement with social change is the deployment of communication for the purposes of change in social systems (Gumucio-Dagron & Tufte, 2006; Rogers, 1962, 1973; Schramm, 1964). Social change communication, therefore, foregrounds the role of communication solutions in addressing social problems. Worth emphasizing here is the framing of social change issues within a broader communicative lens, and it is within this communicative frame that solutions are proposed for bringing about change in the social systems.

What is the relevance of looking at social change from a communicative standpoint? What can a communication perspective provide us in addressing issues of social change? What are the differences between the various approaches to communication for social change, and what is the political economy of these approaches? What are the underlying political agendas in communication for social change? How do the different approaches to social change go about achieving these agendas? Understanding the different bases of communication for social change is foundational in setting up the criteria for evaluating these different approaches to social change, and connecting them to the praxis and politics of social change. The Marxist foundations of the culture-centered approach, alongside the postcolonial and subaltern studies emphasis of the culture-centered approach, situate the culture-centered approach as a political process of social change that resists dominant structures in globalization politics and seeks to change these structures. It is precisely because of the politically driven nature of the culture-centered approach to social change communication that it is imperative to delineate among the different approaches to communication for social change.

We begin the chapter by looking at the definitions of social change. The definition of social change offers the basis for exploring the different conceptual frameworks of social change, followed by an explication of how these conceptual frameworks get constituted in the theory, methodology, and application of social change communication. An overview is offered for the development communication, participatory development, Marxist, and culture-centered approaches to social change communication. Subsequently, theoretical rationale is offered for adopting the culture-centered approach to communication for social change, noting the roles of culture, structure, and agency in disrupting contemporary global structures and in seeking spaces of social change.

The second half of the chapter sets up the context for looking at the need for social change. In order to do so, the chapter provides a theoretical summary of social structures and the ways in which these structures create conditions at the margins. The discussion focuses on the constructs of power and control and the role of communication in supporting the status quo, particularly against the backdrop of contemporary globalization politics. It is in the area of this discussion of the marginalization processes in mainstream social systems of globalization that the chapter introduces the communication processes that offer openings for disrupting the status quo. Here it demonstrates the communicative nature of marginalization processes in contemporary global structures and the resistance that is constituted in the realm of the dominant structures. In order to do so, this chapter heavily draws upon the literatures in postcolonial and subaltern studies theories, thus setting up a theoretical base for the chapters to appear in Part I. Ultimately, by connecting theory and praxis, the chapter will demonstrate the role that communication theorists, researchers, and practitioners can play in the realm of social change interventions.

What is Social Change?

Historically, communication scholars have been involved in the field of social change under the broader framework of development communication programs. These programs conceptualized social change within the goals of modernization. The goal here was to change societies based on top-down interventions so that these societies would be modernized. The problems identified in the Third World were framed as problems of underdevelopment, and therefore, interventions targeting the Third World were framed as solutions to the problems of underdevelopment. The focus therefore is not on changing the existing structures but on creating behavioral and lifestyle changes in target communities in order to bring about development. The status quo, comprising of the existing set of institutions, and their rules, roles, and infrastructures, is engaged with in order to find spaces of change. Change is typically thought of in terms of individual-level behavioral or attitudinal modifications that operate within the broader structures that exist in society.

As opposed to the development-based view of social change, Marxist theorists conceptualize social change in terms of the necessity to bring about structural transformations in order to address the inequalities in society. Based on the concepts of class struggle and surplus labor that feeds into the profits of the capitalists, a Marxist view of social change therefore engages with the revolutionary possibilities of structural transformation. Change is achieved through trans-formations that are brought about in the existing structures. In this sense, social change is constituted in the changes in existing systems of production, and in challenging the relationships that constitute the status quo. Power becomes central to processes of social change and is theorized in terms of its relationship with social structures in bringing about openings for change and in fundamentally changing the political economic structures. Here, social change is theorized in terms of the capacity of the proposed framework of social organization to differ substantially from the existing structures of organizing.

These two concepts of social change presented here diverge widely from one another. In the conceptualization of social change as development, social change initiatives are carried out with the goals of enacting and reproducing the power and control of global power structures. The principles of social change are dictated by the agendas of international donor agencies (governments, private foundations, etc.) and international organizations (United Nations, World Health Organizations, World Bank, etc.), and are oriented toward addressing problems within recipient societies. In the Marxist approach, emphasis is placed on the material inequities that are perpetuated by political and economic structures, and the trajectory of social change is played out through the transformation of social structures and systems of political-economic organizing. Therefore, social change in the Marxist approach is situated structurally and is brought about through transformations in social and economic structures that perpetuate the marginalization of the subaltern classes.

Conceptualizing Communication for Social Change

What then is social change, and what is the meaning of communication that is situated in relationship to projects of social change? Communication is con-ceptualized in two fundamentally different frameworks: message-based framework, and process-based framework. The message-based framework of communication scholarship, also referred to as the transmission view of communication, operates on the basic model of the sender and the receiver, where messages of change are sent out to receiver populations with the goal of persuading these populations to engage in the proposed behavior. The message-based framework therefore emphasizes the creation of effective messages that are able to reach the desired target audience, and have a large impact on the population. The process-based framework to communication for social change, also labeled as the ritual view of communication, focuses on the shared spaces of interpretation and meaning making through which communication comes to constitute social realities. Communication is seen as constitutive, as an active process of meaning making through which individuals and communities come to understand their contexts and act upon them. The process-based framework emphasizes the cultural processes through which individuals and collectives enact their agency, in their relationship to social structures.

There exists a wide range of approaches to communication for social change, and these approaches operate on the axes of two dialectical tensions that have been historically theorized in the study of social change processes. In this section, we focus on the many definitions of communication for social change and then articulate the points of similarities and departures between these definitions. In doing so, we establish a theoretical framework for studying social change communication, with the definition of the key tensions that constitute this framework. Thus, we pay attention to the different entry points for praxis in projects of communication for social change, based on the theoretical conceptualizations of the tensions between individual-level approaches versus structural change approaches on one hand, and top-down approaches versus participatory approaches on the other hand. The individual-level versus structural change tension differentiates between communication programs that emphasize individual-level changes in beliefs, attitudes, and behaviors, and communication programs that focus on structural redistribution and redistributive justice (see Dutta, 2008c). The top-down approach focuses on using mediated networks to diffuse messages of social change as opposed to the participatory approach, which focuses on creating participatory spaces for local community members (Freire, 1970, 1973; Schramm, 1964). The intersections of these two dialectical tensions produce four different approaches to communication for social change: development approaches, participatory development, Marxist approaches, and culture-centered approaches (see Figure 1.1).

Whereas the differences between the individual-level versus structural-level changes in communication for social change are articulated on the basis of the locus, focus, and goals of change, the differences between the top-down versus participatory methods of social change are articulated on the basis of the conceptualization of communication, communicative processes, tools and strategies used, and the modes of communication deployed by the social change processes.

Individual Approaches. Starting with the early theorizations of communication for development, individual-level approaches to social change dominate much of the mainstream literature on communication for social change, arguing that

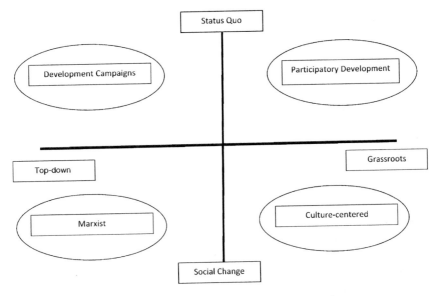

FIGURE 1.1 Theoretical framework for social change communication.

changes in knowledge, attitude, and behavior (KAB) at the level of the individual would bring about changes in individual behaviors and practices, which in turn would constitute broader societal-level change (Lerner, 1964; Schramm, 1964; Schramm & Lerner, 1976). These social change campaigns were constituted under the framework of development communication projects that were directed at changing primitive Third World societies by targeting individual members. Pathways of influence were developed for shifting the beliefs, attitudes, and behaviors of target populations in the Third World, with the goal of aligning them with modernist principles of development that were presented as universal desirable markers of development. For example, Schramm (1964) discusses the role of mass media in teaching modernizing skills at the individual level:

> [A]ny social change in the direction of modernization requires a program in teaching the necessary skills. Some of these are general skills; for example, no society will modernize very far until a substantial proportion of the population can read and count. Others are quite specific—for example, repairing radios and farm machinery, operating machine tools, bookkeeping, surveying, medicine and pharmacy. Almost invariably, skills like these are in short supply when development begins, and one of the great tasks of smoothing social change is to make technical skills and technical development march at the same pace, so that technology does not wait for workers, nor skilled workers for machines and jobs.
>
> *(Schramm, 1964, p. 28)*

The focus of the individual-level approaches is to operate from within the status quo, and further perpetuate the status quo through an emphasis on modernization as a panacea to the constructions of underdevelopment. The articulation of modernization as solution emphasizes the training of skilled workers to participate in the labor processes of the capitalist economy, to serve the interests of the status quo in generating profits for the owners of the capital. The emphasis is on maximizing the profit margins of the owners of the capital, which in turn is perceived to bring about development, as opposed to addressing issues of redistributive justice.

Since the early years of social change campaigns developed by communication scholars under the framework of development communication projects, the emphasis has been on using mass-mediated messages to target audience members, with the goals of modifying their beliefs, attitudes, and behaviors (Lerner, 1967, 1976; Rogers, 1962, 1973; Schramm, 1964). Schramm (1964), for instance, discusses the role of the mass media in widening horizons, focusing attention, raising aspirations, conferring status, helping form tastes, teaching, educating, and training individuals. He further discusses the active role that the mass media can play in creating a climate for development (Schramm, 1968). Similarly, Lerner (1967) discusses the role of the mass media in cultivating the mobile or empathic personality, the capacity to see oneself in another's situation, as the precursor to development by orienting Third World subjects toward modernization projects. Ultimately, the individual-level approach to social change is carried out through information campaigns that seek to build awareness in target communities, and persuasive campaigns that seek to bring about transformations in attitudes and behavioral intentions. A wide variety of information-based social change campaigns have been carried out since the 1950s, covering areas such as family planning, immunization, use of mosquito nets, condom use, and sanitation practices, with the goal of bringing about individual-level change in order to develop societies. In summary, social change in such traditional approaches to development communication continues to be seen as an aggregate of individual-level changes in the community.

Structural Approaches. Founded on the principles of dialectic materialism in Marxist theory, the structural approaches to social change fundamentally note the presence of inequitable structures across the globe that underlie the marginalization and erasure of the subaltern sectors from the discursive and material spaces of social systems (Cloud, 2006; Dutta, 2008a, 2008b, 2008c). The roles of access to economic modes of production and ownership of capital are underlined in theorizing of social change. Social change here is written into the class conflict and class antagonism that are symptomatic of capitalist systems of production, drawing upon the concept of exploitation of labor that drives the profits of the capitalist system. The very existence of class differences in contemporary capitalist societies is the breeding ground for the praxis of social change. Here unpaid labor is the profit of the capitalist classes, and therefore, the struggles of the proletariat are defined in terms of the struggles to seek ownership of the systems of production. These approaches highlight the fundamental inequities in social structures that produce and reproduce cycles of marginalization, exploitation, and dispossession. As Melkote (2000) argues:

> As long as societies distribute needs and power unequally between populations, it is unethical for communications and human service professionals to help solve minor and/or immediate problems while ignoring the systemic barriers created by societies that permit or perpetuate inequalities among citizens. Real change is not possible unless we deal with the crucial problem in human societies: lack of economic and social power among individuals at the grassroots.
>
> *(Melkote, 2000, p. 46)*

Therefore, the structural approaches to communication for social change pay critical attention to the underlying economic inequalities and imbalances in society (see Figure 1.2).

Social change communication is directed at attempting to transform these very structural inequalities, fundamentally transforming the structures through projects of redistributive justice. Scholars such as Dana Cloud (2006) and Lee Artz (2006) foreground the role of the material in processes of social change. Cloud (2006), for instance, argues that the efficacy of resistive practices depends upon their ability

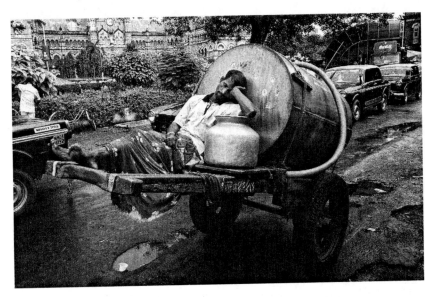

FIGURE 1.2 An Indian man leans on a water container while he sleeps on a water cart in the streets of Bombay, September 6, 2004. (Rob Elliott/AFP/Getty Images)

to collectively disrupt systems of production. Without the threat of the material intervention to fundamentally strike at the economic base of capitalism, the legitimacy of communication for social change is limited to the realm of the symbolic (Cloud, 2006). Therefore, she discusses the role of the material in its relationship to the symbolic as an entry point for social change. Along similar lines, scholars taking the structural approach to marginalization across the globe pay attention to the large-scale data about inequalities, putting forth arguments about the role of neoliberal policies on poverty and inequalities. Social change communication once again is thought about in terms of specific interventions that are directed at addressing issues of redistributive justice. Social transformation and redistributive justice become the focal points of structural approaches to communication for social change.

Top-down Approaches. As noted earlier, the traditional approaches to social change are based upon mainstream ideas of development and modernization, drawing upon the fundamental idea that underdevelopment is a deficiency and a product of backward cultural traits that act as barriers to progress (Lerner, 1968; Schramm, 1964; Schramm & Lerner, 1976). Modernization, based on universal values attached to economic growth, growth in mass media, growth in capitalist opportunities, and technological progress, is the goal of top-down approaches to development. Here is an excerpt from Lerner's (1968) classic, *The passing of traditional society*, that captures the position of universalism as the fundamental tenet of the modernization principle in the context of the Middle East:

> Whether from East or West, modernization poses the same basic challenge—the infusion of "a rationalist and positivist spirit" against which scholars seem agreed, "Islam is absolutely defenseless" . . . millions throughout the Middle East are yearning to trade in their old lives for such newer ways is what modernization promises to most people . . . the Western model of modernization exhibits certain components and sequences whose relevance is global. Everywhere, for example, increasing urbanization has tended to raise literacy; rising literacy has tended to increase media exposure; increasing media exposure has "gone with" wider economic participation (per capita income) and political participation (voting) . . . The point is that the secular process of social change, which brought modernization to the Western world, has more than antiquarian relevance to today's problems of the Middle East tradition. Indeed, the lesson is that Middle Eastern modernizers will do well to study the historical sequence of Western growth.
>
> *(Lerner, 1968, pp. 45–46)*

Based on the core idea that Western-based modernization principles define the universal markers of progress and development for humankind, development communication campaigns are run via mass media to diffuse the messages of enlightenment. Development is achieved through urbanization, literacy, development of media exposure, greater economic participation, and voting, all of which are treated as markers of modernization in the West. Through the principles of modernization, Western values are placed as the universal aspirations for cultures and societies across the globe. The treatment of these values as secular values, removed from their Western roots and situated more in the context of universal human values, serves to support the agendas of top-down development campaigns. Funding structures such as the United States Agency for International Development (USAID) and the Bill and Melinda Gates Foundation determine the agendas, objectives, and goals of the development projects; networks of expert campaign developers from academe, civil society, as well as the private sector team up to develop the interventions based on pre-existing problem configurations and solution frames; the solutions are implemented as strategic persuasive campaigns through mass-mediated, interpersonal as well as community channels. The campaigns are then evaluated for their effectiveness, thus continuing the cycle of development campaigns. Often, local elites representing government, civil society, etc. are involved in the development of tactics, implementing campaign messages, and managing the campaign process at the local level. To the extent that local communities are involved in such vertical campaigns, the involvement is as resource for data to assist with campaign design and development.

Participatory Approaches. In response to the observation that most development communication efforts strategically diffused through the mass media used the one-way communication model that conceptualized linear flow of communication from the sender to the receiver of development messages, Latin American scholars noted that such conceptualizations of development perpetrated the domination of certain classes over the majority of others within nation states, and the domination of the United States over the Latin American states externally (Beltran, 1979). Development communication campaigns then served to carry out the agendas of the powerful actors in the global landscape. It was in articulating this criticism to the classical pedagogy of what he termed as "banking education" that Paulo Freire (1970, 1973) articulated the notion of the "pedagogy of the oppressed" that emphasized dialogic forms of communication built in mutual trust and respect. It is also along these lines that in responding to the traditional domain of top-down development communication campaigns, Robert Chambers (1983) noted the importance of listening to the poor as the starting point for developing solutions:

> Respect for the poor and what they want offsets paternalism. The reversal this implies is that outsiders should start not with their own priorities but with those of the poor, although however much self-insight they have, outsiders will still project their own values and priorities. In what follows, I too am trapped, an outsider asking what poor people want. All one can hope is that the effort of trying to find out, of asking again and again and

doubting the outcomes, will check some of the worse effects of core-periphery paternalism, and the more the priorities of the poor are known, the easier it will be to see what it is best to do.

(Chambers, 1983, p. 235)

Framework for Social Change Theories

The intersections of the two dialectical tensions produce four different approaches to communication for social change. Development in social change uses top-down communication for change projects that are focused on individual-level changes in attitudes, beliefs, behaviors, etc. Participatory development approaches use participatory communication processes and strategies in order to achieve social change at the individual level, with the ultimate emphasis on bringing about changes in individual beliefs, attitudes, and behaviors in the community. Marxist approaches to social change examine the transformative capacity of social change processes, and use communicative processes and channels as avenues for achieving structural transformation.

Development in Social Change

Social change has been traditionally conceptualized under the framework of development communication projects (Gumucio-Dagron & Tufte, 2006; Melkote & Steeves, 2001). In this framework, traditional mass media are typically used to send out persuasive messages of development based on universal notions of development situated in Western hegemony (see Schramm, 1964; Schramm & Lerner, 1976). The underlying idea is to emphasize the modernization of Third World spaces and to carry out development through the diffusion of behaviors at the individual level that are identified as problematic, and hence in need of change. Persuasive campaigns are strategically developed with the goals of changing individuals, which then would lead to aggregate-level societal changes. The emphasis is on developing the scholarly "science" of persuasion that would guide the strategies used in the development campaigns. For example, the Avahan campaign run by the Bill and Melinda Gates Foundation uses principles of social marketing and persuasion to develop strategic messages deployed with the goal of promoting safe sexual behavior (Acharya & Dutta, 2010).

Participatory Development

In response to the criticisms of the one-way flow of communication in development campaigns, participatory development campaigns developed as means for including local communities in processes of social change. The genre of participatory development campaigns use participation as a strategic tool for the purposes of achieving the development agendas of the funding agencies and campaign planners. Initially, participatory mechanisms are involved in the inclusion of the community in formative research to gather data about audience characteristics. This helps improve the effectiveness of the campaign as it takes into account the inputs of the local community. Subsequently, participatory channels are utilized as mechanisms for diffusing the messages of development carried out by the campaign planners through group meetings, forums, performances, etc. Often, participatory communication channels are combined with entertainment-education (EE) programs to achieve development objectives. For instance, the radio soap opera *Taru* was created as an EE campaign to create awareness about the value of gender equality, small family size, reproductive health, and caste and communal harmony in the northern Hindi-speaking region of India (Harter et al., 2007). Folk performances were used a week before the launch of the radio drama to prime the audiences to the drama and to create awareness about the drama, covering the issues that would appear in *Taru*, and were used to form radio listening clubs. These radio listening clubs were later involved in putting together participatory performances on self-identified issues that emerged from within the groups. Here EE was used along with participatory principles, strategies, and tactics to carry out the broader agendas of development. Another often cited example of this genre of participatory development projects is the Radio Communication Project (RCP) in Nepal that used EE along with participatory communication strategies to diffuse the agendas of family planning as determined by the funding agency and the campaign planners (Storey & Jacobson, 2004).

Marxist Theories of Social Change

The classical work of Marxist theorists focus on achieving social change through revolutionary processes, and communication played a key role in the organizing of the social change processes. The emphasis of Marxist praxis therefore is on organizing workers, drawing attention to the inequalities, oppressive conditions, and the fundamental class antagonisms that exist in capitalist forms of production. Social change projects based on Marxist ideals involve efforts of structural transformation, and therefore, communicative practices are deployed toward the goals of developing identities of the organizing effort, identifying and mobilizing resources, creating educational and awareness programs for the education of the proletariat in Marxist principles, and organizing the proletariat to participate in revolutionary practices.

Culture-Centered Approaches to Social Change

The culture-centered approach to social change envisions the capacity of communicative processes to transform social structures, and in doing so, it attends to the agency of the subaltern sectors in bringing about social change. Noting that communicative erasures go hand in hand with structural erasures, the goal of the culture-centered approach is to create avenues and spaces of social change by listening to the voices of subaltern communities that have historically been marginalized. Participatory spaces are created so that these spaces offer co-constructive openings for listening to subaltern voices, foregrounding these voices in the discursive spaces of knowledge production. At the heart of the culture-centered approach is the theorizing of the intersections between culture, structure, and agency as the tripods that offer the base for meaning making and communicative enactment. Structure refers to the institutional roles, rules, practices, and ways of organizing that constrain and enable access to resources. Culture constitutes the local contexts where meanings are continuously negotiated. Agency is the capacity of individuals and collectives to enact their choices as they negotiate structures. As noted in the Introduction, the culture-centered approach builds upon subaltern studies and postcolonial theories to disrupt the hegemonic spaces of knowledge production with dialogues with the subaltern sectors that have historically been erased from the mainstream discourses of development and progress.

Postcolonial Theory and Globalization

Postcolonial theory examines the symbolic representations and material relationships that underlie processes of colonization, offering openings for emancipatory politics that challenges the systematic erasures of the narratives of oppression and exploitation embedded in colonial and contemporary neocolonial configurations, and creating spaces for listening to the voices of the subaltern sectors of the globe that have hitherto been treated as subjects to be scripted, coded, and worked over within the dominant knowledge structures. Central to the articulations of postcolonial theory, then, are the possibilities of transforming those very epistemic structures that sustain and reproduce the agendas of colonialism and neocolonialism in the realm of modernity, rendering knowledge as an inherently political entity embedded within the politics, history, and geography of modern knowledge structures and their colonial agendas.

A postcolonial lens lends itself particularly well to theorizing communication for social change as it explores the ways in which, first, communicative practices serve the interests of transnational corporations and the free market logic that upholds the dominance of these transnational corporations; second, communication theories maintain the hegemony of West-centric articulations of modernity and development, thus contributing to the hegemony of Western configurations in the global landscape; and third, resistive politics among the subaltern sectors seek to transform the global inequities in knowledge production, participation, and resource distribution, even as these opportunities for transformative politics are continually threatened by the co-optive politics of transnational hegemony. Given the fluidity of the global processes we are experiencing today even as global structures are continuously seeking to consolidate their powers, multiple dialectical tensions play out in the theorization of communication for social change in the backdrop of globalization (Pal & Dutta, 2008a, 2008b). For instance, the post-colonial context of communicative practice is rife with tensions between the local and the global. Globally situated policies and practices of transnational corporations continually negotiate with the local cultural contexts of dispersed yet inter-connected global spaces. Similarly, tensions emerge in the centralization of power/control and the opening up of resistive possibilities that seek to transform the structures of inequality and injustice. We specifically examine the geopolitics of global communicative practices that continue to serve the agendas of neoclonial-ism, and the ways in which these geopolitical institutions are resisted by activist politics.

Power, Control, Postcoloniality, and Globalization

Postcolonial theory primarily engages with the dominant power of the West that imperializes developing nations by advancing the modernist logic of progress and development to justify global capitalism. It questions the idea of linear progress by drawing attention to the differences that have emerged economically and politically in the global situation. Identifying capitalism as central to Eurocentricism, post-colonial theory interrogates issues related to inequality and exploitation in the capitalist world order (Dirlik, 2000; Shome & Hegde, 2002). Fundamental to the new form of global capitalism is "transnationalization of production" (Dirlik, 2000, p. 224), where technologies provide a new temporal and spatial dimension to production with the goal of seeking maximum benefits for capital against labor. This new phase of global capitalism is driven by transnational corporations that are at the center of economic activities (Dirlik, 2000; Miyoshi, 2005).

Postcolonial theory is committed to developing a critique of colonialism and imperialism. While colonialism typically is defined as overt coercion in the form of territorial occupation, imperialism is an act of economic and political domi-nation. Generally speaking, postcolonial theory argues that under global capitalism the Western power seeks to establish its hegemony not only politically, militarily, and economically, but also culturally and ideologically (Prasad, 2003). The author argues that postcolonial theory is thus rooted in decolonizing the mind at political, economic, and cultural levels with the goal of achieving an equitable global system. Such a project of decolonizing the mind is committed to disrupting Western categories at an epistemological and ontological level.

Some of the foundational concepts in postcolonial theory can be attributed to several influential theorists. Said's (1979) *Orientalism* deconstructs Western dis-courses or cultural representations of the Orient. Arguing that the Orient is not Oriental in the commonplace sense, but it was made to be Oriental, Said dislocates the "familiar" concept of the Orient to expose how the other helps define the West via contrasting languages, experiences, and images in "a relationship of power, of domination, of varying degrees of a complex hegemony" (Said, 1979, p. 5). Bhabha (1994, p. 67) points out that the idea of otherness is an ambivalent simultaneous production of "an object of desire and derision." On one hand, colonial discourse suggests that the non-West is a category that is radically situated as the other outside of the West. On the other hand, it draws the non-West into the West by way of Western epistemologies. Hence, Bhabha (1994) forwards the concept of ambivalence in defining postcolonial subject positions. Articulating the division between the West and the non-West as the fundamental epistemological and ontological basis of the relational space within which the West and the Orient are projected, Said (1979) writes:

> Orientalism depends for its strategy on this flexible positional superiority, which puts the Westerner in a whole series of possible relationships with the Orient without ever losing him the relative upper hand. And why should it have been otherwise, especially during the period of extraordinary European ascendancy from the late Renaissance to the present? The scientist, the scholar, the missionary, the trader, or the soldier was in, or thought about, the Orient because he *could be there*, or could think about it, with very little resistance on the Orient's part. Under the general heading of knowledge of the Orient, and within the umbrella of Western hegemony over the Orient during the period from the end of the eighteenth century, there emerged a complex Orient suitable for study in the academy, for display in the museum, for reconstruction in the colonial office, for theoretical illustration in anthropoligical, biological, linguistic, racial, and historical theses about mankind and the universe, for instances of economic and sociological theories of development, revolution, cultural personality, national or religious character.
>
> *(Said, 1979, pp. 7–8)*

Essential to the political economy of Western epistemology is the creation of the dichotomy between the West and the non-West that serves as the ontological basis of Western knowledge, which in turn is mobilized as the rationale for Western interventions. For Fanon (1963), this differentiation between the haves and have-nots in the colonial context is inflected by race:

> this world cut in two is inhabited by two different species. The originality of the colonial context is that economic reality, inequality and the immense difference of ways of life never come to mask the human realities. When you examine at close quarters the colonial context, it is evident that what parcels out the world is to begin with the fact of belonging to or not belonging to a given race, a given species. In the colonies the economic substructure is also a superstructure. The cause is the consequence; you are rich because you are white, you are white because you are rich. This is why

Marxist analysis should be slightly strecthed every time we have to do with the colonial problem.

(Fanon, 1963, p. 32)

Gayatri Spivak (1999, 2003) interrogates the colonial histories and geographies of disciplinary structures and institutional knowledge that constitutes the Anglo-European academy and reinforces the transformative impulse of postcolonial studies. Her scholarship has charted an intellectual trajectory that covers feminist deconstruction, Marxist critiques of international divisions of labor and the global flow of capital, critiques of imperial and colonial discourses, and critiques of race in the context of the intersections among nationality, ethnicity, and the politics of representation in a neocolonial world (Landry & MacLean, 1996). The provocative works mentioned above provide rich theoretical linkages between colonialism and knowledge. It is this transformative impulse of postcolonial scholarship that situates it in tension with institutionalized knowledge, making us recognize that forces of geopolitics and colonial history are fundamental to constructing knowledge (Shome & Hegde, 2002). The authors also argue that it is this engagement of postcolonial studies with issues of race, class, gender, and sexuality in relation to geopolitical arrangements of nations and international histories that sets it apart from other forms of critical scholarship.

It is also this demonstration of the structure of world power relations as a legacy of Western imperialism that makes postcolonial studies relevant in the context of globalization. Globalization has led to a number of situations—migration of people, blurring of boundaries, simultaneous homogenization and fragmentation within and across societies, and the interpenetration of global and local among other phenomena (Appadurai, 1995; Dirlik, 1994, 1998). A postcolonial lens critically explores these phenomena and argues that global capitalism manipulates the local for the interest of the global. Dirlik (1998) writes:

What is ironic is that the managers of this world situation themselves concede the concentration of power in their (or their organizations') hands; as well as their manipulation of peoples, boundaries and cultures to appropriate the local for the global, to admit different cultures in the realm of capital only to break them down and to remake them in accordance with the requirements of production and consumption, and even to reconstitute subjectivities across national boundaries to create producers and consumers more responsive to the operations of capital.

(Dirlik, 1998, p. 466)

The local has emerged not only as a site of manipulation for operations of capital that needs to be assimilated with global culture, but also as a site of resistance. In other words, the local becomes a site of complex forces. Postcolonial theory powerfully reminds us that such complexities need to be situated within the context of imperial centers, and the present and historical moments. Hence, as Shome and Hegde (2002) suggest, a postcolonial intervention enables a more "socially responsible problematizations of communication" with the goal of eventually producing "a more just and equitable knowledge base about the third world, the other, and the [rest] of the world" (Shome & Hegde, p. 261).

As noted in the Introduction, postcolonial theory concerns itself with the presences and absences in dominant epistemic structures, and the ways in which these inclusions and omissions serve the agendas of colonial and neocolonial entities. Postcolonial theory creates discursive openings for examining the political nature of knowledge production, and urges us to disrupt the neocolonial interests of transnational hegemony by taking an activist stance in our articulations of knowledge. Given the spatiality of power and control in the ways in which resources are distributed and exploited, it is essential to explore the symbolic representations of the "West" and the "Third" that sustain colonial and neocolonial processes.

Imperial Knowledge Structures of Control

Knowledge of and about social change is a political entity that is quintessential to the project of neocolonialism under the aegis of contemporary globalization. Central to the circulation of colonial and neocolonial practices is the symbolic representation of the necessity for colonization, justifying the violence of occupation, control, and exploitation carried out by the centers of knowledge production. Any colonizing mission is justified rhetorically by the mantra of lifting the "burden of the soul," of delivering the primitive people of a primitive space from their savagery through the messages of enlightenment. The existence of colonialism is predicated upon the dominance of the epistemology of colonialism that sets up the dichotomy of the primitive and modern, and operates on the very basis of that dichotomy. Modernity is juxtaposed in the backdrop of the primitive spaces of the "Third World" that need the mantra of enlightenment. Knowledge of and about the "Third" plays a critical role in marking out, mapping, representing, and offering strategic entry points for the colonizing mission.

Structures of knowledge (universities, research centers, grants, think tanks, etc.) are created and supported for the purposes of carrying out the interests of colonialism and neocolonialism under the rhetoric of social change. Knowledge structures are situated politically and economically as truth-producing bodies that legitimize the political economy of neocolonialism. Therefore, an entire industry of academic, development, and marketing practices are manufactured to ensure the production and perpetuation of symbolic resources that are at the core of colonialism and neocolonialism. These practices circulate the dichotomies of developed and underdeveloped to justify colonialism and the exploitation of the "Third" under the guise of offering aid and bringing about enlightenment. The articulation of the primitive cultural practices in the "Third" serve the basis for occupation and control.

Historically, as demonstrated by Edward Said (1979) in *Orientalism*, West-centric productions of knowledge were quintessential to the colonialist enterprise. Knowledge served as the primary tool of colonialism, gathering data about the colonies, mapping out colonial spaces, and developing hierarchical units in the colonies to be brought under the control of colonial empires. Knowledge also offered the rhetorical base that served as the human face of colonialism, rhetorically positioning a violent occupation as an act of benevolence. Furthermore, knowledge was continuously deployed to bring the colonies under control, to civilize the subjects in the colonies, to teach the subjects the "civilized" ways of the colonizers, and to systematically erase ways of knowing that were native to the colonized spaces. This erasure happened through the portrayal of indigenous ways of knowing as primitive, as opposed to the modernity of the colonizers. The hegemony of West-centric ways of knowing was often accomplished through the languages of rationality, science and medicine, positioned as the antithesis of the irrationalities of the natives.

Inherent in West-centric knowledge structures is the political economy of such knowledge structures situated in the realm of the materiality of colonialism and neocolonialism. In contemporary discursive spaces, the interests of knowledge structures are weaved in with the interests of modernity. Knowledge, therefore, is intrinsically linked to the mercenary interests of the dominant institutions of capitalism. In their articulations of what does it mean to know the world, what are the acceptable tools for knowing the world, and what are the acceptable applications of knowledge, dominant knowledge structures continue to serve the interests of the status quo, further identifying markets and pockets of labor that carry out the interests of the status quo. In doing so, they validate, privilege, and foreground certain forms of knowing that continue to celebrate the dominance of the West and Western institutions over other forms of knowledge from the "Third." Even as standards are put forth regarding what it means to know the world, those ways of knowing are erased from the discursive spaces that fall outside the normative ideals of Western hegemony. As a result, power differentials are continuously maintained in the realm of who comes to know the world, and who gets to be scripted as the subject of studies, as an artifact to be captured in mainstream narratives as constructed by the dominant knowledge structures.

Capitalism, Modernity, and Neocolonial Agendas

As outlined in the previous section on production of knowledge that sustains the dominant interests of colonialism and neocolonialism, one of the core elements of colonialism is the economic gain attached to the occupation of a Third space. Occupied colonies offer cheap resources and labor for the production of commodities of modernity that then are sold to the markets created in the colonies, thus generating systems of profit for colonial institutions. Configurations of colonialism developed hand in hand with the interests of capitalist institutions to make profit, offering cheap sources of labor and ready-made markets for the commodities manufactured in the Empire. This linkage between colonialism and capitalism is aptly noted by Hegel:

> Through a dialectical impulse to transcend itself that is proper to it, such a society [capitalist market society] is, in the first place, driven to seek outside itself new consumers. For this reason it seeks to find ways to move about among other peoples that are inferior to it with respect to the resources it has in abundance, or in general its industry . . . The development of relations offers also the means of colonization towards which, in either an accidental or systematic way, a completed civil society is impelled.
>
> *(as quoted in Beverley, 1999, p. 121)*

At the heart of colonialism then is its attachment with the market and its consensual relationship with the flow of capital; it offers the basis for the operation of capitalism (Marx, 1970, 1975). Colonialism supplies the raw materials, labor, and market for the operation of capitalism. Therefore, for the unfettered operation of capitalism, colonialism is a necessity. In the contemporary global configuration, the modernist tropes of capitalism are circulated through mainstream mediated and other communication channels, through knowledge structures, and through the public relations practices of TNCs, IFIs, and nation states that operate through their claims of legitimacy on knowledge structures.

It is in this realm of the flow of the capital then that colonial agendas enjoy a two-way relationship with modernity and modernist institutions. On one hand, the economic base of modernity is served by colonial agendas; on the other hand, the symbolic representation of modernity serves colonialism by making colonial interventions appear necessary. In representations of the logic of capitalism as the marker of modernity and as the only desirable economic form of organizing, colonialism erases alternative forms of social and economic organizing that challenge the commodity-based articulation of individual identity, lifestyle, consumption, participation, and existence. Modernity is carried out through the consumption of goods and services produced by modernist institutions; therefore, in order to perpetuate this logic, subjects in colonies are turned into mass consumers of products and services manufactured by the modernist institutions. Articulations of development and underdevelopment are continuously mobilized in order to serve the interests of neo-imperial powers and transnational hegemonies. The economic logic of profit-making institutions gets circulated globally without being challenged, continually opening up spaces for transnational corporations to do business, operate in markets across global borders, and continue to make profits across global borders. Profit-making gets tied to notions of development; whereas development offers the rationale for neocolonial interventions, profit-making remains the ultimate objective. This consensual relationship between development and profit-making is well articulated in the following policy report of the United States Agency for International Development (USAID, 2002b):

> Successful development abroad generates diffuse benefits. It opens new, more dynamic markets for U.S. goods and services. It generates more secure, promising environments for U.S. investment. It creates zones of order and peace where Americans can travel, study, exchange, and do business safely. And it produces allies—countries that share U.S. commitments to economic openness, political freedom, and the rule of law.
>
> *(USAID, 2002b, p. 2)*

Development here serves as a strategic tool for opening up the markets of the so-called "underdeveloped" economies to transnational corporations. Through the language of development, the United States finds a way to intervene, colonize, and ultimately create markets for US investments, goods, and services. Most importantly, development offers the mechanism for spreading the mantras of neoliberalism through educational initiatives, public outreach, government lobbying, funding of favorable civil society organizations, development campaigns, and a wide variety of media relations activities.

In the contemporary global configuration, neocolonialism takes up various faces ranging from direct occupation of land that is similar to past forms of colonialism, to indirect occupation through the manipulation of nation states to buy into the economic agendas of neocolonialism. Contemporary forms of neocolonialism transcend the historic location of power and control in the hands of a nation state to clusters of power and control located in the hands of clusters of transnational corporations and nation states. These clusters of transnational corporations, nation states, civil society organizations, and global agencies are broadly referred to as transnational hegemony. Although transnational hegemony enacts its power beyond the traditional boundaries of nation states, nation states continue to be relevant as they serve as the key players in co-creating the agendas of transnational hegemony and in carrying out these agendas globally.

Neoliberal Control and Transnational Corporations

Postcolonial theory is particularly relevant in the context of contemporary globalization processes as it offers a theoretical lens for examining the ways in which the intersections of transnational corporations, nation states, global policy organizations, civil society and local elite work hand in hand to perpetuate their interests of neoliberalization. The interplay of power and control are at the core of the workings of neoliberalism, as power and control are applied through multiple interweaving mechanisms in order to create and foster markets for transnational corporations. Commenting about neoliberalism, Harvey (2005) notes:

> Neoliberalism is in the first instance a theory of political economic practices that proposes that human well-being can best be advanced by liberating individual entrepreneurial freedoms and skills within an institutional framework characterized by strong private property rights, free markets, and free trade.
>
> *(Harvey, 2005, p. 2)*

Inherent then in the neoliberal configuration is the protection of the interests of private property owners, multinational corporations, and financial capital. Accordingly, the impetus is on channeling the influences of local, national, and global policies to facilitate the operation of free markets and free trade, with minimal state intervention. The role of the state then is to ensure the operation of the free market, at the same time intervening minimally once the market has been created in order to ensure that this market operates smoothly under its so-called "free market" logic. The paradox of neoliberalism lies in the very role of the state in enacting violence to ensure the smooth running of the transnational corporations; as Jones (2003, p. 268) notes, "the state is becoming the primary disciplinary mechanism for global capital." This is well articulated by Harvey (2005):

> The role of the state is to create and preserve an institutional framework appropriate to such practices. The state has to guarantee, for example, the quality and integrity of money. It must also set up those military, defence, police, and legal structures and functions required to secure private property rights and to guarantee, by force if need be, the proper functioning of markets. Furthermore, if markets do not exist (in such areas as land, water, education, health care, social security, or environmental pollution) then they must be created, by state action if necessary.
>
> *(Harvey, 2005, p. 2)*

Contrary then to the rhetoric of the free market, neoliberalism operates on the very basis of state power that works continuously to bring about the marketization of economies across the globe. The state serves as a tool for the use of power and control in the interests of multi-and transnational corporations in order to create and foster markets that serve these profit-making entities. The military, police, and legal structures are deployed in order to ensure that economic bases are created for the operation of free markets that ultimately serve the political economic needs of private corporations (Mychalejko & Ryan, 2009).

In the backdrop of these state-sponsored systems and mechanisms of power and control that lie at the base of neoliberalism, the core of the neoliberal logic perpetuates the idea of minimal state intervention, deregulation, privatization, and the withdrawal of the state from many areas of social provision that were previously considered the responsibilities of the state. Harvey (2005) goes on to note:

But beyond these tasks the state should not venture. State interventions in markets (once created) must be kept to a bare minimum because, according to the theory, the state cannot possibly possess enough information to second-guess market signals (prices) and because powerful interest groups will inevitably distort and bias state interventions (particularly in democracies) for their own benefit.

(Harvey, 2005, p. 2)

Worth noting here is the irony in the conceptualization of the state in its relationship to multinational and transnational corporations. Therefore, whereas the state serves as a mechanism of exerting power and control for ensuring the creation and maintenance of markets, the role of the state is simultaneously omitted in the realm of regulating the profit-making ventures of private corporations. As a result, the state becomes a colonizing tool that continually serves the interests of the dominant social classes to enjoy profit and to maintain class power (Harvey, 2005).

Intrinsic in the processes of globalization is the formation of a social class that enjoys maximum power and control over social, economic, and political processes across the various sectors of the globe, and the simultaneous disenfranchisement of the lower classes from social, economic, and political processes where policies are made, debated, and implemented. As a result, globalization is marked by increasing inequalities locally and globally, with a limited number of people having access to the majority of the resources of the globe, as a large majority of others struggle to barely make a living. A postcolonial lens applied to these increasing disparities between the haves and have-nots brings to the fore the necessity for looking beyond nation states to examining the ways in which processes of exploitation and control play out globally; simultaneously, a postcolonial stance also calls for a reading of the global processes of power and control in terms of the agendas carried out by dominant nation states at the center to continue to oppress and control nation states in the periphery, utilizing the same colonial logics of development and enlightenment that have been historically used in the context of colonization. Nation states continue to serve the logics of colonialism; neocolonial and neo-imperial agendas continue to be carried out by a small number of nation states at the center who continue to use the rhetoric of bringing about enlightenment in order to serve their economic interests and the economic interests of the transnational corporations. Worth noting here is the clustering of transnational corporations within a certain configurations of nation states, and the continual utilization of national agendas and resources in the international arena to secure the interests of the transnational corporations.

In the most recent example of Iraq, the penetration and the subsequent occupation of Iraq by the United States under the pretext of bringing freedom to the people of Iraq (through the unjust occupation of their land) served as the perfect set-up for establishing a neoliberal dream project in Iraq, a kind of state apparatus that Harvey (2005, p. 7) calls a *neoliberal state*, embodying the interests of private property owners, businesses, multinational corporations, and financial capital. Paul Bremer, head of the Coalition Provisional Authority that was set up to run the newly occupied state spelled out four orders, including

> the full privatization of public enterprises, full ownership rights by foreign firms of Iraqi businesses, full repatriation of foreign profits . . . the opening of Iraq's banks to foreign control, national treatment for foreign countries and . . . the elimination of nearly all trade barriers.
>
> *(Harvey, 2005, p. 6)*

These orders were to be applied to all areas of the economy including public services, the media, manufacturing, services, transporation, finance, and construction. This mandate on neoliberalization was accompanied by strict regulation on labor, forbidding strikes and the right to unionize. Also, a flat tax plan was introduced into the economy, The rhetoric of freedom and freeing the Iraqi people served as the facade for the neo-imperial interests of the United States and the political-economic interests of transnational corporations. What was framed as freedom was really a reflection of the interests of transnational hegemony; as Harvey (2005, p. 7) notes, "Bremer invited the Iraqis, in short, to ride their horse of freedom straight into the neoliberal corral." Serving as an apt example of the nexus between the neoliberal nation state and transnational corporations, the case of Iraq demonstrates the central role of public relations in reframing neo-imperial agendas under the guise of liberation, freedom, democracy, and nation building. The conglomeration of terms such as democracy and freedom ultimately serve as justifications for the penetration and occupation of Third World spaces.

Furthermore, in the global politics of neoliberalism, those nation states receive aid that agree to adjust their economic structures along the lines of the dictates laid out by the International Monetary Fund, the World Bank, and the World Trade Organization. The WTO and the World Bank serve as the primary channels for securing global markets for transnational corporations, dictating national policies and exerting power and control over these policies to align them along the agendas of the transnational corporations. National policies across global spaces have often been shaped by the World Bank and its structural adjustment policies, dictating that national spaces open up to foreign investments, privatize public resources, and remove trade barriers to transnational corporations. Monopolistic control over international policies held by private corporations becomes evident in the shaping of the Uruguay Round of the General Agreement on Trade and Tariffs, which later led to the formation of the WTO, by agricultural giants such as Cargill and Monsanto. Similarly, the agreement on Trade-Related Aspects of Intellectual Property Rights (TRIPS) serves neoliberal interests through the hijacking of indigenous resources that belong to the subaltern sectors of the globe by transnational corporations, by allowing biopiracy, by not recognizing already existing indigenous knowledge as "prior art" so as to prevent the exploitation of such indigenous knowledge by transnational corporations, and by not taking into account the spatial ownership of genetic resources in privileging technologies developed by transnational corporations (DeSouza et al., 2008). As DeSouza et al. (2008) point out, biopiracy is constituted and facilitated by TRIPS through its policies favoring transnational exploitation of subaltern resources, and operates with relative ease on the basis of differentials in power and control in the neocolonial space, with the transnational corporations in the developed countries staking their claims on indigenous germplasm that was developed originally by farmers in the subaltern sectors of the globe. DeSouza et al. (2008) demonstrate, with the case of Basmati, that articulations of knowledge claims and ownership of knowledge of indigenous resources offer the legal framework for the exploitation of the subaltern sectors, playing out as a new form of colonialism. Knowledge here is critical in carrying out the neocolonial interests of global corporations.

Also critical to the global penetration of transnational hegemony is the role of civil society organizations in carrying out the agendas of transnational corporations, in opening up markets to foreign investments, liberalizing local economies, privatizing the public sectors, and in creating public opinion that is supportive of the broader goals of transnational corporations (Dutta-Bergman, 2005a, 2005b). With the widespread effect of clientelism among non-governmental organizations (NGOs), civil society becomes funding driven, seeking out funding to support the existing configurations and being directed toward meeting the requirements of the funding agencies in order to serve their own interests as economic entities. Veiled under the chador of development aid, public relations tactics are put into place in Third World spaces in order to bring about support for the objectives of transnational hegemony. In Chile for example, US corporations, the Central Intelligence Agency (CIA), and the US Secretary of State worked hand in hand with domestic business elites to undermine the democratically elected government of Salvador Allende, to violently repress all social movements and political organizations of the left, and to sponsor multiple civil society organizations run by the local elite that would carry out the agendas of neoliberalization, opening up the domestic market to foreign (read US) capital and businesses (Dutta-Bergman, 2005a, 2005b). USAID's goal of creating spaces of transnational support through its development aid programs is carried out through the involvement of the local elite and large-scale NGOs, operating to fulfill the funding criteria set out by USAID and to continue receive funding from the organization.

Resistive Politics

Historically, the forces of colonialism have also given rise to forms of resistance that operate across micro-, meso-, and macro-levels locally as well as globally, seeking to challenge the oppressive forces of colonialism, working within them in new ways, and working to transform the oppressive structures of capitalism that limit the opportunities for listening to subaltern voices across the globe (Pal, 2008; Pal & Dutta, 2008b). These forms of resistance are situated locally; they also connect globally across national boundaries in order to influence global policies. Narratives of colonialism coexist with narratives of resistance that seek to rupture the dominant narratives of power and control through which the colonial forces created their systems of oppression. Even as the structures of colonialism and neocolonialism operate through the perpetuation of dominant institutions that exercise their forces globally through the control of transnational, national, and local policies and the ways in which these policies are implemented, they also leave open possibilities of resistance. The very processes of globalization that have perpetuated modes of oppression and control across the globe have also created openings for challenging unequal, unjust, and powerful structures at the center through the creation of solidarity networks across global borders (Moghadam, 2009).

Take for instance the protest organized by the residents of the Bolivian city of Cochabamba in 2000 against the high cost of privatized water sold by Aguas del Tunari, a subsidiary of Bechtel (Olivera, 2004). Even in the face of state-sponsored violence that sought to thwart the protest and unleashed terror on the citizens, the protests continued, ultimately forcing the government to cancel the contract. Similarly, in Dabhol, India, women led the protests against the construction of the Dabhol Power Plant, a collaborative venture among three US-based multinational corporations (Enron, General Electric, and Bechtel). It is in these spaces of resistive practices that alternative imaginations of communication becomes possible, as a field of engagement that imagines the possibilities of structural transformation and the ways in which such transformation might be brought about through communication (see Figure 1.3).

Global resistance constituted and organized against the hegemony of neoliberal politics has been discussed under the framework of "globalization from below," "transnational activism," "transnational social movement," "grassroots organizing," etc. (Ganesh et al., 2005). Noting the lacuna in communication scholarship that studies the communicative processes of organizing and transformative politics, the scholars discuss the relevance for communication studies of resistance at the micro-level to move toward the study of macro-level communicative processes that seek to transform structures. Here, they outline the importance of examining the transformative potential of communication and delineating the precise ways in which communication can bring about transformation. The essay lays out key questions for communication scholars studying "globalization from below," such as (1) what norms, structures, power relations, and practices are targeted by resistance efforts, (2) to what extent does the resistance effort embody the capacity to disrupt the dominant hegemonies, (3) what is the relationship between the resistive processes and democratic outcomes, and (4) to what extent do resistance efforts target multiple forms of inequalities that are perpetrated by neoliberalism? In terms of the praxis of social change, Ganesh et al. (2005) note the relevance of working with resistance movements in challenging the dominant discourses of

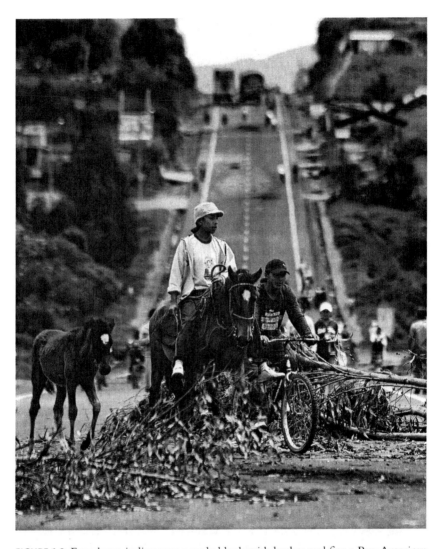

FIGURE 1.3 Ecuadoran indigenous people block with bushes and fire a Pan-American Highway stretch next to their village during a protest against a bill to regulate water resources in Ecuador on May 13, 2010, in San Rafael, Ecuador. Indigenous groups say the law could set the stage for privatizing water supplies, diverting resources that local people have depended on for generations. (Patricio Realpe/LatinContent/ Getty Images)

neoliberalism, engaging with the discursive processes through which organizing gets constituted, developing new forms of organizing globalization from below that offer new ways of challenging the neoliberal structures, working with alternative forms of organization structures in achieving social change, and developing specific tactics and communicative practices for transformative politics.

Along similar lines, in their review of the communication literature on resistance, Pal and Dutta (2008b) emphasize the transformative potential of communication scholarship in engaging with the processes of global networking, transnational flows, and grassroots organizing in local-global partnerships in bringing about social change. They further suggest the relevance of focusing contemporary theorizing in communication of resistance on the complexities of the intersections and interplays between the material and the symbolic realms of organizing. Emphasis is placed on understanding the communicative processes in issue identification and resource mobilization as local and global resistance collectives organize in spaces of change with the goal of transforming the inequitable global structures perpetuated by neoliberalism. Both Ganesh et al. (2005) and Pal and Dutta (2008b) issue a call for communication scholarship of resistance in the neoliberal landscape that is directed toward bringing about transformations in neoliberal structures, both theoretically as well as in terms of praxis. This book seeks to respond to this call by first exploring the discourses and materialities of neoliberalism in the context of marginalization of the subaltern sectors, and then examining in detail the communicative processes through which the transformative politics of resistance in constituted in the global landscape.

Subaltern Studies, Globalization, and Resistance

The subaltern studies project is concerned with writing history from below (Chatterjee, 1983; Chaturvedi, 2000; Conquergood, 1986; Guha, 1981). The very essence of writing history from below is to challenge the dominant constructions of knowledge, with specific focus on that which is left out of such dominant constructions. Subaltern studies as an intervention in South Asian scholarship came into existence to interrupt Indian historiography dominated by "colonialist elitism and bourgeois-nationalist elitism" (Guha, 1981, p. 1). The objective of subaltern studies was to document the historiography of the people by documenting their agency and politics, which had always been left out of colonialist and nationalist histories of India. Prakash (1992, 1994) and Lal (2001) provide a detailed backdrop of what led to the emergence of subaltern studies. Prakash writes that following India's nationalist struggle against British rule, the state adopted capitalist modernity to establish its legitimacy with relentless coercive measures that enhanced the inequities. Several historiographies followed that emphasized nationalist elite achievements. But none of these recognized the history of the masses. Though the Marxists contested such historiographies and celebrated the history of the sub-ordinated classes, their accounts of the masses, as Prakash (1994) notes, are also questionable as these accounts overlooked the contexts of the oppressed classes and regarded them as a stage in the process of their development. It is here that subaltern studies makes its contribution. Subaltern studies contested the colonialist, nationalist and Marxist representations of the common people and claimed a distinct position in scholarship by its new approach toward writing history, an approach that acknowledges the agency of the common people and celebrates their lived experiences while writing their history.

In the preface to the first volume on subaltern studies that came out in 1981, Guha describes the subaltern as subordinated in terms of "class, caste, age, gender and office or in any other way." Drawing from Gramsci, the themes of subaltern studies pay considerable attention to the dominant class, as the subaltern exists in a binary relationship with the dominant. Built on Marxism and poststructuralism (Prakash, 1992, 1994; Spivak 1988), subaltern studies is a complex critique of modernity. Subaltern politics engage with the conditions of exploitation to which people are subjected with the goal of acknowledging the agency of the subaltern. In Guha's words, the subaltern politics during the colonial period of India was "parallel to the domain of elite politics" (Guha, 1981, p. 4) that originated on its own and the contribution of the people to nationalism was made "independently of the elite." In this sense, spaces of subaltern dialogues existed beyond the realm of the mainstream public sphere that played out colonialist and nationalist elitist agendas. In his essay "The prose of counter-insurgency," published in the second volume on subaltern studies, Guha (1983) offers a critical analysis of historical writings on peasant insurgency in colonial India that demonstrates the presence of subaltern consciousness and its omission from the pages of history. Guha (1983) writes:

> Insurgency . . . was a motivated and conscious undertaking on the part of the rural masses. Yet this consciousness seems to have received little notice in the literature on the subject. Historiography has been content to deal with the peasant rebel merely as an empirical person or member of a class, but not as an entity whose will and reason constituted the praxis called rebellion.
>
> *(Guha, 1983, p. 2)*

Hence, the primary concern of subaltern studies is to restore the history and recover the subaltern consciousness. But the issue of recovery of the subaltern brings with it other tensions.

Problematizing the idea of recovering the subaltern voice, Spivak (1988, p. 10) argues that the intention to "investigate, discover, and establish a subaltern or peasant consciousness seems at first to be a positivistic project." Spivak suggests that because of the use of the word "consciousness," the subaltern studies group generates confusion over the treatment of subaltern consciousness. Is this the collective consciousness in the classical Marxist tradition or is this an essentialist understanding of consciousness that treats a certain subordinated political species as subaltern consciousness? Or is the use of essentialism "strategic" in a political interest? The other issue Spivak (1988) raises, over which there has been adequate tension in subaltern studies, is the possibility of recovery of the subaltern consciousness outside the elite discourse: "there is always a counterpointing suggestion in the work of the group that subaltern consciousness is subject to the cathexis of the elite, that is never fully recoverable" (Spivak, 1988, p. 11). Hence, can the subaltern be represented by academic knowledge? Despite the impossibility of recovering the subaltern subjectivity, as Spivak herself suggests, scholars must pursue their efforts of engaging with the subaltern voice and hence exploring possibilities of dialogue. While conflicts and differences have grown over these issues, subaltern studies has grown in its expanse too with more scholars from South Asia and Latin America embracing the scholarship (Prakash, 1992, 1994; Beverley, 2001). The appeal of the subaltern studies project is captured by Said (1988) in the foreword of the book *Selected Subaltern Studies*, co-edited by Guha and Spivak (1988) (see also Chatterjee, 1983; Chaturvedi, 2000):

> As an alternative discourse then, the work of the Subaltern scholars can be seen as an analogue of all those recent attempts in the West and throughout the rest of the world to articulate the hidden or suppressed accounts of numerous groups—women, minorities, disadvantaged or disposed groups, refugees, exiles, etc . . . This is another way of underlining the concern with politics and power.
>
> *(Said, 1988, pp. vi–vii)*

Its interjection with issues of power makes subaltern studies a paradigm that radically challenges modernist epistemologies by interrogating the violent erasures inherent in these epistemologies. Evident is the influence of postcolonial thinking in subaltern studies (Beverley, 2001; Lal, 2005; Prakash, 1994). Since the effort of the subaltern scholars is to recover the history of the marginalized "other" against the institutionalized system of knowledge constructed by the West and the national elite in postcolonial states, it becomes a critique of the dominant system of knowledge production itself, legitimized by the West. At the same time it is postmodern as it endeavors to bring about "epistemological rupture" (Beverley, 2001, p. 15) or what Lyotard regards as interrupting grand metanarratives. Dynamic in its multidisciplinarity, subaltern studies allows for studies in different colonial situations. Establishing its relevance across territories, Guha (2001) elucidates that though subaltern studies was theorized on the basis of South Asian experience, it informs the experiences of any subordinated history that is silenced across regions. Dominant historiographies have always been guided by rationalist discourses, where the primacy of the state gets glorified and experiences on the peripheries of the civil society remain omitted. "Our project calls upon us to unshackle the critique of reason from its tutelage to statism" (Guha, 2001, p. 45). Those foundations of civil society are interrogated that we take for granted as the democratic spaces of civil societies, and as platforms for dialogue. As demonstrated by Dutta-Bergman (2005a) in his analysis of democracy promotion efforts in Chile, Nicaragua, and the Philippines, the very networks of civil societies become the oppressive structures that limit the opportunities for subaltern participation through their requirements for language, literacy, and procedural skills necessary for so-called dialogue; these networks and structures are brought under review.

The project seeks to "displace the question of power" (Beverley, 2001, p. xvi) from the elitist agenda by drawing attention to the "other." It envisions chronicling those histories that are not foretold. It formulates the complex relationship between "subalternity and representation" (Beverley, 2001, p. 1). Thus, subaltern studies offers challenging ways to rethink about dialogue from a highly political and complex position and with an emancipatory ideology. This exhaustive survey of subaltern studies is provided to delineate its potential to open up discursive spaces for marginalized voices in the discipline of communication. Underscoring the meanings that are constructed by people within their cultural politics, it necessitates dialogic encounters with subaltern positions. Such an approach to understanding dialogue opens up new vistas of research in the discipline of communication, and opens dialogue theory to its emancipatory possibilities.

For the purposes of this book, we situate subalternity in terms of marginalization and marginalizing practices. Acknowledging the debates that note the conceptual differences between subalternity and marginalization, it is agreed that not all forms of marginalization refer to the conditions of being subalternized, particularly in the contemporary postmodern landscape of theorizing where marginalization is often theorized to discuss the experiences of individuals and groups at the outskirts of the status quo, therefore locating discussions of marginalization in the realm of identity politics. For the purposes of this book and according to the framework of the culture-centered approach to marginalization, marginalization is constituted at a structural level, connected to the articulations of material deprivations of the poor from the fundamental spaces of production and participation that define the contemporary mainstream. Therefore, the concept of marginalization as is used throughout this book refers to the structural and symbolic deprivations faced by the poorer sectors of society in the contemporary neoliberal landscape. It is through processes of marginalization that subaltern spaces are created across the globe; and it is also in relationship to these marginalizing practices of the status quo that possibilities of structural transformation through subaltern participation can be imagined. The culture-centered approach offers a conceptual framework for understanding the intersections of the structural and cultural processes of marginal-ization, as well as the cultural frameworks through which agency is enacted in challenging dominant structures and in creating new cultural scripts of engagement (Dutta, 2008c).

Culture-Centered Approach, Structural Transformation, and Participation

As noted in the Introduction, the culture-centered approach to communication for social change is founded on the two key concepts of structural transformation and participatory communication (Dutta, 2006, 2007, 2008a, 2008b, 2008c; Dutta-Bergman, 2004a, 2004b). Rooted in the materiality of marginalization, and drawing upon the basic concepts of dialectic materialism and class conflict in

Marxist theory of the 1870s (Marx, 2007), the approach notes that inequities in access to power result from the basic economic inequalities in society, and these inequalities result in epochal clashes (Artz, 2006; Cloud, 2006). This inequality in distribution of power, in turn, creates fundamental inequalities in access to a wide variety of resources, and the communicative inaccess to mainstream platforms in marginalized societies. In other words, marginalized societies are situated at and remain at the margins through their economic and communicative inaccess. Subaltern cultures as constructed as pathologies and as passive target audiences for development communication interventions that are created and directed by more powerful centers of knowledge production in the global landscape.

The condition of subalternity, as noted earlier in this chapter, is materially situated at the margins, and is carried out through discursive erasures that render the subaltern unheard. These communicative erasures are just as important as the material erasures, and serve as the foundation for the material erasures. If the subaltern could speak, she/he would no longer remain the subaltern. The role of communication scholars participating in the politics of social change communication is to deconstruct the communicative erasures, and to seek out spaces of social change through collaborative communicative processes of social change. The voices of the subalterns in alternative discursive spaces challenge the mainstream and the hegemonic assumptions that circulate in the mainstream.

Globalization Policies, Subalternity, and Violence

Globalization policies continue to perpetuate subalternity through the oppression of the poorest of the poor, often threatening to erase them from dominant discursive spaces, spaces of policy-making, and spaces of policy implementation. Structural violence is defined in terms of the violence enacted in the form of inaccess to resources and the fundamental inability to have access to the basic capabilities of life. These forms of inaccess are located structurally, in the form of the inequalities in distributions of resources at the structural level. Structures impede access to basic resources, and operate as continually reinforcing systems that carry out the cycles of poverty. Structures create highly concentrated clusters of risk that are often tied to the projects of industrialization and development, forcing the poorest sectors of the globe into serving as laborers in neoliberal projects, with high levels of exposure to physical, chemical, and environmental risks. Consider for example the structural violence carried out on the *maquiladora* workers in Mexico, who work in the manufacturing shops of large TNCs, in poor working conditions with minimum labor laws/regulations and high levels of exposure to chemical and industrial wastes (Brenner, Ross, Simmons, & Zaidi, 2000).

It is violence when a child does not have enough food to eat. It is violence when the basic access to healthcare is not available in a community. It is violence when families have to live on the streets. These forms of violence are structural because they are rooted in the social structures that define the terrains of society.

Structural violence is deeply embedded in historically perpetuated oppressions that have often been carried out across generations, maintaining the realms of inaccess to basic resources. As neoliberalization policies come to be universally implemented across the globe in the form of structural adjustment programs, the poorest of the poor, already at highly elevated risks of exposure to a wide variety of diseases and inaccess, are further marginalized, uprooted from their spaces of livelihood, displaced from their homes, and further detached from sources of earning income. The already existing forms of structural violence are further deepened as the poorest sectors, a large proportion of them belonging to the indigenous tribes, are displaced from their lands and their sources of livelihood, forced into the capitalist economy as cheap transitory labor for the very projects of industrialization that have displaced them. For example, mining projects all across the globe are being constructed on tribal lands, often depleting the forests where the tribals live, thus uprooting and erasing the tribal from her/his home, and setting her/him up as a displaced laborer in the neoliberal economy, further exposed to the structural violence of neoliberalism.

Farmer (1999) notes that structural violence is perpetrated on all those whose social status denies them access to the basic capabilities of life. Sickness here is located structurally and is driven by the structures, a product of historical oppressions that are often economically driven. He explains how the differential political economy of risk plays out in the case of HIV infection in the poorer sectors of the globe:

> If we are to present meaningful responses to AIDS, we must examine the differential political economy of risk. Structural violence means that some women are, from the outset, at high risk of HIV infection, while other women are shielded from risk. Adopting this point of view—that we can describe a political economy of risk and that this exercise helps to explain where the AIDS pandemic is moving and how quickly—we begin to see why similar stories are legion in sub-Saharan Africa and India, why they are fast becoming commonplace in Thailand and other parts of Asia. The experiences recounted here may be textbook cases of vulnerability, but their moral is deciphered only if we clearly understand that these women have been rendered vulnerable to AIDS through social processes—that is, through the economic, political, and cultural forces that can be shown to shape the dynamics of HIV transmission.
>
> *(Farmer, 1999, p. 79)*

Violence here is politically and economically situated, in the structural configurations that constitute the threats of disease and illness. Violence is constituted in the everyday lived experiences of the poorest of the poor, who continue to be further marginalized with the projects of modernization, development, and urbanization that have been ushered globally ever more powerfully under neoliberal hegemony.

The neoliberal hegemony, however, does not only exert its power and control through shifts in local policies and economic modalities; it further consolidates its power through the violence perpetrated through the military-police complex of the nation state. The state, in much of a departure from the rhetoric of neoliberalism that projects the image of minimal state involvement in the free market, fundamentally serves to create markets for neoliberal configurations through the use of police force and military sponsored violence. Violence here is enacted in the form of police atrocities, firings, arrests, kidnappings, rapes, and tortures that are carried out in the name of development and industrialization (Padhi et al., 2010; Pal, 2008). In the state of Orissa in India, for instance, police oppression in the tribal areas has increased exponentially as tribal people have started protesting the occupation of their lands, their displacement as a result of mining and development projects, and their marginalization from the mainstream (Padhi et al., 2010). This landscape of global violence perpetrated by transnational hegemony also creates spaces and opportunities for resistance from below.

Subaltern Agency in Transformative Politics

One of the main concepts in the culture-centered approach is the articulation of subaltern agency as an entry point for social change (Dutta, 2006, 2007, 2008a, 2008b, 2008c). Theoretically, the culture-centered approach makes the argument that the exhumation of subaltern agency from dominant discursive spaces lies at the heart of the rhetoric of development, thus shaping the praxis and materiality of development communication programs across the globe. The quintessential paradox inherent in the programs of development lies in the structural violence, displacements, and marginalization caused by the very projects that are portrayed as the solutions to global poverty and marginalization. This paradox operates effectively through its construction of the subaltern sectors as passive and without agency; it is on this palette of agency-less target audiences that programs of development are carried out. As Escobar (1995) notes in his critical interrogation of development discourse unleashed on Colombia:

> The messianic feeling and the quasi-religious fervor expressed in the notion of salvation are noticeable. In this representation, "salvation" entails the conviction that there is one right way, namely, development; only through development will Colombia become an "inspiring example" for the rest of the underdeveloped world . . . Before development, there was nothing: only "reliance on natural forces," which did not produce "the most happy results." Development brings the light, that is, the possibility to meet "scientifically ascertained social requirement." The country must thus awaken from its lethargic past and follow the one way to salvation, which is, undoubtedly, "an opportunity unique in its long history" (of darkness, one might add).
> *(Escobar, 1995, p. 26)*

The articulations of the subaltern sector as lethargic, as reliant on natural forces, and as unproductive serve to justify the political economy of development projects that are then carried out as justifications for modernizing the subaltern sectors. In other words, the epistemological exercise of removing agency from the realm of subalternity justifies the top-down campaigns that make the decisions for the subaltern sectors, deciding what is good for them, and utilizing the language of "doing good" to carry out the agendas of the dominant power structures. In its co-construction of culturally centered narratives, the culture-centered approach resists the dominant narratives of the status quo that continue to reiterate global inequalities. Alternative entry points are created for engaging with the agency of the subaltern sectors, thus fundamentally revolutionizing the dominant con-structions of the subaltern in development projects.

One of the excellent examples of subaltern agency in the backdrop of neoliberal hegemony is the Zapatista movement, often cited as the first postmodern rebellion against neoliberal globalization (Burbach, 1994; Ross, 1995). As discussed in the Introduction, the Zapatista rebellion in Chiapas, Mexico, reflected in the uprising that brought large parts of the Las Canadas and Selva Lacandona regions under the control of the Zapatista Army of National Liberation (Ejército Zapatista de Liberación National, or EZLN), embodies the enactment of agency among indigenous communities who created the EZLN as their project, thus noting the indigenous ownership of the project as a site for individual and collective actions of social change. In resisting the global forces of neoliberalization, the EZLN created a global space for transformative politics and alternative rationalities by working through networks of solidarity with activists and mediated sites of change across the globe.

Similarly, in India, large sectors of the indigenous populations in the Eastern states of Bihar, West Bengal, and Orissa have taken up arms in resistance to the contemporary projects of neoliberalization in the form of industrialization and mining that threaten to displace large sectors of the indigenous populations from their spaces of livelihood (De, 2009). Subaltern agency here is constituted in challenging the state apparatus and in interrupting its hegemonic narrative of development by foregrounding the plight of the indigenous populations in India as new projects of development continue to displace them, simultaneously depriv-ing them of the benefits of the modernization projects (Dutta-Bergman, 2004a, 2004b). For example, the *adivasis* (tribal people) of Lalgarh in the West Midnapore district of West Bengal, India, have organized themselves into a collective to resist police atrocities, state-sponsored violence and projects of neoliberalization in the form of the special economic zone (SEZ) to be set up by the Jindal Steel Group in the region (Bhattacharya, 2009; De, 2009; Mike, 2009). The community organ-ized into a collective, called the People's Committee Against Police Atrocities (PCPA), in order to resist state-sponsored violence. Similar tribal movements are emerging all around India, voicing their protests against state violence and global agendas of neoliberalism, played out through the displacement of tribals from their lands and forests, which constitute their primary form of livelihood.

Negotiating the Symbolic and the Material

The overall meta-theoretical framework adopted in the culture-centered approach notes the dynamic relationship between the symbolic and the material. The symbolic refers to the constitutive realm, the realm of communication and meaning making, and the material refers to the economic structures and resources. As noted by Cloud (2005, 2006, 2007), a large proportion of the critical approach to communication scholarship utilizes the postmodern turn to examine the fragmented sites of power, and to locate power communicatively, often divorced from the discussions of the material inequities and the politics of the economic that drive the lived experiences of oppressions and the resistance to oppressive forces in the subaltern sectors. Cultural studies projects of communication, in their emphasis on floating meanings and interpretive frames, lose the fundamental impetus of critical theory to seek social change, and more dangerously, end up reifying and propagating the status quo through their lack of attention to issues of class, class antagonisms and material oppressions in society.

The emphasis often in these cultural studies approaches to communication is on interpretive frameworks and culturally situated contexts of meaning making, without attending to the material bases and the structural inequities that continue to influence the geopolitics of global oppressions, and reifying the fundamental class differences in neoliberal hegemonies. Meanings are important in projects of critical theory, but only when they are examined in relationship to class structures, material inequities, and structural oppressions. What is problematic with the postmodern turn with critical theory is that in its foregrounding of the meaning-making processes, it fails to articulate the role of material interventions in shifting the material structures and in challenging material terrains. Discourse, discursive spaces, and discursive enunciations become the sites for negotiating power, and discussions of material change in dominant structures are backgrounded or erased from the discursive spaces that discuss power.

The notion of fragmentation of power is articulated to draw attention away from the realities of power differentials that have real and tangible outcomes in the lives of the poor across the globe. The inaccess to food, education, health services, and shelter are material realities, and have to be understood as such. In a world where neoliberal forces have continued to reify, recreate, and deepen the class divides, the critical project is necessary as a site of intervention and transformative politics. In the midst of the globally increasing inequalities across the various sectors, the political interventions of critical theory lie in challenging and seeking to transform these inequalities. Without engaging with the material, the project of critical theory loses its transformative capacity. Therefore, the culture-centered approach foregrounds structure as an entry point for understanding oppressive global forces, and situates structure in relationship to culture and agency. Agency is enacted in response to these structures, and is expressed through cultural symbols, tools, and resources. The expression of agency and the circulation of cultural tools are materially situated, and draw upon material resources to disrupt global structures.

Conclusion

This chapter provided an overarching theoretical framework for understanding and locating the different approaches to communication for social change, taking into consideration the divergences and convergences in the theoretical traditions and the ways in which these theoretical traditions play out in the praxis of social change. One of the primary lessons learned in this chapter relates to the goals and objectives of communication for social change processes, and the ways in which these processes vary with respect to their relationship with dominant structures. Also, attention is drawn to the differences in communication for social change projects based on their conceptualization of the nature and role of communication in the social change initiative. After having laid out the basic structures of the development campaigns, participatory development, Marxist, and culture-centered approaches to social change, most of the book will focus on the culture-centered approach to social change, with an emphasis on understanding the intersections among culture, structure, and agency in processes of social change, especially as they relate to the possibilities of structural transformation.

PART I
Structures and Marginalization

2

POVERTY AT THE MARGINS

One of the core elements in the constitution of the margins is the absence of material resources that define the very capacities of human life. Poverty then is articulated in terms of the ability to meet basic needs, experienced at the individual, collective, and state levels (Burkey, 1993). At the individual level, poverty is defined economically, as a marker of individual and household incomes. Furthermore, it is defined in terms of access to the basic needs for resources such as clean air and water, sufficient and balanced food, appropriate clothing and shelter, physical and emotional security, and physical and emotional rest. At the community and state levels, poverty is defined in terms of the absence of basic infrastructures of communication, resources for maintaining the health and well being of community members in order to sufficiently maintain the community, political systems for leadership and decision-making, educational systems for learning, information sharing and continuing the culture of the community, and physical and cultural security (Burkey, 1993). Essential to these definitions of poverty is the conceptualization of basic resources that make up the necessities for human life, both economically as well as politically.

The discussion of poverty as a site of social change is relevant both historically and also in terms of the contemporary geopolitics of poverty. Across the globe, the number of people living in poverty and in extreme poverty is increasing, accompanied by increasing inequalities at the local, national, and international levels (Hubbard, 2001). Similarly, urban poverty as a proportion of total poverty in some developing sectors of the globe is on the rise (Amis, 2001). The advent of neoliberalism, played out through the structural adjustment programs across the globe have contributed to the increasing structural marginalization of farmers, unemployment, and increasing inequalities between the haves and have-nots across the globe. Furthermore, geographical disparities have widened, with poverty increasing in Africa, Latin America, and the Caribbean (Chalmers et al., 1997; Gershman & Irwin, 2000). The implementation of the structural adjustment programs (SAPs) in Latin America, Caribbean, and Africa, for instance, have resulted in increasing marginalization of the poorer sectors and the rising inequalities within countries (Chalmers et al., 1997; Gershman & Irwin, 2000; Inter-American Development Board (IDB), 1997, 1998a, 1998b; Lucero, 2008). The rising unemployment in these regions, accompanied by the absence of social safety nets and public spending on social services, resulted in further marginalization of the poor. Even in regions where economic growth has increased at the national level, the poorer sectors have been increasingly marginalized. Analyzing the widening social inequalities across the globe against the backdrop of the neoliberal discourse of economic growth, Gershman and Irwin (2000) note that the framing of poverty in terms of economic growth instead of redistributive justice reflects the wider political realm of policy-making.

Chapter 2 is organized around the concept of poverty and the ways in which poverty is constituted through policies in mainstream social structures. Attention will be paid to the global, national, and local constructions of policies related to poverty and the conditions of the poor. Empirical data from macro-level studies will be utilized to descriptively document the nature of poverty within and across social systems; this description will be juxtaposed in the backdrop of communicative processes, discourses, and messages in mainstream societies that create and sustain poverty. Of particular focus here are the questions: What are the ways in which poverty is articulated in mainstream public spheres? How is poverty discussed in dominant discursive spaces? What are the key narratives of poverty in mainstream platforms and how do these narratives shape policies around poverty? What are the inter-linkages between the material and the symbolic in the context of poverty? How does the materiality of the lived experiences of the poor get constituted within discursive structures and processes in the mainstream?

The culture-centered approach to marginalization offers a theoretical lens for understanding the political economy of global poverty, and suggests an entry point for praxis in projects of structural transformation (Dutta, 2008c). A culture-centered lens to poverty suggests that the deconstruction of the symbolic markers that circulate in mainstream platforms needs to serve as an entry point for actually listening to the voices of the poor that have otherwise been erased from the very platforms that talk about them, evaluate them, make policies about them, develop interventions targeting them, and then evaluate these interventions (Dutta, 2008a, 2008b, 2009). Voices of the poor co-constructed in ethnographic and cultural projects will provide entry points for developing an interpretive frame around poverty and for understanding the possibilities for enacting agency in the realm of the social structures. This discussion of agency will offer a launching pad for looking at the role of communication in poverty-related social change projects in Part II of this book. Throughout the chapter, the intersections of structure, culture, and agency equip us with theoretically rich understanding of how poverty is constituted within social systems and the ways in which it is perpetuated in these systems.

Conceptualizing Poverty in a Neoliberal Landscape

At its conceptual foundation, poverty is defined in terms of the economic resources that are available to an individual. In other words, the income that is available to an individual is used to operationalize poverty, based on the idea that one's ability to secure the basic resources necessary for life depends upon the economic access she/he has in order to purchase these basic resources. Income-based measures of poverty therefore are utilized to draw a poverty line which serves as an ontological and epistemological framework for defining people living below poverty and for creating policies around poverty. The poverty line is a key indicator in the global politics of poverty as it defines the development, implementation, and evaluation of policies related to poverty, guiding the initiatives, aid programs, and interventions run by global institutions. The measures of the poverty line serve as key tools of evidence making and argumentation in the articulations of certain sets of structures, institutions, and processes that are set up to address poverty. Furthermore, in the politics of globalization, the poverty line is used as a crucial marker to enunciate the incidence of poverty, which in turn, is utilized to generate political and economic support for the neoliberal policies of globalization.

Table 2.1 presents data on the percentage of population living below poverty, based on the World Bank Development Indicators and the latest World Bank estimates of the poverty line to be established at \$1.25/day at 2005 purchasing power parity.

What we observe in Table 2.1 is the dramatic change in the percentage of people to be considered living in poverty depending upon where the line is drawn. So whereas the percentage of people living under poverty is at around 12 percent when considering the \$1/day mark, it changes to 22 percent with the

TABLE 2.1 Percentage of People Living at Different Poverty Levels in the World (World Bank Development Indicators 2008)

Poverty Line[a]	Percentage below
\$1.00	12
\$1.25	22
\$1.45	28
\$2.00	40
\$2.50	48
\$10.00	80

Note: [a]Calculated at US\$/day at 2005 purchasing power parity latest World Bank poverty line of $1.25 a day. When considering the $10 per day mark, which is the level that would be considered as appropriate for a wealthy country such as the United States, the percentage of people living in poverty changes to approximately 80 percent of the world population. Therefore, the marker of poverty that is used to define the poverty line plays a critical role discursively, serving as a key sign in the articulations of poverty-related policies, politics, and interventions. Ultimately, the materiality of the politics of poverty is dependent upon the markers of knowledge that are mobilized in defining and determining poverty, and in making specific arguments about the nature of poverty in the world. The symbolic lies at the heart of the global processes that shape the material, thus drawing attention to the communicative constructions of poverty in justifying global policies. Discourses of poverty articulated at the level of the World Bank shape global policies, the implementation of these policies, and the ways in which these policies are evaluated across the globe. Discourse here operates in the arena of the political, with the political objectives of the dominant global power structures determining the ways in which poverty-related policies are developed and implemented, and the relationships of these policies to broader economic programs in nation states across the globe. For instance, the symbolic articulations of certain markers of poverty and the deployment of certain sets of tools evaluating this poverty are then politically utilized to make the argument that neoliberal policies have contributed to the decline in poverty, although other sets of indicators point otherwise.

At the level of nation states, poverty is also defined in terms of the growth in the per capita gross domestic product (GDP) of a country, based on the argument that the increase in the per capita GDP of a country is also reflective of a healthy economy, serving as a sign that the country is developing (Sachs, 1992; Sen, 1988; United Nations Development Programme, 2004). Here, the emphasis is on the notion that national development leads to the reduction in poverty as resources secured in a nation state diffuse to the sectors living under poverty, leading to the economic development of these sectors. The "trickle down" philosophy under-lying the logic of economic growth assumes that economic progress made by the nation state would then play out in the amelioration of poverty. The emphasis is on retaining the dominant structures of organizing rather than on programs of redistributive justice that seek to meet the needs of the poor. The nation state data, although reflective of the overall economic growth at a national level, does not really narrate the story of distribution of wealth within a nation state. This is especially worth noting, given the empirically documented large-scale disparities within countries and across the different sectors of the globe.

Challenging the definitions of poverty in strictly economic terms, economists and policy-makers have suggested the need for a broader approach to poverty that looks at poverty in terms of capability and human development. In addition to being defined on the basis of economic indicators, poverty is also defined in terms of other indicators of basic access such as education, health, and food, specifically with an emphasis on children (Sen, 1992, 1999). Therefore, the prevalence of hunger among children and the child mortality rates of a country are also used to describe its poverty. Sen's approach to poverty notes the necessity to broaden the traditional concepts of poverty in terms of economy, income, and wealth to include a plethora of other factors that constitute basic human development such as illiteracy, ill-health, and poor education. Suggesting the capability approach, Sen (1988, 1992, 1999) articulates the relationship between poverty and human rights, constructing poverty as the fundamental denial of human rights. Capability is defined as the opportunity to achieve the necessary combinations of human functionings, defining what a person is able to do or be. Poverty, in other words, is the deprivation of these basic capabilities, the lack of alternative possibilities (Sen, 2005a, 2005b) (see Figure 2.1).

Inequality

Inequality refers to the differences in the socioeconomic status that exist within a nation state, as well as between nation states in a global landscape (Coburn, 2000, 2004). Studies of globalization document the increasing inequalities between the various sectors of the globe, both reflected in the inequalities between geographic regions and nation states as well as within nation states. Noting the inequalities that have developed across the globe, Coburn (2000) suggests that the principle of neoliberalism operates on the basis of inequalities, seeing inequalities as tools for promoting worker motivation, participation in markets, etc. By taking an individual-level approach to poverty and to public services, neoliberalism takes an individualistic stance in attacking various types of collective or state action, further reinforcing the inequalities between the rich and the poor (Coburn, 2000, 2004). It further reinforces inequalities by minimizing the ability of workers to organize through weakening unions and simultaneously minimizing the access of the poor to public services such as education and health.

Neoliberalism and Poverty

As noted throughout this book, neoliberalism refers to the constellation of global policies represented in privatization of economies, accompanied by the opening up of these economies to international trade in capital, goods, and services; minimizing tariff and non-tariff barriers; reducing or eliminating government subsidies; and minimizing state control over the free flow of goods, capital, services, and domestic labor markets (Gershman & Irwin 2000; Harvey, 1995). The neoliberal configuration was globally disseminated and implemented through the workings of three key international organizations: the World Bank, the International Monetary Fund (IMF), and the General Agreement on Tariffs and Trade, which later evolved into the World Trade Organization. The combined agendas of these three international actors can be framed in terms of monitoring global markets,

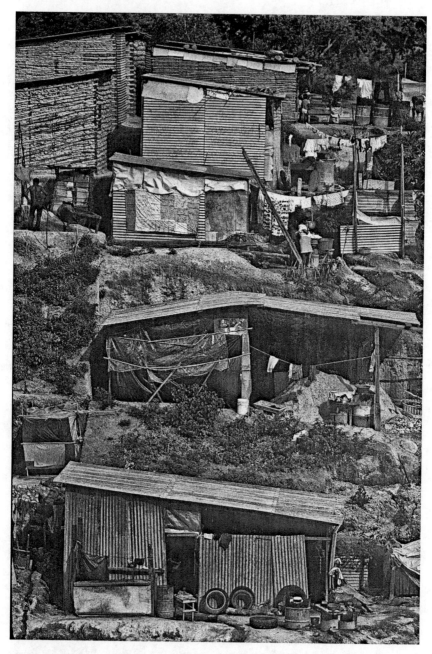

FIGURE 2.1 A view of a poor area of San Salvador. (Cindy Karp/Time & Life Pictures/Getty Images)

encouraging free trade at the global level, nurturing growth in the underdeveloped world, and at the same time, maintaining the interests of the dominant capitalist powers (Gershman & Irwin, 2000). This form of global liberalization was seen as the solution to preventing the incursions of communism by maintaining relative peace between labor and capital, and thus minimizing class antagonisms while simultaneously serving the interests of the capitalist classes. The solution to poverty under the agenda of neoliberalization was the achievement of economic growth in the underdeveloped sectors and not the development of economic policies of redistributive justice.

One of the key features of neoliberalization is structural adjustment. In the face of the large-scale debts faced by several Southern states of the globe, structural adjustment programs were pushed by the World Bank and the IMF as conditions for the allocations of loans offered by these international financial institutions to nation states. During the debt crisis of the 1970s and 1980s, when a large number of Third World countries were unable to continue making their debt payments to commercial banks in wealthy countries that had given vast amounts of loans to the developing countries, the global financial system was threatened with a collapse. In order to prevent the collapse of the global financial systems, wealthy countries intervened through the IFIs, and established clauses of economic restructuring of the developing countries through the SAPs. The SAPs, therefore, emerged as mechanisms of global economic restructuring, played out through the control of IFIs in the hands of the most powerful shareholders in the World Bank and IMF, United States, UK, and Germany. Neoliberal principles were imposed on Third World countries as conditions for loans given out to these countries, thus serving as the primary forces behind economic restructuring across the Third World.

The minimization of trade-related barriers opens up economies and local markets to competitions from TNCs, thus resulting in the weakening of the local industries as they start competing with commodities manufactured by the TNCs. The emphasis on privatization and profits minimizes the organizing ability of unions to negotiate wages, and workers become vulnerable to the movements in the economy, often being the first ones to lose their jobs or experience cuts in wages, in the face of financial crises. The link between poverty and neoliberalism becomes even more clear when countries pursuing neoliberal policies are compared with more social democratic nations (Coburn, 2004). It is observed that countries actively pursuing neoliberalism are more likely to report higher levels of absolute and relative poverty as well as higher levels of inequalities as compared to countries that pursue a more social democratic system of governance.

Neoliberalism and Unemployment. With the implementation of the structural adjustment programs, large tracts of farmland throughout the globe started coming under the control of industrialization projects, thus displacing farmers and rural communities, and leading to the rise in unemployment in the rural sectors (Gershman & Irwin, 2000). In addition, with the opening up of the agricultural sector through privatization, deregulation, and liberalization, the local agricultural sector came in competition with cheap food commodities marketed by TNCs, also leading to the loss of economic forms of subsistence in the farming communities. Small-scale farmers became uncompetitive in the markets flooded by the imported food commodities. In order to remain viable in the changing economy, the farmers were persuaded through agricultural extension programs and government-sponsored initiatives of the economic value of switching from internal-input driven multiple crop farming to external-input driven monoculture farming of hybrid (genetically modified) crops purchased from the TNCs (Shiva & Bedi, 2002). The economics of agriculture shifted from self-sustainable farming where farmers saved the seeds from one year to plant the next year to a commoditized form of agriculture where farmers depended on TNCs to purchase their seeds every year, in addition to needing to purchase fertilizers, pesticides, and even water. Large numbers of farmers who could not generate the capital to continue participating in the com-moditization of agriculture quickly became unemployed, thus becoming prospective migrant labor for the rapid industrialization projects under the SAPs. Similarly, in the industrial sector, as economies across the globe started facing financial crises, the industrial sectors sought to maintain their profit margins by minimizing labor inputs, thus creating a highly volatile economic scenario where workers are vulnerable to the agendas of TNCs and to the fluctuations in global capital. The onset of the financial crisis across the globe resulted in loss of jobs, and therefore, in increasing global unemployment. Neoliberal policies such as the lifting of import regulations and the privatization of the public sector led to public sector layoffs, increasing numbers of unemployed, and high demands for jobs, which in turn resulted in increasing control of labor markets in the hands of TNCs (Millen & Holtz, 2000).

With the increasing privatization and deregulation of markets across the globe, economies across the globe have left workers unprotected in their relationship with management (Escobar, 2003). The "flexibilizing" of labor markets was dictated by the IFIs, with the goal of pushing governments to create more friendly business environments in their countries by minimizing job security protections and minimum wage laws (Millen & Holtz, 2000). This has resulted in greater vulnerability of workers in various industries across the different sectors of the globe, as well as with limited bargaining power in their negotiation of rights with the government. In Chile, for instance, the neoliberalization of the country resulted in poor working conditions for workers, increasing vulnerability of workers as well as low wage levels that leave workers unable to meet their basic needs. Neoliberalism operated as a mechanism for the reproduction of poverty, leaving workers vulnerable and creating conditions for low wages for workers that were not sufficient in helping them satisfy their basic needs and the needs to support their family (Agacino & Escobar, 1997; Escobar, 2003). In 1998, the minimum wage for Chilean workers was 47.7 percent of what was required and therefore was below the minimum cost for the reproduction of the workforce

(Escobar, 2003). Escobar further notes that at least half of the Chilean workers did not earn enough to be able to escape poverty. Neoliberalism in Chile operated as a site of power and control, operating on the basis of the exploitation of workers. The ability of the neoliberal economy to accumulate capital is based on the overexploitation of the workforce. Furthermore, referring to the later period of the effects of the world crisis on the Chilean economy, Escobar (2003) documents that those principally affected were the workers, with rising unemployment and decline in real wages. Therefore, just as the overexploitation of the workers is necessary for the accumulation of capital in neoliberalism, the workforce becomes an expendable element of adjustment in order to defend profits during times of contraction.

The effect of neoliberalization on the deterioration of working conditions is evident in the creation of export processing zones (EPZs) that are no longer confined to the regulations of the border (Brenner, Ross, Simmons, & Zaidi, 2000). In Mexico, the *maquiladora* program was established with the goal of attracting foreign investment, and foreign companies were allowed to import raw materials duty free and had to pay export taxes only on the value added (Brenner et al., 2000). With the signing of the North American Free Trade Agreement (NAFTA), an increasing number of TNCs established their plants, known as *maquiladoras* in Mexico, employing mostly Mexican workers. The weak enforcement structures for environmental and labor laws in Mexico makes the *maquiladoras* particularly attractive to TNCs. *Maquiladora* workers either have no union representation or representation by a union that is government controlled. In spite of the rhetoric of the North American Agreement on Environmental Cooperation (NAAEC) and the North American Agreement on Labor Cooperation (NAALC) accompanying NAFTA, little enforcement has been made of environmental and labor standards, thus making the *maquiladoras* attractive spaces of production for US-based TNCs, who can generate high profits through overexploitation of workers and pollution of the environment. The wages of *maquiladora* workers does not match up with the high cost of living along the borders, and are typically not enough to sustain the families of workers. In addition, the weak implementation framework of labor laws leaves the space open for the use of coercive and violent strategies such as legal maneuverings, firings, and police violence by the government and manufacturing companies. Occupational health and safety conditions are poor, with high rates of occupational injury and illness, and high levels of exposure to chemical, physical, and ergonomic hazards (Moure-Eraso, Wilcox, & Punnett et al., 1994, 1997). Furthermore, the *maquiladoras* produce large levels of toxic chemical wastes, releasing these into the broader region's air and water, causing environmental accidents and polluting the Rio Grande, thus posing short-term and long-term threats (Lewis, Kaltofen, & Ormsby, 1991).

Neoliberalism and public services. The neoliberalization of the globe also plays out through the privatization of the public sectors that offer basic public services to the population (Dagdeviren & Fine, 2004; Kessler, 2003, 2004). The rationale offered here has been that the privatization of state-owned enterprises would increase efficiency and incentivize innovation. Public sector resources such as water, education, and health are turned into the realm of the private sphere and are opened up by national and local governments for private investments and profiteering. This has led to the increasing prices of public services (which are no longer public services but private commodities) for poorer households as well as less coverage for the poorer sectors. In Bolivia, for example, after the privatization of mines and much of the nation's economy, the neoliberal project focused on privatizing the water resources, thus raising the cost of water and making it largely inaccessible to the nation's poor (Oliviera, 2004; McKinley, 2004). The privatization of land in the name of boosting efficiencies in countries such as Cambodia and Mongolia has led to increasing disparities in the distribution of land and landlessness among the poorer sectors (Dagdeviren & Fine, 2004; Nixson & Walters, 2003).

The politics of neoliberalism not only plays out in the existing commercial and industrial sectors, but also has been extended to include the basic services at the local community level. One of the ways in which neoliberalization plays out in the global scenario is through public-private partnerships that are created with the goals of meeting the needs of the poor in an efficient and effective manner. Therefore, many of the sectors that have traditionally been managed by the state are managed by the private sector. These private-public partnerships (PPP) have been conceptualized by development agencies such as the United States Agency for International Development as a key mechanism for delivering services to the underserved sectors of the Third World (USAID, 2002b; see also Fiszbein & Lowden, 1999). For instance, in South Africa, the housing policy for serving the poor adopted PPPs in order to mobilize resources across the private and public sectors to deliver a large number of houses to the disadvantaged families. The PPPs are seen as a collaborative process engaging the local communities, private sector as well as the state. The policy has achieved limited results, unable to produce the number of houses necessary to meet the needs of the poor, delivering units of poor quality, meet and located at inaccessible locations (Miraftab, 2004; Tomlinson, 1999). Miraftab's (2004) analysis of the PPPs in South Africa situated the failure of the PPPs in the framework of unequal power relations between the community and the private partners, thus noting the importance of the mediating role of the state to ensure that local community needs are met and adequate infrastructures are available for the community.

Poverty in the Indigenous Sectors of the Globe

Indigenous communities continue to constitute the poorest sectors of the globe, facing limited access to resources of food, health, water, and shelter (Dutta-Bergman, 2004a, 2004b; UN Department of Economic and Social Affairs (UNDESA), 2010).

Historically, indigenous communities have been constituted at the global margins of development programs that have created systems for exploiting these communities with minimum benefits of development available to the communities. Under the implementation of neoliberalism with the deployment of structural adjustment programs across the globe, these communities face some of the greatest threats of displacement as indigenous lands are brought under state control and sold off to private corporations for the purposes of mining, plantations, tourist resorts, and other projects of industrialization (UNDESA, 2010). The large-scale displacement of indigenous communities from the very spaces they call home has resulted in the fundamental disruption of indigenous lifestyles, cutting off connections to the resources of economic productivity that support indigenous communities. Projects of development have used the rhetoric of development in order to sell off indigenous spaces for the purposes of corporate profit, thus leading to the unemployment of indigenous populations and alienation from the natural resources that constitute the indigenous cosmology. For instance, Santali community members in Eastern India note their loss of health at the hands of deforestation projects that have disrupted their relationship with nature: "Then everything was healthy because they [referring to the ancestors] respected nature. They offered their prayers to nature. They lived a full life. Roaming the mountains and the forests, they were happy. They were healthy because they respected nature" (Dutta-Bergman, 2004a, p. 248). Similarly, indigenous knowledge has been subjected to bio-prospecting and commercialization, with private corporations paying teams of experts to gain access to indigenous knowledge of medicinal plants and herbal remedies, and then to use this knowledge for the purposes of profiteering. The neoliberalization of global economies has reduced the indigenous sectors to sites of profiteering, simultaneously resulting in large-scale unemployment and poverty, as indigenous communities have been increasingly cut off from their traditional forms of sustenance (UNDESA, 2010).

Theories of Poverty

Theories of poverty offer a wide range of explanations for the occurrence of poverty across the various sectors of the globe, thus also offering different entry points to policy-making and intervention development (Melkote & Steeves, 2001). In the realm of poverty, knowledge production is directly linked with the praxis of development, with knowledge occupying a key space in the development of policies, implementation of these policies, and in the carrying out of specific interventions, projects, and programs that are directly linked to addressing issues of poverty.

Modernization Theories

The various modernization theories of poverty are based upon the conceptualization of dichotomies that differentiate between the developed and underdeveloped sectors of the globe. Development is measured on a socio-evolutionary scale in terms of the extent of modernization that is achieved in a society, and poverty reduction is seen as synonymous with development. In other words, development theories operate on the assumption that the greater the development in a society, the lower the extent of poverty in that society. Therefore, the emphasis is on creating an ontology that creates categories of development, and then defining the praxis of development in the form of development policies and development interventions.

Modernization is defined in terms of certain sets of indicators such as economics, industrialization, technology, capital investments, and population growth, thus drawing the line between the modern and the backward. Poverty is situated in the backdrop of underdevelopment and therefore against is connected to the lack of modernization in some societies. A wide net of reasons is cast on the landscape of poverty, drawing upon the underlying theme of backwardness of some societies in comparison to other societies. Based on this theoretical explanation of backwardness that maps out the contours of poverty, interventions are carried out by elite and powerful states in the form of development initiatives, directed at addressing poverty in the underdeveloped sectors of the globe.

Economically Based Explanations.   Under the modernization framework, the primary emphasis has remained on the economic growth of the "underdeveloped" sectors of the world, articulated in terms of the productive resources of a society and the economic institutions that guide the use of these resources, differentiating between traditional and modern economies (Melkote & Steeves, 2001). The economic indicators of poverty are typically measured in terms of the growth of output (i.e., GNP) of the nation state, based on the assumption that an overall increase in GNP would also minimize the poverty trends in a nation state (Rahnema, 1993). Explanations for poverty are offered in terms of the economic indicators of poverty, and are articulated in the realm of the backwardness of the poorer sectors of the globe (Lerner, 1958; Portes, 1976; Rahnema, 1993; Rogers, 1974; Weber, 1988).

In modernization theories, the output of the goods and services of a system is based on the input of labor, capital, infrastructure, natural resources, technology, and entrepreneurship. Labor is measured in terms of its capacity to participate in the industrialized economy, tied to the skills and attitudes necessary to serve as productive resources for the needs of modern industry. Capital is conceptualized on the basis of its relationship to the industrialized sectors, putting forth the argument that the greatest allocation of capital needed to be made to capitalists and entrepreneurs, the success of whom would then lead to a trickle-down effect, with benefits then flowing to the rest of the population.

Land and other natural resources are conceptualized within the modernization framework in terms of their relationship to an industrialized economy, mediated through mass-scale technologies of production that turn these resources into high-yield products. In the conceptualization of land as resource, modernization-based development theories on one hand focus on increasing the outputs from the agricultural uses of land through investments in capital-intensive technologies of agriculture, and simultaneously emphasize the reappropriating of land resources for uses in industrialization projects (Shiva, 1988, 1991). Resources are constituted in their relationships with technologies of modernity; for instance, in agriculture, development initiatives in the form of the Green Revolution were introduced into the Third World that emphasized the introduction of technologically modified seeds, chemical fertilizers and pesticides, farm machineries, and intensive irrigation, thus redefining agriculture within a capitalist framework (Shiva, 1991). One of the key markers of development, the building of dams in the Third World for instance, has been played out under the modernist logic of modernizing agriculture. Similarly, the displacements of rural and indigenous communities across the globe have been carried out as justifications for industrialization projects or mining projects that in turn feed the industrialization projects (Pal, 2008).

Yet another core indicator of development in the modernist framework is the availability of technology, based on the argument that technology brings about development in the agricultural and industrial sectors by increasing production (Abramovitz, 1956). Technology is seen as a catalyst of development, and therefore, the emphasis is placed on knowledge transfers of technological know-how from the developed sectors to the underdeveloped sectors of the world. Jeffrey Sachs (2005) notes in his book *The end of poverty*:

> The real story of modern economic growth has been the ability of some regions to achieve unprecedented long-term increases in total production to levels never before seen in the world, while other regions stagnated, at least by comparison. Technology has been the main force behind the long-term increases in income in the rich world, not exploitation of the poor. That news is very good indeed because it suggests that all of world, including today's laggard regions, has a reasonable hope of reaping the benefits of technological advance.
>
> *(Sachs, 2005, p. 31)*

Therefore, the increase in production brought about by the advances in technology is seen as the primary reason underlying development. Technology is seen as a solution to poverty by its contributions to the overall economy through increases in production; it serves as a point of differentiation between the developed and the underdeveloped sectors of the globe. Yet another indicator of development is the entrepreneurial attitude in a society that opens up possibilities for innovations (Lerner, 1958; Rogers, 1962, 1974; Weber, 1988).

In addition to the resources outlined above, modernization theories underscore the relevance of economic systems in national cultures in determining the allocation of resources and the policies that are put in place to govern the economy.

Based on the foundations of capitalist principles of development, modernization theories emphasize the diffusion of *laissez-faire* principles of economic development that favor complete independence of the private sector, where the capitalists and entrepreneurs are to be left alone by the government, with minimum interventions from the state.

The requirements of the capitalist paradigm that is presented as the paradigm of development, include the following clauses: first, private ownership of all means of production; second, the establishment of an interrelated market system of labor, land, and capital for output; third, an independent and private capitalist firm with no external control operating rationally to generate maximum profit; and fourth, free trade at the local, national, and international levels that would catalyze the free operation of the market. The underlying principles of the minimal economic intervention model emphasize the facilitation of free market conditions locally, nationally, and globally for the minimization of barriers to the global operations of transnational corporations. The goal therefore is to find resources to facilitate the transition of societies and economies to capitalism, which is in turn seen as the basis for bringing about development in the Third World.

Based on the capitalist model of economic development in the United Kingdom and United States, the laissez-faire model operates on the assumption that national economic development works at its best when private corporations are able to operate with minimal state intervention, and these national-level aggregate benefits trickle down to the poverty trends. Global institutions such as the Bretton Woods institutions, IMF, and the World Bank were therefore created to manage and guide the use and distribution of economic resources across the globe, shaping and monitoring national policies and bringing these policies into compliance with global articulations of development.

The privatization and free market models of development and poverty reduction continue to operate globally today, articulated in the form of international policies such as NAFTA and GATT. International organizations such as the WTO, IMF and the World Bank continue to carry out the goals of international capitalism, framed within the realm of development (Harvey, 1995). The World Bank for instance carries out its poverty reduction programs and funding strategies in conjunction with the imposition of structural adjustment programs that seek to move the economies of Third World markets toward a free market framework, with minimum state involvement and minimal barriers to free trade.

Cultural Explanations. Cultural explanations depict poverty as a product of the backwardness of cultures, in terms of the values, beliefs, worldviews, and institutions that circulate in the culture (Portes, 1976; Weber, 1958). Culturally based explanations therefore focus on the ways in which these values, beliefs, and worldviews impact the lives of community members, placing them in paths of underdevelopment. Conceptualizing poverty as a social disorder, models from Europe and North America are utilized to set up the standards of modernization, and to depict the processes of change through which cultures adapt to standards of modernization as achieved in the Western hemisphere. Enlightenment thinking dominated the cultural worldview, differentiating between traditional cultural configurations that were irrelevant to progress and modern values that were quintessential to scientific progress.

At the heart of the culturally based theories of development is an understanding of the cultural processes involved in the transition of Europe and North America from largely traditional feudal societies to fairly complex and highly differentiated industrial-capitalist societies (Portes, 1976). Based on the conceptualization of development as social evolution, poverty theorists in this paradigm discuss the movement toward development in terms of evolution, noting that the highest state of evolution was reflected by European nations in the nineteenth and early twentieth centuries (Melkote & Steeves, 2001). Noting the movement of human societies from simple and traditional configurations to more complex entities that were industrialized, Herbert Spencer believed that Western societies were more likely to survive as compared to more backward Third World cultures because they were better adapted to the shifting environments in the process of modernization of societies.

In culturally based modernization discourse, the Third World is located in the realm of backwardness and incompatibility of its values with the project of modernity as reflected in Western Europe and North America. For instance, Weber's (1964) work on the cultural markers of modernity emphasized the Protestant ethic in European cultures that lent itself to industrialization, capitalism, and the modernization project as opposed to the backwardness of Third World cultures that prevented modernization, often reflected in their religions. For Weber, Islam harbored tradition-bound rigidity, Hinduism prescribed asceticism, and Buddhism emphasized otherworldliness, all seen as barriers to modernization. In the lens of modernization then, these religious values were obstacles that needed to be overcome for the cultures to develop.

Individual-Level Explanations. Whereas the economically driven explanations are typically offered at a macro level and the cultural explanations locate the locus of poverty in the realm of the community, the individual level explanation focuses on individual characteristics and dispositions underlying underdevelopment and poverty (Inkeles, 1996, 1969; Lerner, 1958; Rogers, 1971, 1974). The argument here emphasizes certain dispositional patterns that are perceived to be the causes of underdevelopment. Societies are seen as underdeveloped because they are aggregates of these individual traits of backwardness, manifested in terms of cultural markers, religiosity, and beliefs and attitudes toward modernization. The emphasis then is on targeting the individual-level dispositions which are seen as the root causes of poverty and underdevelopment. This is accomplished through the deployment of campaigns and interventions that target the individual-level characteristics of the primitive or backward audiences located in the Third World.

For instance, based on his research in six developing countries, Inkeles (1966) proposed a model of individual-level modernity that tapped into the likelihood of individuals to adapt to modernity. He defined these characteristics as attitudes toward modernity, and suggested that these were psychological constructs that tapped into the spirit of modernity (see Melkote & Steeves, 2001). The nine attitude items that were utilized to characterize the modern person were openness to innovation, likelihood of forming and holding opinions, orientation toward democracy, habits of planning, belief in personal and human efficacy, belief that the world is calculable, emphasis on personal and human dignity, faith in science and technology, and belief in distributive justice. In this line of work, the psychological construct of modernity was conceptualized as a desirable outcome as well as a mediator in the pathway toward development. Therefore, interventions were proposed that sought to cultivate these personality characteristics in target populations.

Along similar lines, the work of Daniel Lerner (1969) focused on the individual characteristic of empathy, describing the capacity of a person to identify with the new aspects of one's environment. Describing the concept as empathy, he notes that individuals with empathic capacity are more likely to modernize because of their openness to identify with changing aspects of the environment. Further noting that empathic capacity is more likely to be found in Western cultures, where individuals are also more likely to be industrial, urban, literate, and participant, Lerner (1969) suggests the necessity of cultivating empathy in developing and underdeveloped contexts.

Rogers and Svenning (1969) studied peasants and subsistence farmers in Colombia, India, and Nigeria, observing that these farmers lived a traditional lifestyle, and this lifestyle needed to be transformed if they were to be modernized. The emphasis at the individual level was on changing the individual attitudes, beliefs, and behaviors of the peasants that then contributed to the collective level of development of the agrarian communities that constituted the majority of these countries. The individual-level traits of underdevelopment observed by Rogers and Svenning (1969) included fatalism, familism, limited aspirations, limited view of the world, perceived limited good, mutual distrust in interpersonal relationships, lack of deferred gratification, dependence and hostility toward government authority, lack of innovativeness, and low empathy.

Population-based Explanations. Drawing upon the Malthusian notion of limits to population growth, a substantive body of work on poverty notes that the root cause of poverty lies in the population growth in certain societies, which then puts a strain on the resources available to the society (Ehrlich, 1968). Modernization is seen as synonymous with population control and management. The high fertility rates in the Third World are defined in terms of crisis, and noted as the primary cause for the degradation and overexploitation of the environment. Therefore, underdevelopment in Third World and the occurrence of poverty in the

Third World are attributed to the inability of the Third World to manage the population problem, thus resulting in an imbalance in population against the backdrop of the availability of resources (Braidotti, Charkiewicz, Häusler, & Wieringa, 1994).

Based on the problematization of population growth as the source of the problem underlying poverty, development initiatives have emphasized anti-natalist programs in the South, with an emphasis on managing the "population crisis" (Melkote & Steeves, 2001, p. 99). This emphasis on population control became one of the earliest behavioral targets of health development campaigns, involving communication initiatives run by the Population Communication International (PCI) that targeted women in the Third World with mantras of enlightenment, packaged in the form of population control and family planning. The United Nations channeled resources through the United Nations Population Fund (UNFPA), which worked hand in hand with state actors to control population growth in the Third World. Development became synonymous with the agendas of controlling population growth in the Third World.

Communicative Explanations. Communicative explanations offered by social scientists studying poverty against the backdrop of the development literature noted the influential role of the mass media as agents of change, based on the argument that literacy, along with exposure to mass media would create the right ingredients for the transition of traditional societies into modern societies (Lerner, 1958; Schramm, 1964). The mass media here was seen as a means for diffusing the messages of development and modernity, thus breaking traditional peasant societies out of their backward beliefs, attitudes, and lifestyles. Rogers (1973) notes that the mass media are able to raise the level of aspiration among the traditional people of developing countries, and thus create a climate for the adoption of innovations. This is well articulated in the following excerpt: "The media preach the gospel of desire by depicting the good life in advertisements and news stories; this raises the wants . . . by increasing the wants, the media are at least contributing toward a climate of modernization" (Rogers, 1973, pp. 48–49).

More specifically, the mass media are seen as playing a pivotal role with diffusion of innovations in developing countries, as channels for carrying messages about the innovations (Rogers, 1962, 1983). The diffusion of innovations theory operates on the basis of the notion that opinion leaders in developing and underdeveloped societies would spread the message of the innovation to the rest of the community. Thus, mass-mediated and interpersonal communication are seen as working hand in hand to carry out the messages of development.

Critical Theories of Poverty

Critical theories of poverty articulate the structural inequities and differential distributions of power that exist within global, national, and local spaces that underlie poverty. They draw attention to the circuits of power that operate in the processes of knowledge production around global economic policies and the ways in which poverty is taken into account in these policies. Knowledge is conceptualized as a political entity that serves the interests of dominant power structures, and is utilized for the purposes of maintaining the status quo. A critical interrogation of the political economy of poverty-related knowledge production specifically highlights the politics of the status quo that guides global policies on poverty and the implementation of these policies across the globe.

Dependency Analysis. Dependency analysis emerged in the 1960s as a critique of the worldview of the UN Economic Commission for Latin America that held to the viewpoint that underdevelopment in Latin America was a product of too little capitalist development and continued feudal backwardness, and instead argued that underdevelopment in Latin America was the result of the development of capitalism across the world, shaping the New World through mercantile relations and direct capital investment (Cardoso & Faletto, 1979). Underdevelopment here is not viewed as a static condition but rather one of the poles of a dynamic historical process that created both development and underdevelopment; the underdevelopment in certain sectors of the globe is caused by the development in other sectors of the globe, and vice versa (Dietz, 1980, 1998).

Dependency theorists draw attention to the global imperialism that plays out in the dominance of the periphery nations by the core nations of the globe, achieved through the cooperation and participation of elite groups within these periphery nations in the processes of exploitation. Underscoring the power imbalances in the dominant paradigm of development, the dependency approach attends to the economic dependencies that are created in the underdeveloped sectors through projects of development, which fundamentally operate to sustain and reproduce the global inequities in distributions of material resources.

More specifically, the surplus generated by the periphery states is extracted by the states in the center for the purposes of development and growth at the center. The questions of poverty, inequality, and development are conceptualized within the broader framework of imperialism, based on the articulation that imperialism creates spaces of poverty through the exploitation of resources and labor in certain sectors of the globe for the purposes of development in other sectors of the globe. Here then the global distribution of poverty is spatially conceptualized, in terms of the relationships of exchange that exist between spaces, and the ways in which these relationships play into the exploitation of labor and material resources to serve the interests of the dominant power structures.

Cardoso and Faletto (1979) take more of a dialectical approach to the question of dependence and development, noting that even as foreign capitalist penetration into Latin America fosters underdevelopment, it also creates conditions for revolutionizing the means and relations of production. Thus, the crux of the position put forth by Cardoso and Faletto (1979) is that development and dependence are not mutually exclusive, based on the observation that Latin American countries show signs of capitalist development even as the same forces operate to reinforce underdevelopment in Latin America. Dependence is conceptualized as a process, constituted in terms of changing class relations both internally and externally. The wide variety of debates and dialogues within the dependency approach emphasize the relevance of interrogating the question of poverty in terms of the relationships between development and underdevelopment, interrogating the explanatory role of "development" concepts and related policies in creating and sustaining under-development across the globe.

World Systems Theory. Similar to dependency theory, the world systems theory makes note of the spatial inequities in distribution of power that play out materially in the realm of development and poverty (Wallerstein, 1974). Poverty is con-ceptualized relationally, understood within the ambits of relationships among the various actors in the world system, and the roles that are assigned to the vari-ous global actors in the capitalist world systems economy. The world system is conceptualized as a singular economic system that is capitalist in orientation, and is a network of multiplex dependent relations among countries (Wallerstein, 2004). In world systems theory, there are core states such as the United States, European Union, and Japan that are economically strong and therefore dominant on the world stage; peripheral states such as Africa, Latin America, and Asia are considered weak; semi-peripheral states such as oil-producing countries and states of South East Asia lie in between the center and the peripheral states (Wallerstein, 1974). The division of the world into the different strata is based on the different roles assigned to these strata in the international division of labor, therefore operating within the realms of the value assignments that are made to capital and labor within the world system. The roles assigned to the various actors within the world system are related to the inequalities among countries in the distribution of resources and power (Rossem, 1996).

Critical Interrogation of the Dominant Discourse. Critical theorists have interrogated the dominant articulations of development, interrogating develop-ment programs for the ways in which they have served the agendas of the status quo. For instance, critical examination of development programs supported by the United States Agency for International Development (USAID) foreground the military, political-economic, and geo-strategic interests served by these programs, continuing to create global markets for US-based TNCs rather than serving the interests of the poor (Dutta-Bergman, 2004c; Fair, 1989; Fair & Shah, 1997). The geo-strategic and market-based interests served by USAID under the public relations frame of development are adequately captured in the following excerpt from the USAID (2002a) report titled *Foreign aid in the national interest: Promoting freedom, security, and opportunity*:

Successful development abroad generates diffuse benefits. It opens new, more dynamic markets for US goods and services. It generates more secure, promising environments for US corporations. It creates zones of order and peace where Americans can travel, study, exchange, and do business safely. And it produces allies—countries that share US commitments to economic openness, political freedom, and the rule of law.

(USAID, 2002a, p. 2)

What becomes evident here is the implicit agenda of developing markets elsewhere that is served within the framework of development. Explicit articulations of development goals are utilized as the rationale for pushing the agendas of neoliberal hegemony, for opening up the boundaries of nation states to TNCs, and for creating new markets across the globe for US goods and services. Development here is framed within the broader agendas of neoliberalism, operating as a justification for neoliberal interventions, and therefore serving as a neocolonial tool that ultimately serves the political economy of TNCs. Furthermore, the very political economy of development actors is also constituted within the logic of creating new markets for development products (Dutta-Bergman, 2004c, 2005a, 2005b).

Similarly, specific neoliberal policies have been critically examined for their influence on poverty-related national policies and their effects on poverty outcomes across various spaces of the globe. Increasingly, critical interrogations of the policies of neoliberal actors draw attention to the ways in which these policies actually serve the interests of the status quo and continue to carry out the agendas of transnational corporations. International structures/organizations such as the World Bank, IMF, and WTO have emerged as the sites of power, with their capability to dictate the economic policies of individual countries, by holding loans and financial assistance to countries on the basis of their willingness to organize their economies according to the principles of neoliberalism (Brock-Utne, 2000; Dutta & Pal, 2010; Mosley, 2001). Once again, the public relations framing of liberalization and privatization as development justifies the support for global policies that continue to marginalize the poor (Dutta & Pal, 2010). The structural adjustment policies promoted by the World Bank and the International Monetary Fund across the globe have been critiqued for their marginalization of the poorer sectors, simultaneously serving the TNCs and the national elites (Olivera, 2004).

For instance, the privatization clauses laid out by the World Bank for Bolivia combined with the political-economic interests of Bolivia's elite led to large-scale privatization of several public sectors in the country, liberalization of the economy, and a concerted campaign by the national elite to delegitimize the union movement, once a key actor in the Bolivian political scenario. This resulted in the rising inequalities in Bolivia, accompanied by rising unemployment, poorer living conditions, and rising poverty. Similarly, structural adjustment programs implemented throughout Latin America have resulted in economic instability, increasing unemployment, increasing income inequalities, and inaccess to basic resources among the poorer segments of society (Algranati, Seoane, & Taddei, 2004; Potter, 2007). Government spending in the public sectors was curtailed; agriculture suffered tremendously; and state industries were sold to the private sectors (Lora, 2001; Lora & Panizza, 2002; Potter, 2007). It is against this backdrop that the World Bank has been critically interrogated for its promotion of structural adjustment programs elsewhere in the globe, which in turn serve the privatization and liberalization agendas of neoliberalism on a global scale. In this sense, the World Bank is a key player in the neoliberal agenda that has contributed to the global increase in disparities and inequalities.

Experiences of poverty are further situated at the intersections of the global inequities in neoliberal policies of migration and the policies governing the flow of capital, products, and services. Even as the IFIs push toward the opening up of countries to foreign capital, goods, and services, global policies in the realm of migration continue to enact forms of control and dominance directed at managing the flow of labor from the global South to the centers of power.

The World Bank and its poverty-related policies have been historically interrogated for the erasure of the poor from the discursive spaces of policy making and for the top-down approach to policy implementation (Shepherd, 2001). In responding to the criticism of top-down interventions, the World Bank has increasingly incorporated the language of participation and empowerment in its rhetoric. Interrogating this rhetoric, Wong (2003) suggests that the conception of power articulated within the domains of the World Bank continue to serve top-down agendas of economic rationality and market efficiency. Along the same lines, criticisms have been offered to the participatory models espoused by the World Bank, based on the argument that participation has traditionally been utilized to serve the economic agendas of the World Bank, and political participation has often included consultation without really locating the decision-making power within local communities (Oakley, Bichmann, & Rifkin, 1999).

The empowerment of the poor has been situated within the neoliberal logic of efficiency, without attending to the inequalities and power differentials that underlie the marginalization of the poorer sectors (O'Brien, Goetz, Schotle, & Williams, 2000; Oakley, et al., 1999). Feminist criticism of the role of the World Bank (more on this in Chapter 5) note the economic rationalities of market productivity and individual responsibility promoted by the World Bank, which further continue to marginalize the poorer sectors by reifying the structural imbalances that lie at the heart of the inequities (F. Cleaver, 1999; Kabeer, 1994; O'Brien et al., 2000). In spite of the rhetoric of empowerment in project life cycles, the institutionalized structures of efficiency within the bank and the instrumentality of the bank as a power structure that enacts control over development projects become obstacles to empowerment, limiting the possibilities of structural transformation (more on this in Chapter 9). Kabeer (1994) criticizes the World Bank's much celebrated micro-credit programs as solutions to poverty, suggesting

that such programs emphasize individual-level solutions through economic participation of women, completely ignoring the structural disparities that perpetuate
the marginalization of poor women.

Culture-Centered Approach to Poverty. The culture-centered approach to
poverty begins with an interrogation of the constructions of poverty in the
dominant discourses of economics and global policy, seeking to examine the ways
in which articulations of poverty continue to serve the interests of neoliberal
hegemony, drawing upon capitalist discourses of development and further undermining the voices of the poor and/or co-opting these voices within a capitalist
agenda (Dutta, 2008a, 2008b, 2008c; Farmer, 1999). Interrogating the symbolic
representations circulated in transnational hegemony in the context of the material
realities of the globe points to the gaps and contradictions in the articulations of
poverty among the dominant power structures, and the ways in which poverty
eradication initiatives are constituted within the broader agendas of the power elite.
Knowledge guiding the theoretical conceptualizations of poverty as well as the
eradication of global poverty lies primarily in the hands of the World Bank, a global
institution that articulates its objectives in terms of developing policy documents
and policy guidelines regarding development, as well as allocating material
resources to projects based on poverty (St. Clair, 2006a, 2006b).

Juxtaposed against the backdrop of the deconstruction of the dominant
discourses of poverty, the culture-centered approach emphasizes the relevance of
co-constructing the narratives of lived experiences of people living in poverty.
These narratives are constituted through participatory dialogues with the
marginalized sectors of the globe, thus foregrounding the voices of the poor within
the discursive space, and disrupting the silences and erasures constituted in
mainstream discourses. The rationalities of poverty articulated in the mainstream
are thus challenged, being brought face-to-face with alternative rationalities
constituted in subalternity. Essential to the dialogic stance of the culture-centered
approach is the emphasis on understanding the agency of subaltern participants in
local communities across the globe as they challenge the inequitable structures,
work within them, and aspire to find avenues of living in their daily negotiation
of these structures. Far from being the passive and backward subjects portrayed in
the mainstream discourses of poverty, the poor across the globe narrate the various
struggles they engage in on a day-to-day basis in their negotiation of the dominant
global structures. Consider the following narrative of a woman from Latvia as she
describes her poverty in the project narrating the voices of the poor, conducted
by Narayan, Patel, Schafft, Rademacher, & Koch-Schulte (1999b): "poverty is
humiliation, the sense of being dependent on them, and of being forced to accept
rudeness, insults, and indifference when we seek help." In her description of
poverty in her life, the participant narrates the ways in which the structure
marginalizes her communicatively; here, poverty is played out in her humiliation
and in being forced to accept the mistreatment that is meted out to her. Similarly,

for a participant from Pakistan, "we poor people are invisible to others—just as blind people cannot see, they cannot see us" (Narayan et al., 1999b, p. 12). Poverty is marked by this sense of being invisible, of not being seen and of not being accounted for in the dominant spaces of knowledge production. In other words, symbolic marginalization works hand-in-hand with material marginalization. Therefore, a culture-centered praxis of social change seeks to fundamentally alter the material inequities across the globe by seeking to create communicative resources, infrastructures, and spaces for listening in subaltern contexts (Dutta, 2008a, 2008b, 2008c).

Values in Articulations

Descriptions and operationalizations of poverty are value-laden processes that are embedded in certain ideological configurations (St. Clair, 2006a, 2006b). Therefore, the ways in which problems attached to poverty are conceptualized, the roots of poverty as noted in the discourse of dominant structures, as well as the solutions to eradicating poverty are value laden, articulating certain narrowly defined sets of ideological positions that serve the interests of transnational hegemony, setting up certain logic linkages and argumentative claims based on the gathering, analysis, and presentation of data within certain frameworks that suit the interests of transnational hegemony (St. Clair, 2004a, 2004b). The material realities of poverty as constructed within the hegemonic structures are built upon certain sets of abstractions that are dictated by the values informing the science, and the agendas that are served by these values and the hegemonic institutions they serve. For instance, the determination of the poverty line is an exercise in abstraction, intrinsically tied to the values involved in the material realities that are produced by the exercise.

The hegemonic role of the World Bank as a site for institutionalizing knowledge about poverty and in shaping the material realities of the poorer sectors of the globe through the allocation of funding resources to a variety of development projects and national actors, the determination of credit scores of nation states, as well as the shaping of the economic policies of nation states is embedded within the specific values of neoliberal hegemony and the audiences of the World Bank such as the International Monetary Fund and client states (St. Clair, 2006a, 2006b). The World Bank draws its legitimacy from those very actors in the neoliberal arena that are themselves legitimized through the practices of the bank. In other words, the World Bank exists in a consensual relationship with other powerful actors on the transnational stage. The values that guide the production of knowledge around poverty also dictate a political economic framework for knowledge production wherein the World Bank emerges as an institutionalized political actor that draws its legitimacy from the expert knowledge of the economists and policy scholars housed at the World Bank.

Erasures

Structural inequities across the globe are perpetuated through the creation of knowledge structures that place value on expert knowledge and simultaneously erase the voices of the subaltern sectors from the discursive spaces where knowledge is produced, implemented, and evaluated (Dutta, 2008a, 2008b, 2008c). Absent from the discursive spaces of knowledge production and solution development in the realm of poverty eradication are the voices of the poor, who become the targets of policy-making and policy implementation. Similarly absent are the voices of the local actors on a broader global platform that privileges the location of expertise outside the local realm of knowledge production. The institutionalization of knowledge structures places privilege on the expert producers of knowledge and on their methodologies of knowledge generation on poverty and poverty eradication, which in turn then shape the landscape of policy-making, the deployment and distribution of resources, the development and implementation of interventions, and the evaluation of these interventions.

Studying the relationships between southern NGOs (SNGOs), international NGOs (INGOs), and northern NGOs (NNGOs) working on poverty reduction in Ghana, a highly indebted poor country, Porter (2003) observes that local knowledge about poverty is erased by dominant articulations by international knowledge-producing bodies. The validity of claims about poverty alleviation is dependent upon their locus outside of the local communities rather than upon their ability to listen to the voices of the poor, shaped within the donor-recipient relationship that marks the terrain. Even in instances where NGOs directly interact with local community members who live under poverty, external epistemologies and ontologies often override the knowledge articulated on the basis of the lived experience of poverty grounded in the day-to-day struggles of the poor (Fowler, 2000; Porter, 2003). The privileging of the external expert voice and the simultaneous erasure of the local articulations from the narratives of development is well noted in the following interview with a Ghanian country director of an INGO:

> Mostly it is ideas being accepted from northern donors by an educated elite—but these types of programmes and proposals are very often very removed from local communities. There are people who can't stay a few days in a village but generate funds . . . There are one man or woman NGOs that supposedly stand for a number of community groups and raise money to support poverty alleviation—sometimes they can be good, many times they can be horrible (Ghanaian country director, INGO, Accra).
>
> *(Porter, 2003, p. 134)*

Porter (2003) draws attention to the departure between the rhetoric of participation and partnership on one hand, and the simultaneous erasure of the voices of the poor on the other hand; calls for participation are ironically issued to support NGO clientelism and top-down control by donor agencies that supports the political economy of development (Edwards & Hulme, 1985).

In the post-Cold War environment, he notes, the language of partnership has become the language of political correctness although the rhetoric is far removed from the reality of partnerships. Further, Porter (2003) notes that the donor relationship between SNGOs and INGOs turns the emphasis of SNGOs on finding partners, negotiating with them, and negotiating with their accounting procedures and demands for professionalization, thus turning the NGOs toward meeting the criteria established by the international donors rather than addressing the needs of the poor. Just as the voices of the poor remain absent from the discursive spaces of the very policy frameworks that are directed toward them, the needs of the poor also become backgrounded in these frameworks. This notion of being absent from the discursive spaces is narrated by a Santali participant in a culture-centered co-construction of narratives of poverty.[1]

> Where do we have anything babu? Where do Santals get to say anything? Wok hard for a job, get scolded by the babus [referring to the middle, upper middle and richer classes sections of society], go to bed hungry.
>
> *(Dutta-Bergman, 2004b, p. 256)*

Structural Absences

Absent from the discourses of the World Bank is the articulation of the structural violence associated with poverty. World Bank reports, for instance, do not really discuss the deaths that are the result of poverty-related causes; premature mortality therefore figures into poverty measurement as an indicator of reducing poverty (Kanbur, 1987, 1990a, 1990b; Kanbur & Mukherjee, 2007). The authors note that World Bank measures of poverty count poverty-related deaths as actually reducing the absolute number of poor people, which the authors argue, violates basic intuitions about poverty counts. How poverty-related deaths are counted within the broader picture of poverty determines the politics and policy-making around poverty and the role of the World Bank with reference to these policies; in this case, becoming one of the markers in the argument that neoliberal policies actually reduce global poverty (Kanbur, 1987, 1990a, 1990b; Kanbur & Mukherjee, 2007; St. John, 2004a, 2004b, 2006a, 2006b).

Also, the cognitive-bias in poverty measures and evaluations mean that poverty is not really understood from the standpoint of the people who are suffering from poverty, neither are the problems understood from the standpoints of the lived experiences of the people experiencing poverty. Similarly, Pogge and Reddy (2006; Reddy and Pogge, 2007) note that the World Bank's estimates are not meaningful or reliable, therefore leading to the underestimation of the number of people living under poverty. Once again, the World Bank, the key policy institution that defines its functions to outside stakeholders in terms of reducing poverty, paradoxically engages in supporting transnational hegemonies and neoliberal structures that operate on the very basis of the oppression of the poor.

Further, in terms of violence, dominant articulations of poverty do not attend to the various forms of state-sponsored violence that are carried out in order to exert the power and control of neoliberalism. For example, in Chile, in order to set up the neoliberal experiment, the United States sponsored national elites and pro-liberalization organizations in the form of aid; furthermore, it orchestrated a coup working hand in hand with the local elite that would overthrow the democratically elected Sandinista government. In Latin America, the state sponsored several forms of violence in order to minimize resistance to neoliberal policies. Currently, in various sectors of the globe, nation states are increasingly utilizing violence in order to exert the control of TNCs or to create spaces for operations by TNCs. As TNCs receive contracts for large-scale mining and industrial projects, local communities are displaced with the use of a wide variety of violent strategies, threatening local livelihoods as well as local ecosystems. When local communities rise in resistance, such forms of resistance are controlled once again through the use of state-sponsored violence. In the state of Orissa in India, for instance, large-scale police and military violence have been deployed by the government to control the resistance offered by indigenous tribes to the building of a bauxite mining project in the Niyamgiri hills of the Koraput district of Orissa (http://radicalnotes.com/journal/author/campaign-against-war-on-people/). Taken-for-granted in the larger rhetoric of the success of neoliberalism in India are the forms of oppression and control carried out by the state to serve the interests of neoliberalism. A culture-centered engagement with indigenous articulations of their displacement and the violence enacted on them by the state disrupt the hegemony of the discursive spaces of neoliberalism.

Interrogating Structures

Given the structural absences in dominant discourses then, the culture-centered approach seeks to foreground the structures and draw attention to the inequities perpetuated by the politics of dominant structures. Listening to subaltern voices creates entry points for constituting the politics of structural inequities into the discursive spaces of knowledge circulation. Culture-centered conceptualizations of poverty interrogate the underlying structural reasons that result in poverty by politicizing the discursive spaces of the mainstream. Questions are raised about the issues of redistributive justice and the interests of neoliberal hegemony in maintaining the power and control of the existing configurations through the rhetoric of economic growth. Consider the following narrative of a participant from Kenya in the "Voices of the Poor" project:

Don't ask me what poverty is because you have met it outside my house. Look at the house and count the number of holes. Look at my utensils and the clothes that I am wearing. Look at everything and write what you see. What you see is poverty.

(Narayan et al., 1999a, p. 26)

Poverty here is narrated in the symbolic markers that disrupt the dominant narratives of human life and human capabilities; it is the departure from these capabilities, the inability to meet the basic necessities of life. The articulation of poverty is narrated in the interruption of the dominant structures and the taken-for-granted assumptions that constitute the privileges amidst these structures.

The existing configurations not only benefit the TNCs and the powerful nation states that control the IFIs and international regulatory networks, but also continue to benefit the local elites who profit from privatization, liberalization, and deregulation. The politics of power and control is dictated by the economic interests of transnational hegemony; simultaneously, the participation of subaltern voices in the discursive space creates openings for social change by attending to the structures, and seeking to find avenues for challenging these structures. Listening to subaltern voices through culture-centered processes draws attention to these very reasons of politics that underlie global inequities, thus creating frameworks for organizing the grassroots in projects addressing inequalities.

Enacting Agency

As noted in the theoretical framework of the culture-centered approach, the structures that constrain human capabilities are also the backdrop for the enactment of agency. In other words, agency is enacted in relationship with dominant structures. Even as structures define the palette on which the terrains of agency are constituted, these terrains of agency create openings for disrupting and transforming those structures. The discursive space in mainstream knowledge enunciations about poverty is marked by the silence of the voices of those individuals, groups, and communities who live in the midst of poverty. So what are the stories of poverty, as narrated through the lived experiences of individuals who live amidst the absence of the basic resources of living? How do the poorer sectors of the globe construct the stories of poverty, and what are the ways in which these stories offer entry points for social change and transformative politics? Listening to the voices of the poor offers entry points to the co-constructions of alternative rationalities and narratives that disrupt the dominant structures of society. The narratives of the poor disrupt the hegemonic discourses of poverty that are articulated in terms of knowledge and policy produced by dominant social institutions across the globe that serve the interests of transnational hegemony.

In the ethnography conducted in the poorer sectors of the globe by Narayan et al. (1999a, 1999b), the poor narrate their stories and life experiences they work with, constituting themselves in the fissures of, and in resistance to the master narrative of development. For instance, in her/his definition of poverty, one of the participants in this project notes, "Poverty is the fact that sometimes I go hungry to bed in the evening, because I do not have bread at home" (Narayan et al., 1999b, p. 53). Here, poverty is defined in terms of hunger, an immediate need of the person living under poverty. Similarly, for another participant, poverty is articulated in terms of having the last meal with whatever resources are left, and not knowing where the next plate of food is going to come from. For a participant from Macedonia, "poverty for me is the fact that we bought some black flour with our last money, some flour cheaper than the rest. When we baked the bread it was not edible. We were speechless and ate it by force since we did not have anything else" (Narayan et al., 1999b, p. 53). A former collective farm worker in Latvia reaching pension age notes:

> Ivan and Lolita now survive on what they can grow in their own garden, on various jobs Ivan finds, and what Lolita can gather from the forest and sell. They live mainly on potatoes, going through last winter without any bread at all. For the last two months they have lived on potato bread— potatoes are ground up, mixed with oil, and baked. Lolita cries when she sees a loaf of bread.

Once again, emergent in this narrative is the story of hunger, of not having enough to eat when faced with poverty, and of the pain associated with the inability to procure food. These alternative articulations of poverty through conversations with people living under poverty draw attention to alternative rationalities that look beyond the economic measures to the pain experienced by the poor.

Conclusion

How we come to look at poverty, interpret it, and develop spaces of policy-making around issues of poverty is fundamentally predicated by the discourses that constitute poverty. These discourses, being both politically and economically situated in terms of being articulated by those in positions of power across the globe, also create material realities through the policies that are created, implemented, and evaluated by global organizations, nation states, and local-level NGOs. The advent of the neoliberal ideology on the global landscape has shaped the global terrains of political economy, influencing the relationships of nation states to TNCs, consolidating global power in the hands of TNCs that are traditionally located in the Western hemisphere, and creating spaces of marginalization across the world by shifting the bases of power from national governments to TNCs. These spaces of marginalization experience the material consequences of poverty in terms of their access to income and other basic capabilities such as food, clothing, water, and shelter. They are also marked by their limited access to communicative platforms amidst neoliberalism, and therefore, mostly remain unheard. It is on this landscape of legitimizing the oppression of and silencing of the economically marginalized subaltern sectors that the culture-centered approach offers a basic framework for listening to the narratives of marginalization that disrupt the hegemonic narratives of the status quo (reflected in the conglomeration of TNCs, nation states, local elites, and international policy bodies such as the IMF and the World Bank). The culture-centered approach creates entry points for social change through the creation of discursive spaces that co-construct alternative rationalities of knowledge claims. Several movements across the globe have been constellated around the poverty and marginalization of the poor brought on by neoliberalism, therefore utilizing poverty as the guiding principle for bringing about social change.

3

AGRICULTURE AND FOOD

Global Inequalities

Agriculture constitutes one of the core areas in which marginalization plays out globally as it revolves around the production of one of the basic capacities of life: food (Shiva & Bedi, 2002). The dominance and control over the agricultural and food sectors is carried out in contemporary neoliberal hegemony through the development and implementation of global policies that continue to reify structural inequities in food production and food distribution. Much of the political economy in the agricultural and food sectors revolve around the influence of global policies and the hegemony of transnational corporations that dominate the production, distribution and exchange of food and food products (Josling, Tangermann, & Warley, 1996). The goal of this chapter is to examine the ways in which the margins are created in the agricultural sector, through the implementation and propagation of neoliberal policies in agriculture. Who controls the sites of agricultural production? Who controls the discursive spaces of policy-making that determines the material bases of agricultural production? Who benefits from the dominant markers of modernity that are mobilized in the agricultural sector with the promises of development? What are the margins that are produced through dominant globalization discourses and interventions?

In this chapter, we review the processes through which global policies create the margins in the agricultural and food sectors. An overview of the political economy of food production and food consumption serves as the basis for exploring not only the inequities in access to agricultural production and agro-markets in the different sectors of the globe, but also the food insecurities that are created in the marginalized sectors of the globe through the deployment of neoliberal policies that are supportive of transnational hegemony. Of relevance here are global policies around trade-related investments in the agricultural sectors, protection of local systems of productions, intellectual property rights, trade and tariff regulations, etc. Special attention is paid to the lived experiences of peasants in the subaltern sectors of the globe as they struggle with the structural violence embedded in contemporary global policies. Simultaneously, the structures of food distribution are discussed in the realm of the experiences of the poorer sectors of the globe in accessing food, elaborating on the questions of hunger and poverty as they emerge in the current global landscape. Questions are raised regarding the influence of global policies on global food supplies, accessibility to quality food, and quality of food available to the subaltern sectors of the globe (see Figure 3.1).

The chapter begins with the discussion of the articulations of agriculture in the development framework, juxtaposed against the backdrop of indigenous systems of knowledge of agriculture that have been branded as primitive in the development discourse. The intersections of the material and symbolic domains of agricultural knowledge are interrogated within the context of questions of marginalization of the subaltern sectors of the globe, exploring the role of knowledge structures in reifying and reproducing hegemonies. Subsequently, it discusses specific agriculture and food-related policies, and follows up this discussion by examining the trends in the distributions of agricultural and food resources in the different sectors of the globe. The chapter wraps up by offering specific examples that discuss the experiences of marginalized communities in the

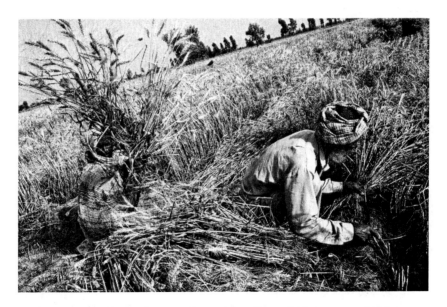

FIGURE 3.1 Indian farmers harvest wheat in the village of Chaina, some 200 km northwest from Chandigarh on April 23, 2008. Thousands of farmers and laborers have killed themselves in the affluent state of Punjab in the past decade because of a crisis blamed on official neglect of the farming sector. Experts say government must pay immediate attention to agriculture if it is to save the situation, even as prices of the food the farmers grow surge rapidly. (Pedro Ugarte/AFP/Getty Images)

agricultural sector, and bringing forth the voices of farmers and farm workers in the co-construction of the narratives of pain and suffering constituted in the realm of agriculture.

Agriculture and Development

A large proportion of the development discourse emphasizes social change in the agricultural sector, with the central idea that revolutionizing the agricultural sector will bring about the necessary growth in food supplies to sustain population growth. The ultimate goal of the development project becomes to increase the agricultural productivity of the large majority of peasants across the country. In terms of agriculture then, the industry of development planning and implementation emphasizes the modernization of agriculture through the incorporation of Western knowledge, the adoption of technologies, and the industrialization and mechanization of agriculture. From a communicative standpoint, the predominant framework for development in the agricultural sector was the diffusion of innovations framework (Rogers, 1995).

Diffusion of Innovations

The diffusion of innovations paradigm was founded on the hybrid seed corn diffusion study by Ryan and Gross (1943). In their study of the adoption of hybrid seed corn in two rural Iowa communities, Ryan and Gross (1943) observed that the adoption rate followed an S-shaped pattern over time; after the first five years of slow growth in the use of hybrid seed corn, the adoption rate "took off," reaching 40 percent adoption within the next three years (Rogers, 1995; Ryan & Gross, 1943). Subsequently, the adoption rate started tapering off. The S-shaped adoption curve, according to Ryan and Gross (1943) was attributed to the different categories of farmers in the target community. Categorizing the farmers into different groups based on their location on the adoption curve, Ryan and Gross (1995) posited that farmers systematically differed in their orientations toward an innovation. The innovators were more cosmopolitan and owned larger farms than the later adopters. Suggesting the critical role of interpersonal networks in the process of diffusion, Ryan and Gross (1943) observed that the early adopters were more likely to hear about the hybrid seed corn from the salesmen, while later adopters heard about the innovation from their neighbors. Communicative strategies were subsequently developed for reaching individuals at different stages of the diffusion curve (Rogers, 1983, 1995).

The knowledge gained from the diffusion of innovations work of Ryan and Gross (1943) was soon to be put to work by the federal government in its agricultural modernization projects. The US Department of Agriculture harvested the knowledge gained from early diffusion of innovations work for spreading the adoption of new agricultural technologies among the rural sectors of the globe

(Rogers, 1983, 1995). Rogers (1995) eloquently pointed out that the diffusion of innovations studies were critical landmarks in speeding up the diffusion process of agricultural revolutions, thus bringing modernization and the promises of higher productivity. Celebrating the miracles of the diffusion of innovations model, he wrote:

> Thanks to Ryan and Gross (1943), the rural sociologists had an appropriate paradigm to guide their diffusion studies. Thanks to the agricultural revolution of the 1950s, these diffusion scholars were in the right place (state university's colleges of agriculture) at the right time. The result was a proliferation of diffusion studies by the rural sociology tradition: 185 by 1960, 648 by 1970, and 791 by 1981.
>
> *(Rogers, 1995, p. 56)*

The successful diffusion of innovations studies were subsequently extended to the developing nations of Latin America, Africa, and Asia (Rogers, 1971, 1995). The US government saw it as a tool for expanding US-style modernity across the globe (Rogers, 1983). Sponsored by the US Agency for International Development and several private foundations, diffusion programs focused on spreading agricultural innovations such as seeds, agricultural equipment, and fertilizers to the Third World (Rogers, 1995).

Definitions and Sources. Quintessential to the diffusion of innovations model is the definition of an innovation (Rogers, 1983, 1995). What is an innovation and who gets to define it? An innovation is an idea, practice, or object that is new to the adopter group (Rogers, 1995). The value of novelty is inherent in this definition; the novel innovations of the sender culture are introduced into the receiver culture in order to emancipate the people of the receiver culture.

Therefore, integral to the definition of the diffusion of innovations process is a sender and a receiver, a subject and an object, and an innovation that links the subject and the object. The sender is the active agent while the receiver is the passive recipient. The sender penetrates, the receiver receives, and through this relationship of penetration and reception, the sender achieves orgasmic heights of success as defined by his/her imperial needs. The receiver culture supposedly achieves development through innovative practices and modernized technologies. Important to note in the diffusion of innovations framework is the argument that both the sender and the receiver of the innovation get spatially located in a relational frame of power difference. Although not clearly spelt out, also implicit in the definition of an innovation is the modernist interpretation of what constitutes an innovation; an innovation is only an innovation to the extent it fits into the criteria defined by the modernist practice of the West. Definition then is intertwined with the definer and his/her relationship with the receiver that is imbued with differences in power and access. The definer in the diffusion of innovations framework is the Western scientist, interventionist, or policy planner that discusses, creates, propagates, implements, reports and trains while the Third World native remains the subject of such diffusion work.

A referential frame emerges in defining what constitutes an innovation, thus reinforcing and propagating the status of the sender and the receiver. The Third World nation continues to be the receiver of innovations sent out by the Western modernizer. Through the mirrors created for them by the West, members of Third World cultures continue to see themselves as underdeveloped and in need of Western innovations (Escobar, 1995; Wilkins, 2000); these Western innovations offer the panacea to their primitive practices and subsequently emancipate them from their miserable plights (Wallerstein, 1997, 2006; Wilkins, 2000). So, for instance, when a new variety of genetically modified seed is introduced as an innovation in Nepal, the fundamental assumption that drives the diffusion effort is that the native seed of Nepal is imbued with problems and hence needs to be replaced by the innovation. Inherent in the definition of an innovation is its conceptualization as a panacea to a pre-existing problem in the target culture. Diffusion is a lens that propagates Western hegemony because the innovation is almost always a creation of the Western mind (Escobar, 1995; Wallerstein, 1983, 1990). What is seen as a problem is based upon the lens of the Western academic. Yet another question often left out of the discursive space relates to the benefactors of the innovation; it is almost always assumed that the Third World benefits from the philanthropic enterprises of the "First World." In the next section, we examine the construction of the Third World as benefactor and the First World as the donor.

Serving Whose Interests? Who gains from the diffusion of an innovation? As articulated in the introductory section on the history of diffusion, diffusion is not a neutral process. A surface-level interrogation of the landscape would perhaps lead us to the conclusion that the diffusion of innovations framework seeks to enlighten the Third World inhabitant when applied to the scenario of development. An examination of texts and research papers would tell us that the ultimate goal of the diffusion of innovations model is to infuse Third World spaces with the mantras of development and progress as envisioned under West-centric knowledge structures (Sachs, 1992; Tomlinson, 1991). Yet a question that often gets left out of the discursive space is, whom does the innovation really benefit? (Escobar, 1995; Esteva and Suri, 1992; Fanon, 1968).

Rogers (1995) fleetingly discusses the importance of the diffusion of innovations model to the US government. Diffusion of innovations served as a conduit for exporting American values to the newly independent nation states of the Third World; the idea situated behind the diffusion model was that the nation states would emulate the values espoused by the United States and hence enlist in the support of American imperialism and US military agendas. These pro-US nation states, it was thought, would be fundamental to the victory of the United States against the

Communists during the Cold War. Third World spaces then could not only be used by the United States for its war efforts, but also provide the labor and markets for American capitalism. They would offer the markets for expanding multinationals. The values of democracy and capitalism, spread through the diffusion of innovations model, would become global values, universal values of humankind.

Discussing the surge in diffusion of agricultural innovations in the 1950s and 1960s, the Indian physicist and eco-feminist Vandana Shiva (1991) forcefully articulates that the export of US agricultural innovations (miracle seeds, fertilizers, pesticides, etc.) to Third World countries were based upon the complicitous interests of the United States and national governments in containing peasant unrest and peasant movements targeted at recovering the land rights of the peasants. The 1950s documented growing peasant unrest in the newly liberated countries of the Third World; this peasant unrest was propelled by the peasants' commitment to regain the lost lands that were concentrated in the hands of the privileged few that served the colonial interests in the pre-independence years (Shiva, 1991). Termed as the Green Revolution and celebrated by Rogers (1962) as one of the miracles of the diffusion of innovations approach, it was thought by the US government and the bourgeoisie national governments that the import of miracle seeds from the United States would solve the food problem and hence stabilize the countryside, prevent peasant unrest, and minimize communist alignments in the rural sectors of the Third World. Shiva (1991) quotes Anderson and Morrison (1982):

> Running through all these measures, whether major or minor in their effect, was the concern to stabilize the countryside politically. It was recognized internationally that the peasantry were incipient revolutionaries and if squeezed too hard could be rallied against the new bourgeois-dominated governments in Asia. This recognition led many of the new Asian governments to join the British-American sponsored Colombo Plan in 1952 which explicitly set out to improve rural Asia as a means of defusing the Communist appeal. Rural development assisted by foreign capital was prescribed as a means of stabilizing the countryside.
>
> *(Anderson & Morrison, 1982, p. 7, quoted in Shiva, 1991, p. 51)*

Although distributive justice in the pre-Green Revolution era produced significant increases in production in postcolonial nations such as India and Mexico, the redistribution of land fundamentally threatened the power and control of local elites and foreign multinationals. Green Revolution, it was conceived, would thwart peasant interests in redistribution of land by generating material prosperity; it would depoliticize the local peasantry (Shiva, 1991). Shiva further quotes Harry Cleaver (1982):

> Food was clearly recognized as a political weapon in the efforts to thwart peasant revolution in many places in Asia . . . from its beginning the

development of the Green Revolution grains constituted mobilizing science
and technology in the service of counter-revolution.

(Cleaver, 1982, p. 269, quoted in Shiva, 1991, pp. 51–52)

Located at the center of the Green Revolution are the interests of the national
elites and US-British capitalism (Shiva, 1991). At the heart of the diffusion of the
miracle seed and the fertilizer to the Third World nation was the marriage between
science and politics. Scientific innovations were proposed as political solutions;
rural development was proposed as an alternative to the spread of Communism in
the rural areas of Third World nations. The political alternatives sought out by the
diffusion of modern agricultural practices to the Third World were intended
to stabilize these spaces; alternatives of redistributive justice were cast out of the
discursive space. Addressing the politics of inequality accommodated by the
goals of the Green Revolution, Shiva (1991, p. 52) writes, "While the Green
Revolution was clearly political in reorganizing agricultural systems, the concern
for political issues such as participation and equity, was consciously by-passed and
was replaced by the political concern for stability." In summary, the political
choices inherent in diffusion of innovations were driven by the political interests
and ideologies of the United States, United Kingdom, dominant capitalist
structures, and local elites. The politics of scientific legitimacy was at the heart of
creating an expanding global market for global agribusiness. The promises of
scientific miracles were constituted within the realm of poverty eradication and
development to open up new markets for the products of TNCs operating in the
agribusiness sector. Science and development joined hands to create the entry
points for the neoliberalization of the Third World, further disenfranchising small-
scale and landless farmers in the Third World.

The introduction of miracle seeds, fertilizers, pesticides, and other agricultural
technologies into the peasant sectors of the Third World also created an entry
point for large US corporations that produced these seeds, fertilizers, pesticides,
and technologies. Thus a new market was created in the agri-business sector
for the global agri-businesses, primarily situated in the United States and UK.
Development, in other words, created new markets for hegemonic agri-businesses,
and offered entry points for transnational corporations into Third World spaces.
Worth interrogating against this backdrop are the taken-for-granted logics of
growth and development in the Third World that are offered as justifications for
the interventions by the global transnational corporations. Development efforts
served as entry points for global TNCs in the agricultural sectors, which continued
to maintain their dominance through the structural adjustment programs, General
Agreement on Trade and Tariffs (GATT), Agreement on Agriculture (AoA), and
Trade-Related Aspects of Intellectual Property Rights. Global agri-businesses, such
as Monsanto, operate through the global structures of policies to continue their
exploitation of the subaltern sectors in order to generate profits.

Effects and Side Effects. Absent from the mainstream discussions of effects and side effects of diffusion of innovations are discussions of the "real" effects of the innovations in the communities in which they were introduced. Absent are questions such as: Did the innovation actually improve the condition of living of the Third World citizen? Did the scientific innovation actually change the life of the peasant to a better state? An interrogation of these questions points out that innovations often, when introduced into local communities, created and subsequently aggravated a plethora of ecological, economic, social, cultural, and political problems instead of solving them (Shiva, 1991). The intended positive effects of the innovation were replaced by negative and regressive effects; situations produced through the adoption of the innovation are more violent and volatile than the years preceding the diffusion of innovation. In order to excavate these real effects, we will specifically engage with the work of Vandana Shiva (1991) on the Green Revolution and juxtapose it against the background of the silenced questions in the mainstream diffusion of innovations literature. Shiva's (1991) critical interrogation of the Green Revolution in the Punjab province of India provides an excellent case study that documents the detrimental effects of innovations introduced by the West in Third World spaces.

As documented earlier in this chapter, Shiva (1991) cogently argues that the Green Revolution was driven by the mutual interests of the bourgeoisie national governments and the anti-Communist British and American governments in depoliticizing the peasant movements of the newly liberated Third World nations. The diffusion of Western scientific innovations was not an objective and value-free process, but a violent exercise of value-laden Western patriarchy; the goals of diffusion scientists was to achieve social peace, the path followed was one of abundant produce through interventions by scientific revolutions (Shiva, 1989, 1991). In her book *Staying alive*, Shiva (1989) writes:

> Modern science is projected as a universal, value-free system of knowledge, which has displaced all other belief and knowledge systems by its universality and value neutrality, and by the logic of its method to arrive at objective claims about nature. Yet the dominant stream of modern science, the reductionist or mechanical paradigm, is a particular response of a particular group of people. It is a specific project of western man which came into being during the fifteenth and seventeenth centuries as the much acclaimed Scientific Revolution. During the last few years feminist scholarship has begun to recognize that the dominant science system emerged as a liberating force not for humanity as a whole . . . but as a masculine and patriarchal project which necessarily entailed the subjugation of both nature and women.
>
> *(Shiva, 1989, p. 15)*

The violence of the colonizing practices imposed on Third World spaces through scientific innovations and the disruption created by the imposition of modern scientific innovations is captured well in Shiva's (1991) discussion of the Green Revolution. Her portrayal of the socio-politico-economic state of Punjab in the post-Green Revolution years fundamentally challenges the typical academic celebration of the innovation as a miracle that emancipated the Third World, as a product of value-free objective science that only reaps benefits for Third World societies. Shiva, Anderson, Schücking, Gray, Lohmann, and Cooper (1991) argue:

> The Age of Enlightenment, and the theory of progress to which it gave rise, was centered on the sacredness of two categories: modern scientific knowledge and economic development. Somewhere along the way, the unbridled pursuit of progress, guided by science and development, began to destroy life without any assessment of how fast and how much of the diversity of life on this planet is disappearing ... Throughout the world, a new questioning is growing, rooted in the experience of those for whom the spread of what was called "enlightenment" has been the spread of darkness, of the extinction of life and life-enhancing processes.
>
> *(Shiva et al., 1991, p. 45)*

At the heart of the Green Revolution were the "miracle seeds" that would break the limits imposed upon seeds by nature, and produce high yields when exposed to a chemically intensive regimen of fertilizers and pesticides; the miracle seeds were conceived as the harbingers of peace and abundance in the rural sectors of the Third World. A narrow genetic base of genetically modified (GM) seeds replaced the crop diversity and rotational agriculture of indigenous populations in the Third World (Lappé & Bailey, 1998; Lappé, Collins, & Rosset, 1998; Shiva, 1991). The intervention of the miracle seeds was accompanied by the necessitation of agrichemicals and machinery produced by transnational corporations to support the high-yield varieties. The Green Revolution thus created a new system of dependence and debt; indigenous Third World peasants needed to purchase their seeds, fertilizers, and machinery from global corporations and depended upon foreign aid to do this (Shiva, 1991). Shiva (1991) argued that the technologies created through the Green Revolution were

> directed at capital intensive inputs for best endowed farmers in the best endowed areas, and directed away from resource prudent options of the small farmer in resource scarce regions. The science and technology of the Green Revolution excluded poor regions and poor people as well as sustainable options.
>
> *(Shiva, 1991, p. 45)*

Interrogating the exaggerated effects of the Green Revolution on Indian agriculture, Shiva (1991) cites Jatindar Bajaj (1986) to argue that the rate of growth of aggregate crop production was higher in the pre-Green Revolution years as compared to the post-Green Revolution years. She further challenges the construction of the Green Revolution as the great miracle that transformed India from "the begging bowl to a bread basket" (Swaminathan, 1983, p. 409, as cited in Shiva, 1991, p. 54). To the contrary, food imports continued to be significant even after the Green Revolution. In addition, the Green Revolution privatized and commoditized Indian agriculture, introduced and supported a system of foreign debt and dependence, reduced genetic diversity by introducing genetically uniform monocultures, fostered deforestation, introduced and catalyzed large-scale spread of diseases and pests, destabilized the farm ecology, and eroded and degraded the soil accompanied by micronutrient deficiencies (Shiva, 1991).

To support the high-yield varieties of crops introduced by the Green Revolution, the farmers needed intensive water supplies and intensive fertilization (Shiva, 1991; Shiva et al., 1991). This increased need for inputs to support the high-yield system in turn led to conflict over the limited resources available to farmers. The exponential increase in water use destabilized the water balance in the region, leading to desertification and salinization of the land, accompanied by the building of dams and displacement of peoples (for an extensive discussion, see Shiva, 1991). In the chapter titled "The Political and Cultural Costs of the Green Revolution," Shiva (1991) pointed out that

> the shift from internal to externally purchased inputs did not merely change ecological processes of agriculture. It also changed the structure of social and political relationships, from those based on mutual (though asymmetric) obligation within the village to relations of each cultivator directly with banks, seed and fertilizer agencies, food procurement agencies, and electricity and irrigation organizations. Further since all the externally supplied inputs were scarce, it set up conflict and competition over scarce resources, between classes, and between regions.
>
> *(Shiva, 1991, p. 171)*

In addition to increased inputs of resources dependent on aid, the Green Revolution needed a centralized system for its success. The centralization needed for the management and maintenance of the Green Revolution marginalized the Punjabi peasants; decisions were made for them by foreign organizations and the national government located at the center. When the returns on investments started falling after the initial years of unstable prosperity, the disillusioned Punjabi peasants found themselves in the midst of high debts. The intense pressure on resources accompanied by the displacement of labor and the marginalization of the lower peasantry further catapulted the peasants toward violence and conflict (Shiva, 1991). Finally, by introducing an externally dependent system, the Green Revolution commercialized the Punjabi culture; interpersonal and community relationships were replaced by the rhetoric of commercialization, creating an "ethical vacuum where nothing is sacred and everything has a price" (Shiva, 1991,

p. 174). "Circulation of new cash in a society whose old forms of life had been dislocated led to an epidemic of social diseases like alcoholism, smoking, drug-addiction, the spread of pornographic films and literature and violence against women" (Shiva, 1991, p. 185). The revival of Sikhism in Punjab emerged as an answer to this moral and ethical vacuum created by the commercial capitalism of the Green Revolution (Shiva, 1991). The economic depravity imposed on the region, the powerlessness of the peasants in the face of the accumulation of power at the center, and the moral–ethical vacuum ushered in by commercialization provided the ingredients for the growth of fundamentalism. Fundamentalism attempted to refurbish the Sikh identity and self-hood that was essentially robbed from him/her through the modernization projects, and was "an ideological crusade against the cultural corruption of Punjab" (Shiva, 1991, p. 185).

The growth in Sikh fundamentalism took a violent turn when the Center interfered with the goals of capitalizing on ethnic identity (led by Indira Gandhi, erstwhile prime minister of India). Gandhi's assassination was followed by anti-Sikh violence; a peaceful peasant culture became the site for gory violence (Shiva, 1991). Challenging the construction of the Punjab conflicts in a purely communalized frame, Shiva (1991) points out that the violence in Punjab was rooted in the Green Revolution, an innovation that was objectively framed by scientists, diffusion workers, Western governments, and the national bourgeoisie as the emancipator of the Punjabi people. Concluding about the violence wrought on the soil of Punjab by this Western innovation, Shiva (1991) writes:

> In the South Asian region, the "most successful" experiments in economic growth and development have become, in less than two decades, crucibles of violence and war. Culturally diverse societies, engineered to fit into models of development have lost their organic community identity . . . The upsurge of ethnic religious and regional conflict in the Third World today may not be totally disconnected from the ecological and cultural uprooting of people, deprived identities, pushed into a negative sense of self with respect to every "other" . . . The Green Revolution was to have been a strategy for peace and abundance. Today there is no peace in Punjab.
>
> (Shiva, 1991, pp. 190–192)

As demonstrated by the Green Revolution project and as attested by diffusion of innovations scholars, one of the critical side effects of the diffusion of innovations model is the increasing disparity it creates between the haves and have-nots of society (Rogers, 2003). The diffusion of innovations has been typically found to widen the socioeconomic gap between the higher- and lower-status segments of society (Rogers, 2003).

In this construction of disparities, it is also worth noting that the discourse of socioeconomic gaps between the rich and poor is built upon the positive value attributed to technology and modernity. The rich are considered to become richer in the realm of their possession of the material goods that define richness by Western standards. A person is considered rich or poor by virtue of his or her possession of a radio, a television, or a computer, indicators that define wealth in strictly material terms based upon an assessment system that values material wealth and technological acquisitions as the indicators of success. In other words, the indicators of wealth and poverty are very much located in the materialist value system of the West.

The ideological bases of the very discussion of increasing gaps in society are tied to the ability of community members to access modern innovations as defined by the West. Therefore, as the richer cross-sections of Third World nations move more toward Westernization in becoming richer, the poorer sections are left behind and are pushed out into the margins in the discursive constructions of modernity. What is problematic in this scenario is not simply the increasing gap between the rich and the poor in material wealth, but the exponential rise in disenfranchisement and marginalization of the poor; the extinction of cultural traditions and practices that define traditional societies. This marginalization and loss of traditional cultural identity in the face of the modernization projects leads to the growth in religious fundamentalism as a struggle against the marginalizing modernization practices. The growth in fundamentalism and the increasing polarization of Third World spaces in turn creates the recipe for violence; not only was this demonstrated by the effects of the Green Revolution in Punjab but is also attested in recent growth in terrorism elsewhere in the world.

The Role of Communication. Communication is seen as a vital element in the diffusion of agricultural technologies to the underdeveloped sectors of the globe (Schramm & Lerner, 1976). Communication was conceptualized as playing two distinct roles in diffusing the agricultural innovations into the Third World. On one hand, communication was seen as a channel for diffusing information about the agricultural innovations into the developing sectors. On the other hand, the role of communication was conceptualized in terms of creating a culture of progress and innovation in rural communities. The mass media were seen as the markers of development, diffusing development messages and seeking to change the traditional attitudes of the agricultural sectors.

Neoliberal Hegemony and Agriculture. Neoliberal ideology manifest in the "new policy agenda" or "Washington Consensus" was first promoted by leading political ideologues Reagan and Thatcher against the backdrop of the global debt crisis, and was used as a framework for utilizing loans channelled through the international financial institutions to restructure economies across the globe. It constitutes a set of economic reforms or policies that usually include cutting tariffs and other trade barriers; reducing government intervention in the economy, cuts in social spending, reducing or eliminating subsidies that provide important benefits for the poor, privatizing public enterprises and services, and emphasizing exports as the engine of growth (Korten, 1995, 1999). Highlighting the inherent superiority of economic liberalism, including the design of an international economic order based on free markets, private property, individual incentive, and a minimal role for the state, neoliberal ideology is furthermore carried out through global trade policies and agreements, constituted under the framework of the GATT and its later version, the World Trade Organization (Farmer, 1988a, 1988b, 1992; Labonte, 2001; Labonte and Torgerson, 2002).

Structural Adjustment Programs. Increasingly, the agricultural sectors across the globe have come under the control of the World Bank through the structural adjustment programs (SAPs). Under the SAPs, Third World countries have been required to open up their doors to transnational seed companies (Josling, Tangerman, & Warley, 1996; Shiva & Bedi, 2002). In this shift from peasant-based systems of agriculture to systems of agriculture that were largely dependent on agri-chemical and seed corporations, the World Bank has played a major role through its loan programs that were directed at making the national seed industries more market responsive (Shiva & Jafri, 2003; Shiva, Jafri, Emani, & Pande, 2002). As a result, the seed sector was privatized; the locally circulated, government-subsidized, and community-based circulations of seeds have been replaced by commoditized purchase of GM seeds manufactured by transnational corporations. Government-sponsored extension programs have on one hand stopped offering government-subsidized seeds to farmers, and on the other hand, have started offering GM seeds to farmers.

Under the structural adjustment programs, specific varieties of GM seeds have been promoted by the government under the premise that these seeds would increase efficiency, optimize pest resistance, and generate maximum yield. These GM seeds respond to fertilizers and pesticides, which are also manufactured by the TNCs, thus leading to an external input-driven system as opposed to the traditional system that was driven by internal inputs. Also, farmer's cropping patterns have shifted from mixed cultivations to monocultures of hybrids that are pushed by external inputs. The emphasis on privatization has also influenced the types of loans available to farmers, shifting from public-sector low-interest loans and extension to high-interest private-sector loans (Shiva, 2002). Overall then, the political economy of agriculture has shifted from traditionally sustainable local forms of agriculture to commoditized forms of large-scale capitalist agriculture brought under the control of TNCs through the displacement of the subaltern sectors from their access to forms of livelihood.

Simultaneously, the emphasis on external liberalization of agriculture has dictated that agricultural subsidies be reduced, which has resulted in the price rise of foodgrains supplied through the Public Distribution System (PDS). The price rise of the foodgrains supplied through the PDS then led to the rise in the market prices of food grains. In order to then address the underserved sectors, the government introduced a specifically subsidized PDS. However, the subsidized products typically do not reach the underserved markets and get leaked into other areas because of corruptions that exist within the structures. In addition, given the distant locations of the underserved areas and the lack of literacy among tribal populations, even when subsidized foodgrains do reach these underserved areas, community members pay prices higher than the stipulated prices. As the government shifted its subsidies from the PDS to subsidies for exporting the grain, the PDS prices were quite similar to market prices, thus making foodgrains fairly inaccessible to the laboring masses. In the case of the Indian states of Maharashtra and Andhra Pradesh, the prices of foodgrains very quickly made them out of the reach of the poorer sectors.

General Agreement on Trade and Tariffs and Agreement on Agriculture.

The formation of the General Agreement on Tariffs and Trade (GATT) in the postwar era was a major landmark in the history of trade liberalization. Immediately following the world wars, the loss of colonies threatened the economies of European nations and the United States predicted significant deterioration in its international trade due to economic nationalism in the postwar environment (Hudec, 1988). There existed the consensus among developed countries that economic growth and reconstruction was essential to prevent further political unrest. The rationale of trade liberalization was simple: if countries specialize in goods that they can produce efficiently, and exchange these goods with other countries, the cost of production will be reduced at the global level, and every nation participating in free trade will benefit with economic growth (Madeley, 1999, 2000). Upon this consensus, twenty-three countries signed a contract with a code of rules for international trade called the General Agreement on Tariffs and Trade in 1947. The GATT centered around three central principles (Hudec, 1988). First, all contracting parties (i.e., the signatory governments of the GATT) were required to eliminate many non-tariff protectionist measures affecting international trade[1]; second, all tariff levels could not exceed the level of those at the time of the agreement and all contracting parties would engage in negotiations to gradually decrease the levels of tariffs; and third, the most-favored-nation principle required all participating governments to eradicate discriminatory trading practices and treat all other contracting parties equally (see General Agreement on Tariffs and Trade: United Nations, 1947).[2]

Critics argue that the GATT was a symbol of the hegemonic leadership of the United States. The specific objectives of the United States in negotiating the GATT were twofold: to abolish non-tariff barriers and to significantly reduce all tariffs to eradicate economic protectionism, and to put an end to the discriminatory trading practices originating from the colonial system (Hudec, 1988). The first objective was achieved in the subsequent decades. Seven rounds of GATT meetings were held between 1947 and 1979 to liberalize trade in manufactured goods, and this resulted in a significant reduction of trade barriers within the framework of GATT (Madeley, 1999, 2000). The second objective of removing discriminatory trading practices was not realized, however. The promise of economic growth proved to be empty as importation and international debts increased in developing countries, and exportation remained insufficient (Hudec, 1988; Madeley, 1999, 2000). Developing countries struggled to protect their infant-industries and to gain special status in the international trade market. There were some amendments made to the GATT in subsequent years, but developing countries soon realized that the modifications, aimed to assist the economic development of developing countries, were merely obligations with no legal binding (Hudec, 1988; Madeley, 1999, 2000).

The need for major trade reforms led to the formation of the World Trade Organization (WTO) on April 14, 1994, when trade ministers from more than 100 countries met in Marrakesh, Morocco to sign the Final Act Embodying the Results of the Uruguay Round of Multilateral Negotiations. The purpose of the WTO was to oversee a new and equitable multilateral trading system, and to administer the trade agreements negotiated during the 1986–94 Uruguay Round of trade negotiations. A key feature added to the WTO was a considerably more effective procedure for the adjudication of legal disputes called the "dispute settlement" procedure (Hudec, 1997). Unlike the GATT dispute settlement procedure, the new GATT/WTO procedure gave governments automatic access to tribunals, made legal rulings by tribunals automatically binding, introduced appellate review, and made trade sanctions automatically available in cases of noncompliance. The Agreement on Agriculture (AoA) came into effect in 1994 as a result of the 1986–94 Uruguay Round of the GATT. The objective of the agreement was to amend the 1947 GATT to include fairer agricultural trade agreements and to establish a "significant first step towards order, fair competition and less distorted sector" (WTO, 2005). Prior to the Uruguay Round, agricultural commodities were largely exempt from the application of GATT requirements, thus developing countries taxed the agricultural sector in order to earn badly needed revenue, while industrialized countries used a number of techniques to promote agricultural production (e.g., export subsidies, import tariffs, import quotas, and other non-tariff barriers). Moreover, under the pre-Uruguay GATT, the United States and the European Union adopted a variety of measures to protect and promote agricultural production, which conferred a big advantage on agricultural producers in industrialized countries compared to their competitors in developing countries. The AoA was significant because it represented the first time since the creation of GATT that agricultural commodities were subject to the multilateral trading rules (Gonzalez, 2002). The Agreement obliged participating nations to provide market access to other nations and to significantly reduce traditionally allowed domestic supports and export subsidies to farmers. Specifically, the AoA obligates WTO members to liberalize agricultural trade in three respects; the expansion of market access by requiring the conversion of all non-tariff barriers to tariffs (i.e., tariffication) and the binding and reduction of these tariffs[3]; the reduction of both the volume of and expenditures on subsidized exports; and the reduction of trade-distorting domestic subsidies.

It is important to note that while the agricultural trade negotiations were meant to remove trade inequities, the AoA was shaped by the intense rivalry between the United States and the European Union for world agricultural markets, and developing countries were almost entirely left out of the negotiating process. The United States called for a phase-out of agricultural export subsidies over a five-year period, while the European Union seeking to protect its Common Agricultural Policy argued for a more modest subsidy reduction proposal designed to preserve status quo.[4] Japan and South Korea, both net food-importing nations, placed great emphasis on the need to support domestic production in order to promote food security. South Korea argued for special and differential treatment for developing countries, including longer timeframes to remove import restrictions, and developing countries (led most often by India, Jamaica, and Egypt) advocated the elimination of developed country protectionism, the importance of agricultural support for the economic development in non-industrialized nations, and the prime importance of food security for developing countries (Gonzalez, 2002). In the end, however, the AoA served only to institutionalize the existing inequities between developed and developing countries by restricting policy options available to developing countries to promote food security; the agreement enabled developed countries to continue to subsidize and protect domestic producers while requiring developing countries to open up their markets to foreign competition.

The repercussions of the GATT/WTO can most clearly be seen in the case of the "banana war" involving Latin America, Africa, and the Caribbean and Pacific (ACP),[5] and US and European stakeholders. The ongoing banana trade war is a result of US and Latin American objections to the European Union's preferential treatment of banana exports received from ACP regions, with the goal of creating greater access to the European Union market for US-based corporations operating in Latin America (Finley, 2003). Preferential treatment by the European Union involved not only limiting Latin America's access to the European market, but also allowing duty-free importation of ACP bananas in the European Union. According to the European Union, the purpose of the duty-free treatment was to make ACP bananas competitive with banana imports from Latin America. Latin American countries have significantly cheaper production costs because several multinational corporations (e.g., Dole Food Company, Inc. and Chiquita Brands International, Inc.) have large capital investments in Latin America's banana industry. As a result, Latin American banana plantations are larger and more efficient than ACP banana production, which suffers from poor soil conditions, independent farmers, natural disasters, and more expensive shipping costs due to the absence of mass production mechanisms. For example, production and transport prices on the Windward Islands in the ACP are 1.5 to 2 times higher than in Latin America.

The dispute was taken to the WTO, which in its newly established role was in charge of overseeing trade-related disputes. In 1996, five countries (Honduras, Guatemala, Ecuador, Mexico, and the United States) lodged a complaint with the WTO against the banana regime, which they considered discriminatory to their interests. The United States became involved on behalf of the multinational companies because it was especially keen to increase its access to the European market. In 1997, the WTO ruled in favor of Latin American and US interests; the WTO adjudicated that the European Union banana regime was discriminatory and ordered it to be amended, authorizing the United States to impose trade sanctions of $191 million against the European Union for not making satisfactory modifications, and finally, in 2001, the United States and the European Union, after protracted negotiations, agreed on a new European Union banana importation regime (Clark, 2002). The new banana importation scheme was designed to abolish all individual country quotas and phase in a tariff-only system by 2006 (Clark, 2002). In other words, the ACP regions could not have preferential access to European markets for much longer.

The new importation scheme, which denies preferential access of ACP bananas to the European Union markets, has already had devastating effects on the economy of ACP regions because a large proportion of the ACP population (i.e., 50 percent of St. Vincent and 30 percent of St. Lucia and Dominica) is engaged in banana production (Banana Link, 2004). A 1997 fact-finding mission by European parliamentarians argued that the loss of the banana trade with the European Union would lead to mass poverty and high levels of unemployment because small farmers in the ACP regions cannot compete on a "free market" (Banana Link, 2004). This has proved true; over the past years, the increased competition from Latin American "dollar" bananas in the European Union has reduced the market share of Caribbean farmers; as a result, many small-scale marginal farmers; in the ACP are abandoning their lands for the only other economic alternatives, which include the cultivation of illegal drugs, emigration, or poverty (Clark, 2002).

Negative repercussions of the banana trade are witnessed in Latin America as well. According to Banana Link (2004), a non-governmental organization, Latin American plantation workers and producers do not benefit from changes to the European Union banana regime. In fact, increased social and environmental deregulation negatively affects their health, and further decreases their share of the benefits. Plantation workers in Latin America earn as little as 1 percent of the final price of a banana, workers in Nicaragua earn as little as $1 a day, and workers in Ecuador earn between $3 and $5 a day; these wages are often insufficient to meet the basic needs of communities at the local level. Furthermore, the establishment of mass-producing plantations results in the displacement of indigenous people; for example, indigenous populations like the Cabecar and the Bribri peoples are seriously threatened by the colonization of vast tracts of land by banana companies, contamination of rivers, and pressure on their lands. The displaced people are either transformed into plantation workers or migratory laborers, who often have no official documents and thus cannot benefit from any medical or social facilities. Thus, the WTO policies produce winners and losers, but the winners are generally large enterprises, such as transnational corporations, while the losers are poor farmers and rural laborers, whose livelihood and health are undermined by falling commodity prices and by the loss of rural employment.

Similarly, the repercussions of the AoA can most clearly be seen in the case of sugar in the Pacific Islands. Pacific Island nations have long sustained their economy by keeping high tariff level and maintaining preferential measures from the previous colonial system. However, as the Islands joined the WTO and adopted the rules of trade liberalization, the economic, social, and political scapes of these Island countries are dramatically changing. Abiding by the rules in the AoA, the entrance to the WTO mandated the nations to significantly reduce tariffs and inhibited their traditional reliance on preferential relationship with a few major trading partners. For example, the sugar industry, the Island nations' primary export sector and income source, was one of the hardest hit by the trade liberalization rules. The Island nations' sugar export to the European Union (for the case of Fiji, see Kelsey, 2005) was interrupted by the AoA; this was because the goal of the AoA was to inhibit any preferential measures that disrupted free market trade. This resulted in the loss of market access from the part of the Island nations. At the same time, the application of the Most-Favored-Nation principle provided other WTO members with access to the Island's economy. The tariff cuts, in the meantime, significantly decreased governmental revenues and increased reliance on imported foodstuffs, and deprived agricultural rural areas of workers (see Kelsey, 2005, for the case of Tonga). A 1999 study by the Food and Agriculture Organization (FAO) reported that agricultural trade liberalization had resulted in a concentration of landholding in a wide cross-section of countries, so while large, export-oriented agricultural enterprises reaped the benefits of trade liberalization, small farmers frequently lost title to their plots of land. Add to that, government cuts in agricultural input subsidies had increased the price of farm inputs, thereby forcing farmers to pay more for agricultural inputs while receiving less for their output.

The application of the AoA is also threatening communities' access to healthy food in the Pacific Islands. The AoA negatively impacts food security and the economic livelihood of small farmers by producing a flood of cheap food imports and restricting domestic food production in developing countries (Gonzalez, 2002; Madeley, 1999, 2000). According to the FAO (1999) report, the AoA resulted in an increase in food imports (e.g., meat and dairy products), which proved a threat to key agricultural sectors important for economic development, employment, food supply, and poverty alleviation. In addition, the AoA resulted in a decline in domestic food production in developing countries. Trade liberalization has led to an increased emphasis on export production, thus developing countries have begun to devote more land and resources to export crops, but due to declining world prices for many agricultural com-modities small farmers do not necessarily receive better prices for export commodities. In the Pacific Islands, cheap but unhealthy import foodstuffs (e.g., mutton flaps) are replacing healthier traditional diets, such as fish, organic chicken, and taro, because they cannot compete with cheap imports.

The lack of importance given to food security in the AoA has had negative repercussions for small farmers, with limited infrastructures for addressing the needs for these farmers both in terms of agricultural policies and also in terms of other public services. The application of the AoA has resulted in reduced access to economic resources, which significantly limits communities' access to healthy food. As farmers have shifted from growing food crops to growing cash crops under the frameworks of economic growth, their ability to secure food has become dependent upon the economic performance of their crops in the international market (Narayan & Petesch, 2002; Shiva, 2000, 2002, 2005). In sharp contrast to this worldview of cash-crop-dependent agriculture, traditionally farmers grew a wide variety of crops that were often grown in rotation in order to feed themselves and their families, thus participating in sustainable agriculture. As demonstrated with the monoculture crop failures in various parts of the globe, the advent of neoliberal principles in agriculture has made farmers more vulnerable to global market trends and to the performance of their crops in the international market, thus also making these farmers food insecure (Shiva, 2000, 2002, 2005).

Furthermore, the principles of liberalization in agriculture have focused on the logic of competitiveness, based on the argument that a nation can increase its efficiency by producing and exporting commodities in which it is relatively efficient, and by importing commodities in which it is relatively inefficient (Shiva, 2002). However, Shiva (2002) demonstrates that the comparative advantage for countries actually turns into absolute advantage for TNCs because as a nation starts importing large quantities of a particular commodity on the basis of the very logic that the commodity is cheaper on the international market, the international prices go up because of the large-scale import possibilities.

Agreement on Trade Related Aspects of Intellectual Property Rights. Trade Related Aspects of Intellectual Property Rights (TRIPS) came into effect in 1995 as a result of the 1986–94 Uruguay Round of the GATT and was seen as a pivotal element in fostering international trade (WTO, 1994). According to the WTO, governments need to ensure that innovators have the right to prevent others from using their innovations and the right to negotiate payment from others in return for using their innovations. However, since the extent of protection and enforcement of these rights varied widely across geographical boundaries, causing much tension, the "new internationally agreed trade rules for intellectual property rights (i.e., TRIPS) were seen as a way to introduce more order and predictability, and for disputes to be settled more systematically" (WTO, 1994). TRIPS covers the following areas of intellectual property: copyright and related rights (the rights of performers, producers of sound recordings, and broadcasting organizations); trademarks; geographical indications including appellations of origin; industrial designs; patents including the protection of new varieties of plants; the layout-designs of integrated circuits; and undisclosed information (WTO, 1994). The agreement stresses fair and equitable action against infringement of intellectual property rights, and the need to make redressal procedures less complicated, less costly, and short in duration.

The repercussions of TRIPS can most clearly be seen in the case of basmati in South Asia. The TRIPS Agreement threatens food security not only by not recognizing indigenous community's rights over their resources but also by enabling biopiracy or the appropriation of local biological resources without consulting the local community or representative state actors. Constituted in the realm of questions of legitimacy of knowledge structures and the political economy of these structures, TRIPS treats indigenous knowledge as common property because it is not patented; the idea here is that if knowledge is not patented, it is not owned and therefore is open to technological modifications, which can then be patented (Bodekar, 2003; Woods, 2002). Woods (2002) and Bodekar (2003) note that the TRIPS Agreement does not extend either patent or geographic protection to the traditional knowledge of indigenous people; for example, the patent laws under TRIPS do not adequately recognize the traditional form of breeding as "prior art" (i.e., the entire body of knowledge available to the public before a given filing or priority date for any patent, utility model, or industrial design). This has thus led to multinational biotechnological corporations success-fully seeking patents on food grains (Woods, 2002), which in turn negatively impacts local economies. In addition, TRIPS enables biopiracy to take place with relative ease, especially in less-developed countries that are rich in genetic resources and low in technology. Access to technology in developed countries allows richer countries to harness and reproduce genetic material for patenting, thereby enabling the expropriation of local resources and bringing them under the instruments of control of TNCs to generate greater global profit.

RiceTec, a Texas-based company that sought to patent basmati rice, is a case in point. Basmati rice is traditional to India and Pakistan, and in 1997 comprised 4 percent of India's export earnings, receiving premium prices in the international market. In September 1997, RiceTec, a US multinational agri-company, successfully applied for several patents on the basmati rice and grain lines. The Pakistani and Indian governments refuted the patents, stating that the plant varieties and grains already exist as a staple in India, and that neither variety of rice can be grown in the United States. The United States Patent and Trademark Office rescinded fifteen of the twenty patents granted. However, the five remaining patents continue to permit RiceTec to exclude others from making, using, and selling its patented basmati rice in the United States until September 2017. What this means is that the rice-producing nations in South Asia will have a smaller (and perhaps non-existent) international market in the coming years. In addition to marginalizing access that developing countries have to international markets, TRIPS also enables biopiracy. For example, the RiceTec's US patent claimed the invention of "novel rice lines with plants that are semi-dwarf in stature, sub-stantially photoperiod-insensitive and high-yielding, and that produce rice grains having characteristics similar or superior to those of good quality basmati rice grains produced in India and Pakistan." However, what the policy does not take into account is that the patent takes ownership of genetic material originally developed by South Asian farmers; the germplasm from these varieties were initially collected in the Indian subcontinent and later deposited and processed in the United States and other places. Add to that, TRIPS also allows the patent holder to usurp the "basmati" name, which itself could jeopardize the sale of basmati from South Asia due to confusion (Trade and Environment Database ((TED) 1998, 2005).

The patenting of food grains can have major implications for the economy and food security in the least developed countries (LDC). In many of the LDCs, food grains such as rice form a vital part of people's diet. According to Owens (2002, as cited in Woods, 2002), Asian rice provides up to 85 per cent of the calories in the daily diet of 2.7 billion people. According to the Trade and Environment Database (TED, 1998, 2005), with the basmati patent rights, RiceTec will be able not only call to its aromatic rice basmati within the United States, but also to label it basmati for its exports. This means farmers that depend on basmati cultivation and export in India and Pakistan will not only lose out on the 45,000-tonne US import market, which forms 10 percent of the total basmati exports, but also lose its position in markets like the European Union, the United Kingdom, Middle East, and West Asia. This would certainly hit the local economy in rice growing regions of India and Pakistan. As farmers lose markets for their crops, their incomes will be hit hard, leading to increased inability to spend on a basic necessity like food. Thus, the very resources that are a part of the day-to-day life of indigenous groups have to be purchased at a price from the technologically advanced countries and from TNCs, creating the scenario for continuous exploitation.

The combination of TRIPS and SAPs in the context of the Third World has resulted in the large-scale co-optation of agricultural spaces as the markets for the seeds and chemicals manufactured by TNCs. Furthermore, TRIPS emerges as a disciplinary site of control for enacting the hegemony of global agri-business such as Monsanto. With 94 percent of the global acreage for GM food in 2000 under the control of Monsanto for instance, large sectors of agricultural land come under the purviews of Monsanto, thus ensuring that the TNC uses the articulations of intellectual property rights to bring additional acres of land under its domain and further establish its dominance in global markets. As local farmers are surrounded by more and more GM seeds in their agricultural lands, the chances of contamination with GM seeds increase, and so do the threats of being litigated by the agri-business giants for the violation of property rights.

The threat of litigation for violating patent laws operates as a site for hegemonic control, bringing additional agricultural lands under the purview of TNCs. For instance, Monsanto sends inspectors into farmlands, investigating the crops and trying to find some of their patented crops; if these patented crops are found not to have been purchased directly from Monsanto, the farmers are threatened with lawsuits (see CBS, 2008). Farmers such as David and Dawn Runyon of Indiana have been threatened with lawsuits of patent infringement as their farm was found to be contaminated with Monsanto's patented "Round-up Ready" soy, which according to the Runyons was probably a product of pollination through wind drafts. In a similar incident, a Canadian farmer, Percy Schmeiser, had been ordered to pay $85,000 to Monsanto for illegally growing its patented Canola, although the farmer claimed that he had not planted the seed, and his farm must have acquired it through cross-pollination from the 40 percent of the surrounding farms that were using the Monsanto variety (Herrick, 2008; Oguamanam, 2007). Furthermore, seed cleaners, who separate the seeds from debris in order for the seeds to be replanted, have been threatened with lawsuits by Monsanto. In one instance, Mo Parr, a seed cleaner from Indiana, was sued by Monsanto under the charges of aiding and abetting seed piracy, and his bank records were subpoenaed to find the names of farmers who were using his services. As Madeley (2000) notes, agreements like TRIPS establish private, monopolistic control over plant resources and lead to dislocation of farmers, loss of food security, and ultimately denial of "the right to survive."

Neoliberalism, Development, and Aid. Development programs serve as the gateway for carrying out the agendas of TNCs in the agricultural sector. TRIPS, working hand in hand with the structural adjustment programs and programs of development, pushes the monopoly of GM crops into the agricultural sectors of the globe. Crops such as Bt. Cotton are introduced as the miracle solutions to development and pushed through the agendas of development programs in the agricultural sector. Simultaneously, under the frameworks of intellectual property rights in neoliberal agriculture, the relationships of farmers to their seeds are changed forever. Farmers no longer can simply store their seeds from one season and grow them in the following year; instead, as seeds become commodities in this new paradigm of agriculture, farmers have to purchase their seeds each year from global agri-business. Therefore, in seasons of crop failure, farmers are forced to go back and take additional debts in order to purchase the seeds for the next year instead of simply saving a part of their seeds. In yet other instances, aid programs in response to famines are used to create markets for GM foods (Herrick, 2008). For instance, in response to the famine in South Africa, USAID donated GM maize in the kernel form, which would then need to be planted, thus threatening to pollute the non-GM varieties and organic crops which constitute the majority of agri-cultural exports in the region. Furthermore, the possible introduction of GM seeds into the system threatened to inject risks into the food chain.

The commoditization of seeds is accompanied by the markets for fertilizers and pesticides that are also created along with the seeds, thus further consolidating the hegemonic control of global agri-business. Simultaneously, water, a key requirement in the cultivation of GM crops, is increasingly privatized, with farmers having to pay money for the privatization of water. The privatization of water has further meant that the small-scale farmers are increasingly marginalized in the agricultural sector, having to purchase each of the components of the inputs into agriculture.

In addition to influencing the agricultural production systems, contemporary neoliberal policies limit the markets for agricultural commodities by minimizing the trade-related barriers and by eliminating subsidies. As we have seen in the case of the banana war between the ACP growers and the Latin American and US growers, when certain trade related preferences for ACP bananas in the European Union were removed, farmers in the ACP regions faced serious difficulties, including poverty and marginalization. Furthermore, the competitiveness of the banana market led to further consolidation of the power in the hands of the multinational banana giants in Latin America, further displacing indigenous populations from their lands, who turned into laborers for the plantations. Simultaneously, social and economic deregulations in Latin America led to the worsening of the working conditions of the plantation workers and producers, reducing their share of the benefits.

Food security across the globe, and particularly so in the Third World, is threatened as development programs are increasingly used as tools of the global agri-business to promote GM crops, which further threaten the sustainability of local farmers by making them dependent on TNCs, and turning them into consumers of products marketed by global agri-business, which they often can't afford (Herrick, 2000; Shiva & Bedi, 2002). Farmers in the global South end up taking large loans in order to purchase the GM seeds from TNCs, accompanied by the necessity to purchase agri-chemicals also manufactured by the TNCs such as fertilizers and pesticides. The water requirements of the GM crops and their sensitivity to irrigation further situate agriculture in the domains of capitalist interests as water across the globe is also increasingly becoming a privatized commodity to be owned and transacted by TNCs. When the GM crops fail (such as in the case of the failure of Bt. Cotton in Gujarat, India), the farmers are left behind with large debts that they can't repay. Furthermore, the ramifications of TRIPS in the agricultural sector imply that the farmers have to go back to the TNCs in order to purchase additional seeds for the following season when the crops fail, thus ensuring a continued cycle of dependence on global agri-business and further indebtedness of farmers in the hands of lenders.

Experiences at the Margins

The culture-centered approach draws attention to the structural constraints, institutional configurations, and boundaries that define the scope of marginalization. It is within the realm of these structures that agency is constituted, and sites of resistance are constituted in response to the dominant structures of oppression. Foregrounding the experiences at the margins, the approach discusses the relevance of participatory dialogues in underserved communities that narrate the stories of the margins, and in doing so, disrupt the hegemonic narratives of the status quo.

It is through these participatory frameworks that alternative sites are created for the enactment of resistance. The listening to the subaltern voices within the dominant discursive spaces ruptures the mainstream narratives of these spaces, opening up the spaces to alternative articulations and stories. Consider for instance, the following narrative of a peasant farmer from Haiti:

> I don't know what is meant by structural adjustment, but it sounds to me like even less for poor people. How could we possibly live on less? If privatization goes forward, they might as well just dig a big pit and shove us all in it.
> *(Farmer & Bertrand, 2000, p. 81)*

What the narrative of the peasant farmer foregrounds here is the articulation of development under structural adjustment as loss to the poor. This framing of structural adjustment from a subaltern perspective challenges the dominant constructions of SAPs as universally good for development.

Along these lines, the story of agricultural development and neoliberalism in the agricultural sector is juxtaposed against the backdrop of the narratives of the poor farmers who have been marginalized because of neoliberal agricultural policies, and have been pushed toward committing suicide in their fight with poverty as their crops, purchased with monies borrowed from lenders, have failed (Sainath, 2010). The narrative of peasant suicides in this case brings forth the violence underlying the mainstream narrative of the Green Revolution and neoliberalism as being the markers of prosperity; Sainath (2010) suggests that the suicides tend to be concentrated in regions of high commercialization of agriculture and accompanying high debts.

In 1998, the National Crimes Record Bureau reported that 1,813 farmers had committed suicide in the Indian state of Andhra Pradesh, and 2,409 in the Indian state of Maharashtra. In contrast, these numbers went up to 2,105 in Andhra Pradesh, and 3,802 in Maharashtra in 2008. Sainath (2010) reports that in 2008, India saw a total of 16,196 farm suicides. Note, for instance, the following narration made by Jeevan, a farmer in Chattisgarh, who refers to the death of his friend Beturam:

> Beturam died due to loans. He had no fight with anyone. He was also not keeping well lately and burnt himself one day. Here every farmer is in debt. I have 15 acres of land but I too have around Rs.27,000 in loans from the bank.
> *(India Together, 31 March, 2009)*

These stories of farmer suicides across India in the face of crop failures attest to the structural violence that is perpetrated by neoliberalism in the agricultural sector. These ruptures and disjunctures in the universal narratives of development further create openings for interrogating the core ideas of agriculture in the mainstream with alternative entry points.

Land as a Site of Contestation

For the subaltern sectors of the globe, land becomes the site of contestation as neoliberal projects continue to encroach on agricultural lands in order to carry out the agendas of the transnational elites. For instance, in the form of development programs, industrialization, increasing privatization, and trade liberalization, agricultural lands are encroached upon in order to carry out the development programs. Structural adjustment programs implemented across the globe have resulted in the loss of agricultural land, as such land has been converted into industrial and manufacturing spaces (Mahadevia, 2002). Across different regions and countries throughout the globe, in the form of projects of building dams sponsored by the World Bank, indigenous and rural communities have been displaced from their agricultural lands. Similarly, mining projects that have come into agricultural communities have taken over agricultural land in order to carry out the mining. Projects of industrialization have displaced farmers and rural communities as spaces have been sought in order to build production and manufacturing facilities.

Listening to the local voices in the political economy of contemporary attempts of nation states to usurp land in the services of TNCs offers alternative rationalities and interpretive frameworks for engaging with the meanings of land for the subaltern sectors of the globe. Participants often discuss the value placed on land not simply as a source of livelihood, but also an integral part of the subaltern cosmology. For instance, references to land as mother reverberate in the discursive spaces of displaced communities or communities being threatened to be displaced; land no longer remains an economic commodity that can be exchanged, but emerges as an embodiment of the Goddess mother Lakshmi, who symbolizes peace, bounty, and prosperity. Therefore, as we will note later in this book, struggles over land emerge as struggles over the modes of meaning making and representation, not only influencing the economic capacity of communities but also fundamentally threatening a way of life.

Collective Properties versus Individual Rights

One of the key spaces for debate in the neoliberal landscape is over the articulation of property rights and the framing of agriculture in the realm of individual poverty. Contrary to the neoliberal articulation of property and ownership as individual artifacts, subaltern frames note the ownership of property as resources in the realm of the collective. For instance, in Cochabamba, Bolivia, subaltern resistance to the privatization of water is framed in the form of the collective ownership of water in the hands of the local community. The articulation of resistance here is fundamentally constituted in the realm of an alternative interpretive frame that takes water as a public resource that belongs to the collective as opposed to the conceptualization of water as a private commodity to be transacted in the marketplace at a price (more on this later). Similarly, subaltern communities across the globe are increasingly resisting the deforestation of lands by putting forth the conceptualization of forest land as collective ownership rather than individual-level ownership to be guided by the profit-making interests of corporations.

Nature as a Site of Control

Yet another contestation that emerges through local participation emphasizes the importance of living in harmony with nature, drawing upon knowledge bases and philosophical traditions that directly contradict the ontological and epistemological foundations of capitalism. For instance, in Shiva's articulation of the Sanskrit verse *vasudhaiva kutumbakam* (the world is a family), she suggests earth democracy as an alternative to the competition-driven market-based logic of neoliberalism. In her depictions of agriculture under the neoliberal framework, she draws attention to the agendas of global corporations of making profits by utilizing reductionist science to gain control over natural resources. Such control, although essential to the large amounts of profits made by global agri-business, is an attack on the right to survival of the two-thirds majority of human beings who depend on nature's capital and do not have the capacity to participate in the global markets because of their poverty (Narayan & Petesch, 2002; Shiva, 2000, 2005).

The control of natural resources in the hands of TNCs is also contested by subaltern sectors across the globe. For instance, Navdanya, a network of seed keepers and organic producers across sixteen states in India, has emerged as a resistive site against the globalizing practices of TNCs that seek to bring more and more agricultural lands across the globe under their control. Navadanya's resistance is enacted in the form of promoting seed sovereignty (*Bija Swaraj*) and food sovereignty among farmers by setting up a learning center on biodiversity and organic farming, training farmers on seed sovereignty and sustainable agriculture, promoting the rejuvenation of indigenous knowledge and culture, running campaigns on the hazards of genetic engineering, and defending people's knowledge from biopiracy (www.navdanya.org/). In its campaign against the approval by the Agricultural Ministry of India for the commercial planting of Bt. Brinjal, Navdanya interrogated the science behind the dissemination of Bt. Brinjal, questioning the claim that without the genetically modified Bt. pests cannot be controlled and citing the evidence of increase in pesticide use in Vidarbha after Bt. Cotton was introduced (Shiva, 2010). This evidence was presented against the backdrop of evidence of the efficacy of toxic-free organic farming as practiced by the Navdanya farmers. Second, questions regarding the safety and risks associated with transgenic Bt. were raised. These questions of safety of GM foods have been also raised in the European Union as well in the United States, where non-profit advocacy groups such as the Center for Food Safety have emerged as sites contesting the control held by TNCs in the agricultural market. Of particular concern are the health effects of GM foods and the question of safety of such foods (www.centerforfoodsafety.org/geneticall2.cfm). Third, Navdanya called for data from studies of self-pollination versus cross-pollination of Bt. Brinjal, along with the maximum distance travelled by the Bt. pollen.

Farmers organized themselves as GMO free Jaiv Panchayats (Living Democracy), with letters being sent from approximately 4,365 Navdanya farmers representing 126 Jaiv Panchayats, declaring *Bija Satyagraha* (non-cooperation) to stop GM foods. References were made to the indigenous culture and to the historic-cultural concept of *Satyagraha* to locate the indigenous movement in the context of the Indian freedom struggle against British colonialism, where *Satyagraha* or non-cooperation was used as a strategy of resistance to the British colonialists by promoting sustainable indigenous forms of production and simultaneously boycotting the products marketed by the imperialists in the indigenous spaces. Based on public hearings on Bt. Brinjal, pressures from farmers, and the declaration of twelve states that they will not allow Bt. Brinjal, the Minister of Environment declared a moratorium on Bt. Brinjal (*Hindustan Times*, February 24, 2010). As the example of Bt. Brinjal demonstrates, culture-centered co-constructions with the margins create opportunities for the development of alternative discourses and rationalities that challenge the reductionist and profit-driven narrative of neoliberalism.

Conclusion

In conclusion, this chapter notes the ways in which dominant structures play out the interests of transnational hegemony, and simultaneously create spaces of marginalization of the poor. Worth noting here are the central roles played by neoliberal structures of oppression. Structures of political and economic interests define the ways in which the agricultural sector is organized under neoliberalism, creating spaces of profits for TNCs and simultaneously marginalizing the individual farmer. It is in this landscape of global inequities that issues are raised, transforming into the foundations for communicative processes of social change.

4

HEALTH AT THE MARGINS

Health is a core area where the disparities between the haves and have-nots in global systems become evident, with increasing health inequalities documented across the various sectors of the globe (Kawachi, Kennedy, & Wilkinson, 1999; Kawachi, Wilkinson, & Kennedy, 1999; UNDP, 2004). The comparative differences in the distribution of economic resources go hand in hand with the absence of the basic structural health resources for the poorer communities of the globe. In other words, there is a fundamental economic base underlying the (in)access to health resources amidst poverty. At an absolute level, poorer communities lack the basic capabilities of health that are considered to be minimal to human life. These basic forms of health capacity are constituted in terms of access to health services and treatments, access to information resources, and access to a wide variety of preventive resources (Dutta, 2006, 2007, 2008a, 2008b, 2008c; Dutta-Bergman, 2004a, 2004b). In this chapter, we examine the intersections of poverty and health, and the ways in which the margins of healthcare are symbolically and materially constructed in dominant discursive spaces of health communication. The overall objective here is to understand the processes of marginalization that create the peripheries of health in contemporary global spaces.

In seeking to understand the ways in which the margins of health are communicatively constructed, the culture-centered approach suggests that communicative marginalization creates and sustains structural marginalization. Communication lies at the heart of the marginalizing process as it is predominantly in the realm of the symbolic that justifications are made for the erasure of the voices of certain sectors of the globe. Culture enters into the domains of scholarship and practice as a category for intervention, further reiterating the marginalization of communities with minimal access to basic health infrastructures (Dutta-Bergman, 2004a, 2004b). The culture-centered approach draws attention to the discursive moves through which the voices of the marginalized communities are erased from the spaces of health policy-making and program implementation, thus putting communities at the margins of health (Dutta, 2006, 2007, 2008a, 2008b, 2008c). How are structures of inaccess communicatively constructed? What are the intersections of culture and structure in the realm of the creation of the margins of health? Those structures of policy-making and policy implementation are interrogated that create and sustain the material experiences of (in)access to health among communities living in poverty.

In addition to the marginalization of communities in their access to basic health capacities, global health outcomes are also influenced by the material inequalities that exist within and across communities (Bradshaw & Linneker, 2001; Kawachi & Kennedy, 1997; Kawachi & Wamala, 2007; Milanovic, 2005; World Bank, 2001). Whereas certain sectors of the globe enjoy continued and increased access to health resources and to the continually reinvented health technologies that promise the miracles of twenty-first century medicine, other sectors of the globe are increasingly deprived of the basic necessities of health, facing issues of inaccess to health services and health programs. Increasing income inequalities are noted for the last two decades in cross-country comparisons of average national incomes; Kawachi and Wamala (2007) note that whereas since the early 1980s, rich countries have grown richer, poorer countries have either stayed poor or become poorer in terms of their per capita income. Furthermore, studying income inequality within countries on the basis of the GINI coefficient, Cornia and Kiiski (2001) reported that between the 1950s and 1990s, inequality increased in 48 of the 73 countries studied. Both cross-country comparisons as well as within-country analyses suggest that income inequality predicts both morbidity and mortality (Kennedy, Kawachi, & Prothrow-Stith, 1996; Wilkinson, 1986a, 1986b, 1992a, 1992b, 1996, 2005). How are these inequalities created and what are the justifications for them? What then are the symbolic markers through which these inequalities circulate globally? (See Figure 4.1.)

Based on the articulations that the global margins in health are created through fundamentally unequal policies of global health, we focus on an examination of global health policies under the dominant framework of health. What are the underlying policies and social structures that govern these disparities? How are health inequalities supported communicatively in mainstream health configurations across the globe? From a communication perspective, how are the margins of healthcare constituted in policies and programs, and how are they sustained through contemporary hegemonic structures? Drawing upon the culture-centered approach, we reiterate the argument that material inaccess to healthcare is mapped out, sustained, and propagated by communicative inaccess to basic infrastructures. The key arguments made in this chapter about the communicative nature of structural marginalization in healthcare are supported through empirical evidence, case studies, and ethnographic interviews of those sectors that are placed at the margins of mainstream healthcare systems. Furthermore, the structures of global

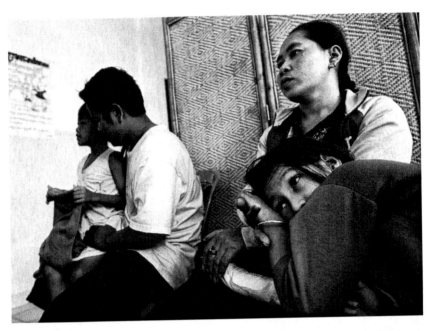

FIGURE 4.1 Children infected with AIDS wait to be seen by a doctor at the National Pediatric Hospital outpatient clinic for HIV/AIDS on February 15, 2010 in Phnom Penh. (Paula Bronstein/Getty Images)

inequality are questioned for their conceptualization of culture and the ways in which culture enters into the discourses of hegemonic structures to justify the creation of the margins of health. We will begin this chapter by discussing the explanations offered for the marginalizing experiences in healthcare, followed by a discussion of the dominant discourses of health and conceptualization of the culture-centered approach.

Theoretical Perspectives

The theoretical perspectives offered in this section offer explanations for understanding the marginalizing experiences in healthcare. Whereas these explanations mostly draw upon a material foundation to explore the role of material structures in the health experiences and outcomes of marginalized communities, they also explore the social, political, and communicative realms in which the margins of health are constructed. Overall, the theories offered in this section of the chapter seek to build a framework for understanding the ways in which marginalization works in creating the subaltern sectors in healthcare.

Absolute Income and Health

The material framework of health inequalities examines the role of absolute income in shaping health outcomes. Poverty here is depicted in terms of the income earned, based on the argument that the absolute income of an individual and her/his family determine the access to health resources, and is the underlying cause of absolute material deprivation. As articulated in the Millennium Development Goals, poverty is a key determinant of health, being particularly evident in child mortality, a health outcome that is most sensitive to poverty (Marmot, 2005). At a national level, in the comparison of countries, there remains tremendous variance in under-5 child mortality; whereas countries such as Iceland, Finland, and Japan reflect less than 6 deaths per 1000 live births, countries such as Sierra Leone reflect 316 per 1000 live births. Furthermore, in some parts of the world, child mortality is on the rise (rising 43 percent in Zimbabwe and 75 percent in Iraq in the 1990s). These differentials in health outcomes are directly situated against the backdrop of the material deprivation in particular sectors, thus directly impacting the ability of community members to access resources.

Within-country comparisons also demonstrate that child mortality tends to be the highest among the poorest sectors (Marmot, 2005). Similar observations are also made in adult populations, with the greatest mortality and morbidity rates being observed in the poorest parts of the globe (Marmot, 2005). At a basic level, material inaccess, articulated in the form of absolute poverty, influences health through the inability to access clean water, nutritious food, and a wide range of medical services. However, at a broader level of social policies across the globe, how these resources are distributed and who gets access to these resources are socially determined, suggesting that inequalities in distributions of power within social systems determine the ways in which health resources get distributed and the absolute material markers of health that become available to the poorer sectors.

The effect of poverty on health outcomes is evident not only in studies of countries at a global level but also in comparisons of the various sectors within nation states. Within the United States for instance, studies have examined the role of health insurance in determining access to care and the subsequent health outcomes. Health insurance is increasingly tied to one's ability to have a job that pays insurance, and therefore is contingent upon one's performance as a worker in the contemporary global economy. Uninsured people in the United States not only face tremendous inequities in their access to health resources but also are marginalized in terms of their access to communication platforms where they might learn health information. The marginalized health experiences of the working poor in terms of the ability to access health services further documents the material effects of structural deprivation. With the increasing neoliberalization of the globe, the labor classes have come under direct control of the capitalist classes, with deteriorating access to healthcare among these classes, and increasing workplace exposure to health hazards. Furthermore, the global control of TNCs in the policy sectors has adversely influenced environmental pollution, further putting the marginalized sectors at health risk (see the example of *maquiladora* discussed in Chapter 2 and later in this chapter).

Not only do the poor have lower levels of access to basic health services as compared to the other segments of the population, but they also report poorer quality of health services as well as disparities in their communication with healthcare providers (Agency for Healthcare Research and Quality (AHRQ), 2008). In the United States, for example, poorer adults were more than twice as unlikely to get timely care as compared to high-income adults. Parents of poorer children reported facing greater levels of problems communicating with their physicians as compared to higher-income parents. Similarly, in the work with Santali communities in Eastern India, Dutta-Bergman (2004a, 2004b) reports the poor quality of health services received by Santalis and the mistreatment by the healthcare providers.

Income Inequalities and Health

Clustered under the framework of the relative income hypothesis, a growing body of research on income inequalities points out that unequal societies are also more likely to face poorer health outcomes (Kennedy et al., 1996; Wilkinson, 1986a, 1986b, 1992a, 1992b, 1996, 2005). When incomes are unequally distributed in a society, the real welfare of the poor may be lower than that suggested by the measures of real income (Waldmann, 1992). Health is perhaps one of the most sensitive social indicators of inequality, pointing out that inequalities adversely affect life expectancy, mortality, morbidity, as well as life satisfaction within communities (Kawachi, Kennedy, & Wilkinson, 1999; Wilkinson, & Kennedy, 1999). In the realm of life expectancy, cross-national studies document the negative relationship between inequality and life expectancy, such that societies with greater levels of inequality in the distribution of resources are also likely to report lower levels of life expectancy, as opposed to societies that are more egalitarian in their distribution of resources, and therefore, are more likely to report higher levels of life expectancy (Rodgers, 1979; Wilkinson, 1986a, 1986b, 1992a, 1992b, 1996, 2005).

In a seminal piece on income distribution and health outcomes across several countries, measured in the form of life expectancy at birth, life expectancy at age 5, and infant mortality, Rodgers (1979) reported that income inequality resulted in approximately five years of difference in life expectancy. Similarly, in his comparison of eleven countries belonging to the Organization for Economic Cooperation and Development (OECD), Wilkinson (1992a) reported a strong correlation between income inequality and life expectancy. Further noting the relative income hypothesis, Waldmann (1992) observes that after controlling for the real incomes of the poor, the indicators of the amount of healthcare available to the poor etc., income inequality emerges as a strong predictor of infant mortality.

Additionally, the relative effect of income inequality does not seem to be diminished when factors such as the number of doctors per capita, nurses per capita, urbanization indicators, female literacy, and gross reproductive rates are taken into account. Waldmann (1992) offers the possible explanation that the higher incomes of the rich are probably associated with the greater importance given by government policies to the interests of the rich at the costs of the poor. Noting a social gradient in health outcomes, extant scholarship documents the drop in health outcomes as relative income diminishes. Therefore, even in the more affluent countries that have some of the highest GNP measures, the poorer social classes have shorter life expectancies and greater number of illnesses as compared to the richer classes (WHO, 2003).

When the relative and absolute markers of income are combined together in examining their effects on national mortality, it is observed that the effects of absolute income in mortality diminish beyond a certain level, although the effects of relative income on mortality continue to be salient. This suggests the importance of investigating the health effects of relative income, above and beyond the influences of absolute income. Summarizing the relationship between income distribution and life expectancy across countries, Wilkinson (1992a) suggests the possible psychosocial influences of income inequality on indicators such as stress, self-esteem, and social relations. He further notes the importance of looking at the ways in which relative poverty influences health by excluding community members, both socially and materially, from the day-to-day spaces of society. The income inequality-health outcome linkage is explained by the mediating role of social capital on one hand, and the political role of neoliberal policy-making on the other hand.

Social Capital and Health Inequalities. Social capital refers to the extent of social cohesiveness experienced within a community (Berkman, 1995; Bradshaw & Linneker, 2001; House, Landis, & Umberson, 1988; Kawachi & Kennedy, 1997; Kawachi, Kennedy, Lochner, & Prothrow-Stith, 1997; Wilkinson, 1996, 2005; World Bank, 2001). That social cohesion and social support relationships are fundamentally health promoting in nature is well documented across a wide range of studies (Berkman, 1995; House et al., 1988). Social relationships promote health because they act as buffers against the deleterious effects of stress and other health hazards, and offer a wide variety of social and psychological resources (Berkman, 1995; House et al., 1998). Individuals that are embedded in intimate relationships and in supportive communities are also more likely to report better health outcomes.

Scholars working in this area have proposed the concept of social integration, which is conceptualized both at an individual level as well as at the level of the collective (Kawachi & Kennedy, 1997). A socially integrated individual is well connected, with a large number of both intimate contacts as well as more distant connections. Extending this conceptualization to the level of the collective, socially integrated societies have large stocks of social capital in the form of networks of trust, reciprocity, and community participation. More socially integrated societies typically tend to have lower rates of crime, violence, and mortality from all causes (Kawachi et al., 1997; Wilkinson, 1996). Across a variety of study designs and frameworks conducted since 1979, researchers report consistent findings regarding the increased risks faced by those who are socially isolated and disconnected (Berkman, 1995). What is highlighted here therefore is the notion that negative health outcomes are attached to social marginalization and isolation. For instance, studies on recovery after myocardial infarction (MI) report that socially isolated patients had higher mortality risk than those who were not socially isolated (Berkman, 1995).

Furthermore, extant research on health epidemiology documents the mediating role of social capital in the relationship between income inequalities and health outcomes (Berkman, 1995; Kawachi et al., 1997). In other words, in responding to the social gradient of health within countries, public health researchers suggest that income inequalities within societies affect health outcomes through their influence on the social capital of communities.

Communication scholars studying the intersections of social capital and health look at a wide range of dimensions of social capital, ranging from interpersonal trust to community participation (Dutta-Bergman, 2005a, 2005b). For instance, the scholarship emphasizing the participatory element of social capital examines the ways in which communities serve as health enhancing resources and as repositories of health information and preventive resources. Marginalization is carried out communicatively through the location of communities at the peripheries of mainstream discursive spaces. These locations at the peripheries then play out in terms of poor access to communicative platforms of policy-making and intervention planning, as well as to the structural resources of health. The absence of social ties and participatory spaces in low social capital communities also weaken the capacity of these communities to participate in processes of change, articulate community specific issues, and seek out resources to address these issues.

Power in Policy-Making. A critical interrogation of the linkage between inequality and health outcomes notes the role of policy-making in the context of health, arguing that the determination of health policies and the distribution of health resources is made at the centers of power (Coburn, 2000, 2004; Daniels, 2008). Those with access to power establish the agendas for healthcare, further determining the ways in which health resources will be distributed, and economically shaping the characteristics of healthcare. Therefore, societies with high levels of inequality also reflect high levels of inequality in the distribution of power, with most decisions being made at the economic centers, directed at benefiting the agendas and interests of the power structures. This leaves large sectors of the population outside the realm of policy articulations and with minimum access to health resources. In contrast, societies with more equitable distribution of economic resources are also more likely to have equitable distributions of health resources, with widely distributed networks of decision-making.

Approaching health inequalities within the framework of power in policy-making examines differences in health outcomes within the population in terms of questions of access to sites of power and policy-level decision-making (Coburn, 2000, 2004). The advent of the neoliberal logic into the delivery of healthcare put tremendous amounts of power for policy-making into the hands of TNCs, who are able to shape global policies about health, and simultaneously continue to influence local policies across the globe through their influences on the IFIs and the corresponding SAPs imposed on countries. As we note later in this chapter, the poorer sectors of the globe, with limited forms of access to dominant policy platforms and with limited power in shaping policy agendas, remain as target audiences of global interventions. The poorer sectors continue to mostly remain marginalized by their limited access to global discursive spaces. Global differentials in distributions of power then dictate the experiences of health that are played out locally at the margins of contemporary neoliberal structures.

Racial Inequalities in Health

According to the Agency for Healthcare Research and Quality (2008), health disparities reflect the gaps in the quality of care received by one population in comparison to another population. The term "health disparities" is used to capture the widespread experiences and perceptions of injustice and inequity in access to, utilization of, and quality of care among certain demographic segments of society (Baquet, 2002; Braveman, 2006). These inequities in experiences with the health-care system also influence health status as well as a plethora of other health outcomes. Within the United States, studies of healthcare disparities point out that ethnic minorities consistently face discrepancies in their health outcomes when compared to Whites (AHRQ, 2008; Baquet, 2002; Dutta, Bodie, & Basu, 2008; Williams, 1999).

These disparities play out in a variety of ways including access to preventive resources and health information sources, access to health services, the quality of healthcare received, access to screening services and other health technologies, the nature of the interactions at points of healthcare delivery, etc. First, these studies document the strong correlation between race and class such that certain races are more likely to be economically deprived and this deprivation then plays out in inaccess to healthcare resources (Williams, 1999). Second, in addition to the effect of class, there seems to exist a racial bias, such that even when belonging to the same social class and therefore able to purchase the same health resources, racial minorities report poorer access, poorer quality of services, and poorer experiences with healthcare interactions as compared to Whites. Summarizing the results of several studies on disparities, Williams (1999) reports that there is a large body of clinical evidence suggesting that even after adjustment of socioeconomic status, health insurance, and clinical status, Blacks are less likely than Whites to receive a wide range of medical procedures.

According to the 2008 National Health Disparities Report, for Blacks, some of the greatest disparities exist in the number of new AIDS cases as compared to Whites (AHRQ, 2008). Also, some other areas with large disparities include the lack of prenatal care for pregnant women and hospital admissions for lower extremity amputations. Asian Americans report high levels of disparities as compared to Whites in terms of timeliness of care, being less likely than Whites to receive care for injury or illness as soon as wanted. For American Indians, women were less likely to receive prenatal care as compared to Whites and adults were less likely to receive colorectal cancer screenings as compared to Whites. Blacks, Asian Americans, American Indians, and Hispanics all experience lower levels of access to screening as compared to Whites. Also, both Blacks and Asian Americans reports disparities in the patient-centeredness of physician-patient communication as compared to Whites (AHRQ, 2008). Overall, across a wide range of indicators, racial and ethnic minorities face lower levels of access, poorer quality of care, and poorer quality of physician-patient communication as compared to Whites. In responding to these inequalities, whereas the cultural sensitivity approach sets up objectives to adapt to the characteristics of the culture, the culture-centered approach interrogates the basic underlying reasons that create these disparities.

Social Determinants of Health

The "social determinants of health" approach seeks to investigate the underlying causes of the poorer health outcomes in the disadvantaged sectors of the globe, both in the comparison across countries as well as in comparisons within countries. It suggests that although it is indeed important to look at the immediate causes of communicable as well as non-communicable diseases, it is further important to investigate the social conditions within which human beings live. The environments in which individuals live have dramatic impacts on human health, playing out in the everyday lives of individuals (WHO, 2003). Summarizing the evidence base on the social distributions of health, Blane (1995) observes that the distribution of health outcomes in society is graded such that for each change in the level of advantage experienced by a group, there is a corresponding change in health outcomes. Therefore, the more advantaged groups in society, expressed in terms of education, income, social class, and/or ethnicity also typically tend to experience better health than other members of society.

Existing evidence suggests that parental disadvantage is associated with low birthweight in the parents' offspring, which in turn is associated with social dis-advantage in adolescence and adulthood, disease risks, and with several chronic diseases in late middle age (Bartley, Power, Blane, Davey-Smith, & Shipley, 1994; Kuh & Cooper, 1992; Kuh & Wadsworth, 1993). The location of an individual and her/his family in the social structure, therefore, fundamentally affects individual as well as family health. Disadvantages typically tend to aggregate in clusters cross-sectionally and accumulate longitudinally. In addition to examining the material outcomes of disadvantage, it is also important to examine the social meanings of disadvantage. Therefore, the WHO (2003) report on social determinants of health points toward the roles of social exclusion, stigmatization, and meanings of poverty in the lives of the poor, above and beyond the material dimensions of inaccess brought about by poverty.

The WHO Commission of Social Determinants of Health (WHO, 2008) observes that it is essential to attend to the broader structural issues underlying the unequal distributions of health opportunities across countries and within countries. According to the WHO report, there is an emerging need for taking into account the unequal distribution of power, income, goods, and services both within countries and across countries globally in understanding the influence of these structural inequalities on poor health outcomes of the poor, health inequalities between countries, and the social gradient of health within countries. The importance of a holistic treatment of broader structural determinants is highlighted, with an emphasis not only on the basic health capacities such as access to schools, education, and healthcare, but also in terms of the everyday living conditions of work and leisure, and the environments in homes, communities, towns, or cities. Poor health here is treated in terms of the political and economic conditions that constitute it, attending to the social policies and the structural conditions that propagate the conditions of poor health.

Dominant Discourses of Health

The dominant discourses of health constitute the mainstream, the collection of ideas and articulations that define the basic ontology and epistemology of health communication, narrated amidst the existing structures. The perspectives that are termed as the dominant perspectives of health are the ideas of the global ruling classes that determine the meanings of health, the problematization of health issues, and the development of health solutions to serve the interests of the status quo. The conceptualization of health problems and the corresponding solutions are constituted in the realm of the logics of the dominant structures of health, serving the agendas of these structures, and dictating the meaning and scope of health programming and interventions.

Health and Development

Much of the global health communication emphasis addressing issues of marginalization has been constituted under the framework of development (Dutta, 2006, 2007, 2008c; Dutta & Basnyat, 2008a, 2008b, 2008c; Dutta-Bergman, 2005a, 2005b). Development communication programs have been globally funded on the basis of the principles of behavior change, identifying the problematic behaviors in target communities, developing a framework for constructing campaign messages directed at bringing about behavior change in target populations, implementing campaign messages disseminated through a strategic combination of media, and evaluating these campaigns for their effectiveness. The entire industry of health development campaigns has been situated within this broader agenda of behavior and/or lifestyle change in target communities, emphasizing individual-level behavior change. In doing so, the dominant framework of development communication campaigns has been constituted within the capitalist logic of health promotion, with an emphasis on producing healthy individuals that can participate as labor in the economy and simultaneously shifting attention away from questions of redistributive justice or structural transformation (Dutta, 2006, 2008a, 2008b, 2008c).

The predominant framework that has been carried out in development communication programming has focused on addressing the knowledge, attitude, and behaviors in the target communities, based on the fundamental assumption of existing problems in target communities that could be solved by campaign messages targeted at these communities. The predominant framework of persuasion operated through the assumption that messages of health disseminated through the strategic choice of media would bring about the desired changes in the target communities. The emphasis on the message assumes that the creation of effective messages would lead to greater likelihood of adoption of the recommended behaviors, and once these behaviors were adopted, the health outcomes of communities would improve.

The dominant framework of health development campaigns works on the basis of certain taken-for-granted assumptions based on West-centric knowledge structures that are assumed as the universal markers of human existence (Dutta, 2006, 2008a, 2008b, 2008c; Dutta & Basnyat, 2008a, 2008b; Dutta-Bergman, 2004a, 2004b). The theories applied in health development campaigns therefore continue to impose the dominant framework of biomedicine as the framework for intervention, simultaneously erasing the discursive space for possibilities of engaging with alternative rationalities such as the harmonious relationship between body and mind or respect for the relationship with nature (see Dutta-Bergman, 2004a, 2004b). Similarly, the framework of health campaigns targeting individual beliefs operates on the reductionist assumption that the disease is located at the level of the individual, thus ignoring the realms of collective decision making and collective responsibility sharing for health. Furthermore, the cognitive basis of health campaign theories does not take into account human emotions and alternative rationalities that exist outside the realm of the mainstream ideologies of campaigns. The family, the community, and the collective as sites of negotiating health decisions are erased from the conceptual bases of individualistically directed theories such as the Theory of Reasoned Action (TRA) and the Health Belief Model (HBM).

Power and Control. The "science" of campaigns serves as the site of power, where knowledge claims made on the basis of access to power at the global centers serve as the foundation for guiding the development of health communication campaigns targeting the periphery. The introduction of health into the logic of development serves to reinforce inequities in the relational positions of the sender and receiver of health campaigns. The Western sender of campaign messages operates on the basic logic of the universality and modernity of Western appeals to reason juxtaposed in the backdrop of the backwardness and primitiveness of the Third World spaces. In other words, the portrayal of the other as primitive is a primary discursive move that underlies the political economy of campaign knowledge and praxis, ensuring the flow of capital into health communication programs directed at bringing about changes in the Third World. At the same time, the use of the "science" of health campaigns continues to justify the inequities in distribution of power, and the discursive power of the West to write over the bodies of the Third World, targeting these bodies as recipients of health interventions.

Implicit Agendas. The broader discursive and material space of development is constituted within the agendas of dominant power structures in the global landscape. The logic of development operates on the marking of the Third World as a recipient space, in need of the intervention. It is this very marking that continues to reify the differentials between the First and the Third Worlds, one as the producer of knowledge and the other as the target of this knowledge production. The political economy of development campaigns is based on the depiction of the Third World in deficits and therefore, in need of First World interventions derived from universal values. Development communication campaigns carry out implicit agendas of reifying certain dominant structures globally. For example, the development projects launched by the Agency of International Development serve as tools of the US government to generate spaces of political and economic support abroad, with the creation of favorable spaces across the globe that would open up their markets to US-based TNCs, offer favorable business climate to the US-based TNCs, serve as spaces of political support for the United States, and serve the geostrategic interests of the United States as well (see Dutta, 2006).

Similarly, when the implicit agenda of the President's Emergency Plan for AIDS Relief (PEPFAR) is considered, what becomes apparent is the political economy of development as a facade for carrying out the neoliberal agendas of the status quo (Sastry & Dutta, in press). PEPFAR emerges as the site for pushing private-public partnerships in the Third World. HIV/AIDS relief becomes a framework for pushing the privatization agenda of the IFIs and WTO. Private corporations and media giants find access into the discursive and material spaces of health through the deployment of partnerships between TNCs, local NGOs and government to solve the issue of HIV/AIDS. Health and development become the sites of intervention for commercial interests, serving the commercial interests of TNCs by creating new markets across the globe. HIV/AIDS moves from the domain of public intervention to the arena of private partnerships to carry out marketing through a variety of media platforms such as video games and entertainment programs. Similarly, driven by widespread clientelism, NGOs in the Third World direct themselves toward the agendas of transnational hegemony,

Policy and Intervention Spaces. The culture-centered approach puts forth the key argument that the structural violence carried out in subaltern contexts is directly related with the absence of the subaltern sectors from spaces of policy making (Basu & Dutta, 2008a, 2008b, 2009; Dutta, 2006, 2007, 2008a, 2008b, 2008c, 2009; Dutta-Bergman, 2004a, 2004b, 2005a, 2005b). The turning of the subaltern into a passive agent is a key discursive move in ensuring the absence and strategic erasure of the subaltern from the expert spaces of policy making and knowledge production. An entire industry of healthcare knowledge producers, program planners, and evaluators is supported on the foundations of the passive body of the silent subaltern, turned into a fixed category with undesirable characteristics such as fatalism, illiteracy, external locus of control, and low motivations for engaging in health behaviors. The fixing of the subaltern is fundamental to the deployment then of instruments of data gathering for identifying beliefs and barriers and targeting these beliefs and barriers for the purposes of producing changes in beliefs, attitudes, and behaviors. In other words, the legitimacy of the entire industry of the science of health campaigns and communication is built on the silencing of the subaltern subject as the object of knowledge articulations, interventions, and evaluations (for an extensive discussion, see Dutta, 2008c).

Cultural Sensitivity Interventions

Increasingly, within the United States and across the various sectors of the globe, there has been an acknowledgement of the large-scale disparities that exist within populations (Kreuter & McClure, 2004). With the goal of addressing these disparities, health researchers have identified the concept of culture as a key construct that needs to be taken into account if culturally diverse populations are to be encouraged to engage in healthy behaviors (Kar, Alcalay, & Alex, 2001). The emphasis is on creating culturally sensitive or appropriate messages that are aligned with the key characteristics of the culture that are identified by the campaign planners and researchers (Kreuter & McClure, 2004; Kreuter & Haughton, 1996). Culturally sensitive health promotion programs operate on the basis of extracting certain sets of tangible characteristics from the culture, closely examining these characteristics and then adjusting the messaging strategies of health interventions to be aligned with the characteristics of the population identified in the formative research.

In one thread of culturally sensitive health promotion programs, the cultural characteristics are identified as barriers to the implementation of the proposed behaviors. Therefore, the intervention focuses on addressing the beliefs of cultural members and in minimizing the barriers to the implementation of the proposed behavior through message strategies. In the United States, targeting the under-served communities entails the investment in formative research to learn about the cultural characteristics of the community, and the subsequent utilization of message development strategies to align the message with the identified cultural char-acteristics. For instance, in the case of health disparities that exist in the domain of cancer (African Americans are more likely to die of cancer than Whites), culturally sensitive messages deliver culturally relevant information with respect to cancer as well as develop culturally based messages that are directed toward instilling motivation to engage in preventive behaviors and to obtain screening. Further elaborating on the cultural sensitivity approach, scholars working with new media technologies in health emphasize the creation of tailored messages that are respon-sive to predetermined sets of audience characteristics. The research on tailoring typically suggests that tailored messages are likely to be more effective than non-tailored messages in producing persuasive change in the target audience.

Neoliberalism and Health at the Margins

As noted earlier in this book, neoliberalism is a political and economic framework that is based on the ideas of economic liberalization through privatization, liberalization, and deregulation (Coburn, 2000). Further building on the social capital and income inequalities linkage articulated by Wilkinson (1996) and others, Coburn (2000) posits the relevance of interrogating neoliberal policies and their adverse influences on health through the promotion of income inequalities, through the weakening of social ties, and through the decline of the welfare state. Implementation of neoliberal market principles has exacerbated income inequal-ities globally, with negative health outcomes for the poorer sectors of the globe (Coburn, 2000; Navarro, 1999). Neoliberal trade agreements have been associated with negative health and dependency patterns in developing regions of the world. Clarkson (1995) concurs that nation states today often find themselves locked into neoliberal principles by structural adjustment programs in the South and by international agreements and international institutions in the North. The growth of neoliberalism based on the principles of the uncharted operation of the market has been accompanied by the commodification of health, minimizing and elimi-nating safety nets in welfare states that have offered basic health services to the poor. Navarro (1999) articulates the importance of locating discussions of health inequalities amidst the issues of power and control embedded in current neoliberal configurations, and the ways in which the agendas of powerful global actors shape global health policies.

Scholars (Farmer, 1988a, 1988b, 1992; Harris & Seid, 2004; McMichael & Beaglehole, 2000; Narayan & Petesch, 2002) argue that the principal promoters of the contemporary market-based economic system advocate development strategies that often impair population health in countries affected by the strategies and reforms, by increasing inaccess to the basic health services and health resources among the poorest of the poor. According to Labonte (2001; Labonte & Torgerson, 2002), globalizing influences such as enforceable trade agreements and various forms of international development affect the national context of health through effects on labor rights, food security, the provision of public goods and services, and environmental protection. Zoller (2003, 2004, 2006) draws attention to the ways in which neoliberal economic organizing consolidates global power in the hands of pharmaceutical corporations, and dramatically reduces the access to basic medical supplies and medical capacities among the global poor (see also Farmer, 1988a, 1988b, 1992; Zoller & Dutta, 2008a, 2008b).

Furthermore, as noted by DeSouza (2008), the negative health effects of neoliberalism are played out among the subaltern sectors through the stealing of subaltern knowledge, the patenting of such knowledge, and the commodification of subaltern knowledge into market-based products sold by TNCs. Neoliberal political and economic policies that lead to the displacement of subaltern populations from their natural resources fundamentally threaten subaltern health, perpetrating multiple forms of physical and structural violence at multiple levels. The growth of global medical industries such as the clinical trials industry is further based on the exploitation of human capital from subaltern contexts, supporting the economic growth of transnational capital through the commodification, marketing, and exploitation of the subaltern subject (Prasad, 2009). As the vocabulary of progress and economic growth launches spaces across the globe on pathways of development, the poorest of the poor are further placed at the margins of contemporary global economies, turned into profitable sources of knowledge and human capital to be transacted for the purposes of profit.

Structural Adjustment Programs. One of the ways in which the neo-liberalization agenda has been carried out globally is through the structural adjustment programs (SAPs) implemented by the World Bank and the International Monetary Fund. By setting specific criteria for the deployment of development aid to specific nation states in the form of the SAPs, these international organizations have ensured their economic control over the markets within these nation states. The SAPs have pushed privatization, liberalization, and deregulation, thus threatening the public sectors in the Third World, as well as leading to the collapse of local industries. Unemployment has mostly increased and the working conditions have deteriorated. The emphasis on minimizing barriers to the movement of transnational capital has worked hand in hand with the limits imposed on labor organizing and in promoting poor labor policies, with the goal of maximizing the profits that are generated by TNCs.

The decline in the agricultural sectors in the global South as these sectors have been increasingly industrialized and commoditized has led to the exclusion of the subaltern sectors from locally situated systems of food production, thus creating food insecurities in subaltern sectors throughout the globe (DeSouza et al., 2008; Dutta, 2007, 2008c, 2009; Dutta-Bergman, 2004a, 2004b). The absence of food supplied from subaltern sectors has fundamentally impacted health through the large-scale creation of hunger and malnutrition. Furthermore, the growth of industry in response to liberalization and industrialization policies has displaced subaltern populations from the land resources that served as the sources of food and livelihood, further impacting health negatively (Dutta, 2008a, 2008b, 2008c; Dutta & Pal, 2010).

WTO, GATT, and TRIPS. The establishment of the agreement on trade and tariffs as well as the trade-related intellectual property rights have on one hand created global markets for pharmaceutical TNCs, and have simultaneously limited the capability of the subaltern sectors of the globe to secure access to health services and healthcare products. As health has been increasingly commoditized with the minimum presence and poor implementation of healthcare programs, inaccessibility to health has grown dramatically, especially in the Southern sectors of the globe. The commoditization of health has been further carried out by the global growth of the insurance industry and by the increasing incorporation of health within the agendas of capitalism. The provision of healthcare resources and services has become the domain of capitalist configurations, having been turned into the domains of profiteering (Dutta, 2008c; Navarro, 1999).

Scholars examining issues of health inequalities and neoliberalism highlight the relevance of interrogating the intersections of power and control that play out in neoliberal governance of global health (Navarro, 1999; Sastry & Dutta, 2010). Critical interrogations of powerful global institutions such as the WHO suggest that the agendas of WHO are constituted in alliance with the interests and agendas of IFIs and powerful transnational actors through the recommendations of global policies that appear "value free" and appeal to the universal discourses of science and technology on the surface. Referring to the hegemony of transnational capitalist discourse, Navarro (1999) notes:

> This discourse and practice (which I will provisionally define as technocratic) quickly becomes the accepted discourse in academia and the guiding force for all the systems of rewards that exist for intellectuals in our societies. One part of their strategy for reproduction, incidentally, is that all critical views are excluded, usually by being ignored. Any reader of most WHO publications for example, knows how rare it is to find in these forums any voices that are truly critical of that conventional wisdom. And multiple examples exist of professionals being vetoed by and excluded from such forums . . . the conservatism, that one detects, for example, in western economic and academic circles—broken by a few, very isolated voices—is constantly reproduced not only in the World Bank and the IMF, but also in many UN agencies.
>
> *(Navarro, 1999, pp. 219–220)*

The economic agendas of neoliberalism move from the domains of the IFIs and diffuse through the practices, knowledge structures, and discursive fields of dominant health structures, institutions, funding agencies, and academic circles. The national and global agendas of health are framed within the conventional wisdom attached to the values and principles of the neoliberal project, treating health as an individual-level commodity to be transacted in the free market.

Furthermore, the global adoption and privileging of TRIPS has led to bioprospecting, and turned indigenous knowledge into an exploitable commodity (DeSouza et al., 2008; Dutta, 2008c; Shiva, 2007). Bioprospecting is the stealing of indigenous knowledge and the patenting of such knowledge so that it can then be turned into a commodity and marketed by TNCs. It threatens the health of subaltern populations in the global South by turning indigenous food sources and health resources that have traditionally and historically been utilized as resources for life among subaltern communities into commodities that are patented and sold by TNCs, further making them inaccessible to the very people that historically have owned these resources and produced the knowledge vital to the utility of these resources toward serving human health (DeSouza et al., 2008).

Culture-Centered Approach to Health

The culture-centered approach to health communication engages with questions of marginalization by interrogating the erasures in the dominant structures of health (Airhihenbuwa, 1995; Dutta, 2006, 2007, 2008c; Dutta-Bergman, 2004a, 2004b). The foundation of the culture-centered approach is situated in subaltern studies theory, deconstructing the absences from the narratives of knowledge production. At the heart of the approach lies the commitment to continually interrogating the dominant power structures for the absences and erasures in these structures, examining the ways in which the poorer sectors of the globe are continually relegated to the peripheries of the discursive spaces of knowledge, and are turned into passive target audiences of intervention messages and programming. The ways in which the cultures of the Third World are constructed as pathologies to be then worked over by the messages of development is of key interest to culture-centered scholars. Making the argument that the symbolic and the material continually intersect in the perpetuation of inequities, Dutta (2008c) observes that it is through the construction of the other as primitive in the realm of the symbolic that material relationships of oppression are justified and reinforced. Historically, colonialism has operated on this primary logic of "lifting the burden of the soul," offering altruism as the veneer for the colonial intervention.

This scripting of the subaltern as the passive recipient of the mantras of development and health is built upon the depiction of the subaltern culture as pathological, and hence in need of interventions carried out by the agencies at the center. Marginalization therefore is constituted within the very realms of access to power based on the control of economic resources. The economically privileged sectors at the center of power play their roles as senders of messages directed toward the recipients in the peripheries.

Why is it that the economically deprived sectors of the globe have minimal access to the spaces of policy-making and policy implementation that discuss them? What are the implications of these absences of the subalterns from the spaces of policy-making and policy implementation? The key argument made by culture-centered scholars emphasizes the absences and erasures that are created in the discursive spaces of knowledge production, legitimizing the structural marginalization of the subaltern sectors of the globe. In essence then, the marginalization of certain spaces of the globe is played out materially, experienced in the form of minimum access to health resources, poor quality of care, and minimum access to health-related communication resources.

Voices from Below

The culture-centered approach resists and transforms the dominant power structures by engaging with the voices in subaltern spaces that have been situated at the peripheries of the mainstream. Listening to subaltern voices is the basic act of resistance that disrupts the status quo through its articulations of alternative narratives. These narratives emphasize subaltern agency and discuss the ways in which this agency is negotiated in everyday practices of living in subaltern communities across the globe. For instance, in conversations with Basu and Dutta (2009), a sex worker community organizer of the grassroots Sonagachi HIV/AIDS Program (SHIP) implemented in Kolkata notes, "We know what is best for us. We go around our community talking to people. They tell us what they need. Here we are in charge of things. We take care of the project that we run here" (Basu & Dutta, 2009, p. 95).

The ownership of subaltern agency is the crux of the culture-centered approach, resisting the dominant narrative of health communication programs that construct subaltern agency as passive. Similarly, consider the following narrative of health and poverty:

> We are all poor here, because we have no school and no health center. If a woman has a difficult delivery, a traditional cloth is tied between two sticks and we carry her for seven kilometers to the health center. You know how long it takes to walk like that? There is nobody who can help here, that's why we are all poor here. Togo, 1996.
>
> *(Narayan et al., 1999b)*

The narrative here discusses the structural inaccess faced by community members and it is against the backdrop of this story of inaccess that the participants discuss the stories of enacting their agency.

As noted earlier in this chapter, the culture-centered approach seeks to disrupt the hegemonic configurations in mainstream discursive spaces by listening to the voices of the subalterns, and therefore by creating possibilities of knowledge creation through the articulation of subaltern agendas as co-constructed with the researcher (Dutta, 2007, 2008c). The core idea is location of the capability of problem identification and solution development within the local communities that have historically been rendered passive as target audiences of policies and interventions. The emphasis on subaltern agency as an entry point of change foregrounds the narratives of structural violence, embodied in the experiences of inaccess and mistreatment among subaltern communities. These narratives of marginalization in healthcare bring forth the hypocrisies of the development rhetoric that pathologize the subaltern sectors and simultaneously minimize their access to health resources and health services (Farmer, 2003).

Engaging with the narratives of subalternity then offer entry points to health policy-making and program development through the co-constructions of problem configurations and solution frameworks by the subaltern participants. In-depth co-constructions in the subaltern spaces of the globe primarily draw attention to the lack of access to the fundamental elements of healthcare within subaltern communities. Here is what Lokkhi notes, discussing her inaccess to health:

> It is very expensive [referring to allopathic medicine]. A visit to Dr. Bera is Rs. 20 just for the visit, Rs. 10 for the medicine. If I get that medicine, I won't have rice at home. I won't have the money to buy anything. You know, I work hard. Day to night. But I can't go to the doctor.
>
> *(Dutta-Bergman, 2004a, p. 254)*

Lokkhi works part time as a farmer in the farming season, and is unable to secure access to doctor and medical treatments with the limited money that she earns. Securing access to health is situated amidst optimization of resources, and in the face of the inability to purchase health, subaltern community members discuss the hard work they do from day to night, and yet can't go to the doctor. In discussing the ineffectiveness of the public healthcare programs, subaltern participants point out that most of these resources are not available to them. For instance, here's the narrative of Nimai describing his decision of not visiting the clinic in spite of his worsening health, and articulating the intersections of the material and communicative marginalization that he faces in his life:

> Who will go to the state hospital? Do you want to go there and stand in line for the whole day? Who cares if the patient is dying? You go talk to the doctor. The doctor says settle down. Can't you see? There are all these people that are waiting. I stopped going to the state hospital. If something big happens, I will sell everything and go to the private doctor.
>
> *(Dutta-Bergman, 2004b, p. 14)*

Worth noting in this narrative is the juxtaposition of inaccess against the backdrop of communicative inaccess. The feeling of not being cared about because one is poor is tied to the experiences of stigmatization and mistreatment in interactions with health providers, further minimizing access to health resources. The hypocrisy of the rhetoric of state-sponsored support is disrupted in Dutta-Bergman's theoretical co-constructions with subaltern participants, who discuss mistreatment, inaccess, and corruption within these structures of health.

Here is another articulation of subaltern inaccess in Zapatista narratives noted by Farmer (2003):

> Health? Capitalism leaves its mark: 1.5 million Chiapans have no medical services whatsoever. There are .2 clinics for every 1,000 people, five times less than the national average; there are .3 hospital beds for every 1,000 Chiapans, three times less than the rest of Mexico; there is one operating room for every 100,000 people, two times less than the rest of the country; there are .5 doctors and .4 nurses for every 1,000 population, two times less than the national average.
>
> *(Farmer, 2003, p. 99)*

The articulation of inaccess creates the entry point for the enactment of agency. The absence of basic healthcare resources as noted by subaltern communities becomes an entry point for mobilizing processes of social change. The positioning of the limited structural resources played out in the form of limited access to health services offers the palette for the enactment of creativity in the subaltern sectors. It is amidst the narrations of structural violence that local subaltern participants narrate the stories of resistance and the hopes for structural transformation. Connecting to the Santali historical story of the *Hul* that was a collective resistance against imperial oppression:

> Can't we do it? They did it . . . You can't listen to the babus. Sidhu and Kanhu led all Santals, in the plains, in the forests, in the mountains to come out and fight. We can do it. But where is the leader? Something needs to happen.
>
> *(Dutta-Bergman, 2004b, p. 17)*

It is through the ownership of agency that Santalis, an indigenous community in Eastern India who have been oppressed historically and continue to be oppressed by the structures of capitalism, co-construct entry points for structural transformation. Agency is constituted in articulations of processes of change amidst a highly engaged sense of political consciousness amidst subaltern communities about the processes of marginalization and exploitation constituted in the dominant structures of development.

Disparities, Inequities, and Co-optation

Increasingly, global, national, and local structures across the various spaces and sectors of the globe have started emphasizing the goal of these structures in minimizing and/or erasing disparities in health; the agendas here are framed in the realm of reducing disparities based on indicators of health within and across communities around the globe (see Kreps, 2005). However, interrogating the symbolic and material constructions within these spaces draws attention to the conceptual gaps between the representations that circulate within the neoliberal hegemonic configurations of health and the inherent agendas that are constituted by these structures. What are the agendas served by funding agencies when they position themselves as working with inequalities? Whose agendas do they serve through these projects? How have they been able to address the inequalities?

Critical interrogations for instance of the five-a-day campaign carried out and supported by the US-based National Cancer Institute and the Centers for Disease Control and Prevention (CDC) under the framework of addressing health disparities raise questions about the effectiveness of messages of fruit and vegetable promotion in addressing the material inequalities in health, and in addressing the structural disparities that exist within the United States in the realm of inaccess to the basic capacities of health (Dutta, 2008c)? Similarly, critical interrogations of projects promoting certain forms of cancer screening among Hispanic communities in the United States raise questions about the effectiveness of these interventions in actually addressing the disparities faced by Hispanic populations, and in materially impacting the structurally situated inequalities in access and quality of health. The culture-centered approach raises the fundamental question about the indicators and measures that ought to be utilized in projects claiming to work on disparities, noting the absence of material indicators and measurements in the planning and evaluation of projects that position themselves as addressing a materially and structurally situated issue (Dutta, 2008c; Dutta-Bergman, 2005b).

The rhetoric of inequality and disparity, in such instances, tends to become co-opted into the status quo instead of exploring the spaces of change in those very structures that underline these inequalities. In other words, the language of disparity and inequity often operates to play out the status quo agendas of dominant social actors rather than interrogating the unequal political structures and the injustices built into the unequal distribution of economic and political resources. To the extent that these projects of healthcare disparity are situated within the broader agendas of the neoliberal project, the emphasis on disparity remains in the realm of addressing individual lifestyles (beliefs, attitudes, and behaviors) rather than on addressing the issues of underlying structures that constitute these very disparities.

Conclusion

In this chapter, we examined the ways in which the margins of healthcare are constituted, drawing attentions to the interplay among culture, structure, and agency in the production and reproduction of the margins. The individua-level emphasis on health perpetuated by the neoliberal logic has framed health as a commodity to be purchased through the free market. This commoditization of health has led to the minimization of basic healthcare services, and in addition, has fostered large-scale health inequalities. In spite of the mounting evidence of the moderate effect of individual-level health interventions, global healthcare policies continue to promote the logic of healthcare campaigns and interventions promoting individual behavior change, and simultaneously ignore the structural issues and issues of redistributive justice that need to be addressed across the globe. The culture-centered approach on one hand critically interrogates the rhetoric of individual-level interventions and policies, and on the other hand, emphasizes the creation of discourse entry points for listening to subaltern communities, and for engaging with subaltern voices to seek structural transformations.

5

GENDERED MARGINALIZATION

Historically, gender has remained a key site of oppression locally, nationally, and globally. What are the ways in which global social and economic systems have reproduced gendered experiences? How have women been constituted in the economic logics of global hegemony, and how have these constructions shaped the materiality of women's lived experiences and women's labor? What are the principles of gendered organizing within which discourses of work have circulated and created the normative expectations around the economic value attached to certain types of work, the devaluation of other types of work, and the corresponding economic and social marginalization of women? What are the structures of governance within which women's lived experiences have been constituted in contemporary global geopolitics, and how have women been erased from these structures of governance?

In this chapter, we explore the interactions among culture and structure that underlie the gendered experiences of women globally, and specifically in the global South. The chapter sets out to understand the experiences of poor women in the South who have historically experienced large proportions of the inequalities against the backdrop of globalization processes. Of interest here are the economic indicators of marginalization, and the experiences amidst poverty that women negotiate as they find themselves in the midst of marginalizing structures of oppression that are both locally and globally constituted. The material exploitation and marginalization of women in the global South are situated amidst the interplays among global policies, agendas of TNCs, national politics, and local processes that are circulated, established, and reproduced through communicative processes that are materially situated amidst dominant global platforms.

What are the symbolic and material processes in globalization politics through which women's experiences have been constructed and constrained? Structural inequities in the global distribution of material resources are played out through the local contexts of culture and patriarchy that define the immediate framework constituting the lived experiences of women (Mies, 1982, 1986; Mohanty, 2006). The larger political and economic ideologies of global capitalism interact with the local specificities of gendered norms and ideologies to constitute the everyday struggles of women. This chapter attends to the specificities of these local margins that are created, enforced, and circulated through the processes of globalization under neoliberalism (see Figure 5.1).

The exploration of communicative processes and strategies in dominant social configurations provides a lens for understanding how women are marginalized in social systems, particularly within the framework of contemporary economic and political configurations that define the realms of labor in which they participate, the value attached to this labor, and the economic markers attached to women's labor. The geopolitical landscape surrounding the exchange of women's labor in the global marketplace is situated alongside the modernist policies of development that have increasingly displaced women from their traditional modes of economic participation and from the sources of food that they have historically produced in local communities across the globe. We examine the experiences of women at the margins of development projects, and the ways in which modernist development has served the interests of the dominant patriarchal structures, simultaneously erasing women from their traditional spaces of production and economic participation.

Furthermore, emphasis is placed in this chapter on understanding the processes of knowledge production through which women are turned into the subjects of

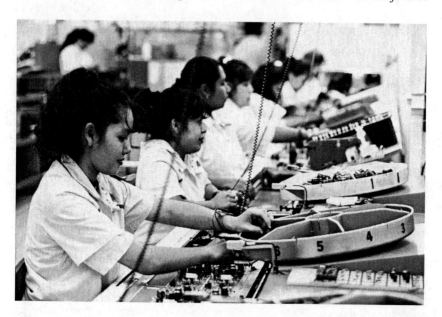

FIGURE 5.1 Women workers at a television assembly line. (Mark Segal/Getty Images)

policy-making and intervention development in spheres of modernization and neoliberalism. Knowledge is understood as a political entity that generates the realms of praxis by defining policies and programs that are carried out by key global actors. It is ultimately through their subject positions as objects of knowledge that women enter into the dominant discursive spaces of knowledge production as bodies to be worked over even as their traditional modes of knowledge get stolen by transnational capitalist structures for the purposes of profiteering.

The chapter delves into those processes through which women are turned into objects of interrogation and the ways in which women's voices are silenced in the various platforms of policy-making, political processes, and economic institutions in contemporary global structures. As noted in the culture-centered approach (Dutta, 2007, 2008c, 2009), the material marginalization of women works hand in hand with the silencing of women from the dominant platforms of knowledge production globally, nationally, and locally. Women continue to be erased from mainstream discursive spaces, as their bodies become the sites of interventions that seek to modify their behaviors, shift their perceptions, and emancipate them in the process of carrying out the enlightenment agendas of modernist development. It is against the backdrop of these silences that women's voices and narratives are presented through meta-synthesis of in-depth interviews and ethnographic projects that have engaged with a gendered lens in interrogating the marginalization of women across the globe. The voices narrate the experiences of structural violence and erasure written into the mainstream public spheres of contemporary policies at local, national, and global levels.

Complementing the emphasis of communication scholarship on gender within localized contexts and spaces, this chapter explores the gendered sites of oppression in contemporary global spaces, articulating the linkages between structure and culture in their constraining and enabling capacities globally. How is the politics of the local shaped by global geopolitics, and what are the entry points for the local specificities in the global landscape? We examine the ways in which the margins of gender are written into the logics of mainstream frameworks of political and economic organizing under neoliberalism. Attention will be paid to the interplay of the material and the symbolic in the perpetuation of the neoliberal framework that oppresses women as sources of knowledge production, labor, economic production, and profiteering.

Gender at the Margins

What are the processes through which gender is situated at the margins of current economic configurations? What constitutes the experiences of women at the margins and how are these margins created by patriarchal structures based on Western ideologies? What are the possibilities of listening to the voices of poor women from the global South amidst structures of knowledge production that are patriarchal in their configuration? What functions does communication play in the creation and reiteration of the margins of contemporary global economies? What are the positions of articulation in global economies and how are these positions situated within the politics and governance structures of neoliberalism?

Although an impressive body of organizational communication scholarship has emerged around the question of gendered work, one of the important criticisms of this line of scholarship focuses on its emphasis on white-collar jobs situated within mainstream organizations, emphasizing the middle class, bourgeoisie spheres of neoliberal organizing, and feeding into the capitalist forces of neo-liberalism that marginalize women across the globe. In other words, the feminist articulations made in this line of work fail to criticize the fundamentally patriarchal nature of neoliberal structures and organizations, and do not attend to the profound forms of material and social marginalization experienced by poor women in the global South that are direct outcomes of patriarchal neoliberal policies. The fundamentally patriarchal nature of neoliberalism that is based on the values of competition, private property, profit, greed, and economic efficiency remains unchallenged as these values get projected as the universal standards for guiding human behavior (Dirlik, 1997; Mohanty, 2006; Shiva, 1989).

This line of scholarship does not question the very nature of gendered organizing underlying the neoliberal policies that produce and recreate global organizations and the margins perpetuated by these organizations. The patriarchal structures of transnational capitalism remain unchallenged as the focus is predominantly placed on the everyday practices of resistance constituted within these structures of capitalism and taking for granted the logics underlying these structures of capitalism. To the extent that contemporary interrogations of gendered workspaces do not attend to the oppressive characteristics of these workspaces within the neoliberal framework and the various rationalities that are erased by the dominant rationalities of capitalism, they fall short of engaging with the deep-seated global structural inequities that are gendered in their existence and violent in their erasures (Shiva, 1989).

Also, the thrust of this traditional domain of scholarship foregrounds the fragmented sites of power and the discursive enactments of power and control within organizational contexts, without really attending to the material bases and material inequities that underlie the unequal distributions of power and resources globally. The notion of fragmented sites of power, although valuable, also stands in opposition to the reality of the material inequities and the effects of these inequities experienced by women in the global South. Approaches that only focus on discursive elements of gendered organizing do not attend to the forces of neoliberal hegemony that seek to take control of the subaltern sectors across the globe by occupying subaltern lands, stealing subaltern knowledge bases, forcing subaltern populations as cheap sources of labor for TNCs, and turning subaltern spaces into markets for the products and services of the TNCs. What is particularly worth noting here is the devaluing, erasure, and theft of knowledge bases that are specifically owned by subaltern women in the global South in order to serve the patriarchal interests and value structures of transnational hegemony.

The focus on primarily the symbolic and the discursive navigates away from questioning the economic bases of the material inequities that are perpetuated by neoliberalism, and the patriarchal nature of transnational hegemony that marginalizes women in the global South. In doing so, the study of the discursive negotiations of gendered oppressions at workplaces ends up serving the status quo, without paying attention to the realm of the material that constitutes the major fault lines of neoliberal oppression. When most of the workers on the other side of the global division of labor are women working in many of the transnational spaces of TNC subsidiaries as cheap sources of labor, earning low wages for the work they participate in and produce, the emphasis on the symbolic as the site of oppression and resistance disappointingly draws attention away from the material bases of collective organizing that are necessary to structurally transform the neoliberal configurations of the globe. Also, the framing of the gendered oppressions as symbolic ignores the essence of material marginalization experienced by the poorest of the poor, a majority of whom are women. The emphasis of this chapter therefore is on understanding the ways in which gendered sites of marginalization are perpetuated through neoliberalism, attending to the material margins of contemporary economic formulations.

The material margins of globalization are intrinsically intertwined with the discursive margins (Mohanty, 2006). Therefore, in order to understand the processes of marginalization of women, communication theorists and activists studying social change ought to engage with the intersections of structures and communicative processes in the perpetuation of the economic marginalization of women. Communicative processes and sites are situated in material structures at the heart of neoliberalism, and the erasure of Third World women from these structures is quintessential to the perpetuation of global inequities through the neoliberal project. This erasure is achieved through the devaluing of Third World women, and through the depiction of their rationalities as primitive and irrational (Shiva, 2001). This depiction of Third World woman as primitive lies at the core of the erasure of Third World women from the dominant discursive spaces where policies are created, interventions are planned, and evaluations are reported. Therefore, an entire knowledge industry of Western patriarchal capitalism exists to manufacture images of the Third World as backward and in need of development. The portrayal and reproduction of this need is essential to the projects of transnational capitalism that are justified as interventions designed to bring the primitive Third World into the folds of civilization as epitomized in neoliberal governance. The marginalization of women in the Third World then is accomplished through their removal from dominant discursive spaces, which serves as the justification for the perpetuation of epistemic and structural violence in the name of development and modernization.

Gender and Development

Historically, women have been configured into the global mainstream as targets of development interventions, framed within the rubric of development, and missing from the spaces of development policy-making, planning, and evaluation. Therefore, whereas on one hand, women were missing from the development processes and configurations in early projects of development, on the other hand, women subsequently were configured into development as targets of interventions. As gender specific analyses emerged into the development discourse, thus moving toward addressing issues of gender inequities in development, it did so by continually erasing the voices and participatory capacities of Third World women.

Women as Targets of Population Control

Women from the Third World have emerged on the landscape of global development campaigns as the markers of the field of interventions, defining the political economy of interventions targeting the Third World, and serving as the targets of campaigns messages. The basic principle underlying the targeting of women is founded on the economic viability attributed to women as participants in the labor forces of the economy, and as the producers of children who would participate in the economy as sources of labor. Therefore, the body of the woman becomes the site of development interventions, and her reproductive capability is framed as a problem in order to justify the intervention. She is discursively constructed as oppressed, passive, and lacking in agency, and it is her emancipation that becomes the basis for the justification of the interventions carried out by the North/West in the global South. This framing is done by powerful actors often situated in the West/North, often removed from the reality of the lived experiences of the women, and situated amidst decontextualized theorizations based on assumptions of universality (see for example Speidel, Sinding, Gillespie, Maguire, & Neuse, 2009).

The problem of population growth in the Third World sectors of the globe is framed in the context of the problems of limited global resources. Population growth is framed as threatening global health and environment by putting pressure on existing limited resources. Discursive deconstructions of the intervention messages and the public policies underlying them demonstrate the focus on the individual Third World women as the locus of the problem, and the simultaneous absence of discussions of structural inequities and issues of redistributive justice underlying the problems of resources inaccess across the globe. Absent from the discourse are discussions of the realities of resource consumption, for the largest proportion of global resources are consumed by the existing resource-rich sectors in the global West/North, whereas the large majority of the world's population struggle with highly limited resources.

The education of the woman offers the altruistic framework within which development is framed as a solution. In problematizing women, efforts of development turn women into nameless, faceless masses of homogeneous bodies to be enlightened. The aggregation of women from the Third World into a monolith is carried out through their portrayal as passive, uneducated, illiterate, and disempowered subjects of interventions. The development industry then exists to empower and educate these women from the global South, who need to be saved through the mantras of development and modernization. In other words, essential to the justification of the development industry and to the allocation of resources to development projects is the communicative erasure of Third World women from the discursive spaces of development. Particularly worth noting here is the systematic absence of women from the subaltern sectors in the global South from policy and intervention platforms that determine the objectives, processes, and strategies of the development programs to be carried out in the South.

Critical interrogations of the rhetoric of development draw attention to the ways in which the altruistic claims of development serve as the cover for political and economic interests of the national elite, campaign planners, and international funding agencies that fund these campaigns. Disrupting the claims of altruism also disrupts the logic of development and the ways in which women emerge as monoliths within this logic to serve the interests of transnational actors. For example, critical deconstruction of the rhetoric of the United States Agency for International Development emphasizes the deployment of population control in promoting US geostrategic and economic interests. The power configurations embedded within these networks of interventions (including funding agencies, program planners, national governments, and elite local organizations) perpetuate the control of the dominant patriarchal configurations that carry out their interventions on women, precisely on the basis of the logic of "doing good" and serving poor women, while actually serving the interests of the status quo both politically and economically (Dutta, 2006). For instance, in depicting the role of population control in serving the political economic interests of the United States, Madeleine Albright articulated the following:

> international family planning also serves important US foreign policy interests; elevating the status of women, reducing the flow of refugees, protecting the global environment, and promoting sustainable development which leads to economic growth and trade opportunities for businesses.
> (Albright, as quoted in USAID, 1998, p. 33)

In this excerpt, population control internationally is seen as a mechanism for promoting sustainable growth, which in turn is seen as a mechanism for promoting trade opportunities for businesses. What becomes explicit here is the linkage between the framing of population control as a problem and the interests of transnational capitalism. Opportunities are created for trading through the creation of economic development, brought about by population control (see also Speidel et al., 2009).

With respect to the problematization of population growth, the framing of population growth as a threat to security exists in the realm of protecting the interests of the status quo under the name of development. Population growth is perceived as disruptive of the status quo and as a challenge to the dominant social actors at the center of patriarchal neoliberalism who consume the predominant proportion of the earth's resources, simultaneously depriving women in the global South from vital resources.

Women and Agriculture

In the economies of the global South, women constitute large proportions of the agricultural sector, participating in the production of food resources and being responsible for putting food on the table (Shiva, 1989). The modernization frameworks of development have consolidated power in the hands of large farms that are traditionally operated by men, and weakening the smaller farms in the wake of the Green Revolution. As an increasing number of government policies worked with the IFIs and international aid to industrialize agriculture, more and more women participating in the agricultural sector were marginalized (Shiva, 1989; Shiva & Bedi, 2002).

With the advent of the structural adjustment programs imposed by the global configurations of neoliberal governance (more on this later), farmers in local economies were pushed by the government to shift to growing cash crops, moving away from their multicrop food-based agricultural production that was directed toward addressing food security at the community level. The seed monocultures promoted by government programs pushed farmers toward buying genetically modified seeds from transnational seed manufacturers, accompanied by the purchasing of fertilizers, pesticides, and water in order to feed the seeds. The agricultural sector transformed from being a self-sustaining, ecologically sound, harmonious system of food production to an industrialized sector dependent on commercial inputs and dependent on the market economy in order to generate revenues to food local communities. The marginalization of women in the agricultural sector happened through the marginalization of their roles as producers of food and through the threats to food security that gradually emerged as the everyday reality of women in agricultural communities. The identities and roles of women as mothers and as providers of food have been violently threatened through the structural adjustment programs.

Furthermore, in subaltern contexts across the globe, women have lived on the basis of locally situated feminine principles of harmony and balance. For example, Shiva (1989) draws attention to the feminine principle of sustaining and nurturing nature. The large-scale industrialization of agriculture has violated these feminine principles of balance and harmony through the penetration of Eurocentric patriarchy of the market principle, embodied in the agendas of transnational agricultural giants such as Monsanto, operating on the principles of conquering and controlling nature to maximize outputs and efficiency.

Women as Labor

Large proportions of workers at the bottom of the global economy are women, serving as laborers to TNCs (Hossfeld, 1990; Katz & Kemnitzer, 1984; Mies, 1982; Mohanty, 2006). The global penetration of neoliberalism through the several SAPs has adversely affected the agricultural sector, forcing women from the rural sectors of poverty-stricken economies to migrate to the global centers of exploitation. The devaluing of women and the devaluing of women's work in transnational capitalism are intertwined with the ways in which economic value is attached to the work done by women, the money that women earn in exchange for the work they do for TNCs, the treatment of women at their workplaces, and the various forms of risks they are exposed to at their sites of work (Mohanty, 2006).

The exploitation of poor Third World women in the global economy is situated at the intersections of the politics of race, class, nationality, and gender that is embodied in the practices and profit-making goals of TNCs, positioned amidst neoliberal global and national policies that facilitate opportunities for the exploitation of workers and for the maximization of profits. These forms of exploitation take place at various sites of global geopolitics including sweatshops, call centers, manufacturing units in specially designated export processing zones, assembly lines that hire immigrant women, agencies that place domestic workers, spaces of global sex trade, and homes that hire domestic help and nannies (Millen & Holtz, 2000). On one hand, sites of global exploitation are locally situated amidst the neoliberal politics of local economies; on the other hand, transnational migrations in the face of neoliberal politics have placed women from local economies across the globe at the global sites of exploitation.

As SAPs under neoliberalism have been adopted full-fledged by global economies, special economic zones (SEZs) and economic processing zones (EPZs) have been created for attracting foreign capital (Brenner, Ross, Simmons, & Zaidi, 2000; Millen & Holtz, 2000). The economic, environmental, and labor policies in these SEZs work in ways that attract global capital, and create economic opportunities for the extraction, processing, and manufacturing units of TNCs, mostly employing women from the Third World. The increasing trade liberalization has created poor working conditions for workers in the processing plants and manufacturing units of TNCs, criminalized trade unions, and has fostered low wages of workers in the EPZs.

On the US-Mexican border for instance, processing plants called *maquiladoras* have been set up by primarily US TNCs, operating under poor environmental conditions and causing serious economic costs to the environment and to the health of the workers being exposed to the toxic chemicals. In addition, the poor implementation of labor laws has subjected the *maquiladora* workers to low wages, workplace harassment, occupational health hazards, job insecurity, and the inability to organize in unions. Specifically in the case of Mexico, in spite of the rhetoric of the North American Agreement on Environmental Cooperation (NAAEC) and the North American Agreement on Labor Cooperation (NAALC) along with NAFTA, the implementation of the environmental and labor laws is weak, and the *maquiladoras* consistently violate these laws. Furthermore, the procedures set up under NAALC require that the complaint be filed in one of the two other NAFTA countries, therefore requiring substantive resources and familiarity with procedures in order to file a grievance. In one such instance of a submission under NAALC's grievance procedure against the Mexican government regarding its inability to enforce labor law on union registration in the case of Magneticos de Mexico, a subsidiary of Sony Corporation in Nuevo Laredo, Mexico, where employees organizing to form an independent union were beaten up and fired, an incessant number of consultations between the US and Mexican governments, international seminars on union registration, and meetings among the Ministry and workers, union representatives, and managers of the TNC subsidiary have failed to rehire or compensate the employees or allow them to organize into an independent union (Brenner et al., 2000).

Women and Displacement

Women make up large sections of the indigenous and rural populations living in the global South that are most strongly affected by the structural adjustment programs (SAPs) and neoliberal policies of development (Kabeer, 1994). With the increasing presence of development projects in the Third World that connect spaces of subalternity to the centers of profit, women have emerged as the "new subalterns" referred to by Gayatri Spivak (1999) in her work on silences in subalternity. These new subalterns are sources of knowledge of biological resources that may now be patented by TNCs in order to generate profit; furthermore, the spaces they occupy are seen as resources of minerals and raw materials that must be exploited by TNCs to generate profits. The displacements of women from the geographic spaces, from economic resources of production, and from locales of knowledge production are intrinsic to the political economy of neoliberalism.

Therefore, on one hand, women are disconnected from the natural and biological resources they have historically utilized as these resources are turned into patentable commodities owned and sold by TNCs; on the other hand, they are displaced from their geographic spaces and homes so that these spaces can be turned into mines, manufacturing units, or sites of other development projects intended to benefit the dominant classes locally, nationally, and globally, situated within the West-centric patriarchal structures of neoliberalism. The global displacement of poor women creates a wide variety of structural vulnerabilities, including the vulnerabilities of exposure to HIV/AIDS, marking the disease as a disease of inequalities (Dutta, 2008c; Farmer, 2003).

Culture-Centered Approach to Gendered Marginalization

The subaltern studies project informs the foundations of the culture-centered approach, with an emphasis on interrogating the dominant structures for the absences and erasures in these structures. The state of being subaltern is reflective of being hidden, under, erased, or absent from the spaces of legitimacy within mainstream frameworks of knowledge production where policies are produced, discussed, implemented, evaluated, and reproduced. Missing from the discourses of development are voices of local women from the Third World who remain scripted within development interventions as data points to be entered into pre and post evaluations measuring the effectiveness and efficiency of the intervention.

The category of the "Third World woman" emerges in mainstream discourse as a category to be worked on as a target of interventions, as a justification for the deployment of the structural adjustment programs, as a data source to be measured through needs assessment programs in order to justify development interventions. The rationale underlying the political economy of neoliberal hegemony operates on the basis of the erasure of the voices of the poorest women from the global South, situating them in subalternity. Therefore, a culture-centered reading of gendered marginalization begins with the deconstruction of the predominant cultural tropes in mainstream structures that subsume the agency of subaltern women.

Structures of Gendered Oppression

In contemporary global frameworks, women's lives are constituted at the intersections of the local and the global, played out in the relationships between patriarchies that are situated locally and the Western patriarchal foundations of the market economics of transnational capitalism. Locally situated patriarchal ideologies take up new meanings through the patriarchal forces of transnational hegemony, ultimately serving the political economy of transnational hegemony. The structures that determine the scope and nature of participation of women are constituted within the agendas of neoliberal hegemony. Therefore, the emphasis of these structures is on constituting women as labor in transnational hegemony and as participants in the patriarchal principles of the market (Mohanty, 2006).

Gendered oppression is fundamentally carried out through the global dissemination of the market as the governing rationality for securing access to resources, forcing women to participate in the market so that they can have access to the basic life-sustaining and life-giving resources of food, shelter, and water, and so that they can support their families. Increasing numbers of women travel from their home countries in Thailand, Philippines, Sri Lanka, Nepal, and Malaysia in search of jobs, working as domestic workers and as nannies at global sites of oppression that have fundamentally created and sustained the inequities in the global South. The forces that push women into the global markets also render them vulnerable to various forms of exploitations as evident in the migrations of women from the global South to the centers of development as domestic workers and as sex workers. These movements and migratory patterns also place women as commodities in the markets of global sex trade, turning desire into a commodity in the free market, and operating on the bodies of women through the marketing of desire as evident in the global sex tourism and sex trade industries. Culture-centered interrogations question the erasures of women's voices and rationalities accomplished through the articulations of specific rationalities within dominant structures, thus creating rallying points for global-local mobilizations and for the politics of change.

The Myths of Development

Culture-centered interrogations question the taken-for-granted assumptions underlying the rhetoric of emancipation and progress embodied in the language of development under neoliberalism. It asks questions such as: Whose development? Development for serving what purposes? Who defines development? and Who benefits from development? The agendas of finding new sources of knowledge that can then be patented accompanied by the quest for new markets for TNCs are carried out through the removal of women from the global South from the spaces of development policy-making. Noting the discursive erasures carried out by mainstream platforms of development, Afshar (1944) observes that the process of development in the Third World has historically marginalized women by not even taking them in account the discourses of development. Women have been largely missing from development planning and implementation processes, as well as from the projects of development that have been targeted toward the Third World. When they are present in development discourse, women have been constituted as passive subjects, as target audiences of interventions directed at bringing about progress in the backward communities of the rural South through the education of the woman in her reproductive capacity, who is seen as the receptacle for the (re)production and nurturing of the healthy child.

Although women continue to constitute the majority of the target audience that are framed as recipients of the messages of development sent out by the capitalist centers of the globe, their voices remain missing from the discursive spaces of development policy-making where problem configurations and corresponding solutions are discussed. Even as approaches such as the Women in Development (WID) approach have emphasized the inclusion of women in the discursive spaces of development policy-making, worth noting here is the absence of the poorest women of the global South from the global spaces of development policy-making, and the co-optation of dialogic spaces of development within the neoliberal market rhetoric.

For example, the roundtable titled "Women Reclaim the Market" sponsored by Women's Global Alliance for Development Alternatives, which is a joint project of Development Alternatives with Women for a New Era (DAWN), WID, National Action Committee on the Status of Women (NAC), Canadian Research Institute for the Advancement of Women (CRIAW), and other organizations, articulated its visions of development within the neoliberal framework of the market although it set out to question the social dimensions of globalization (Runyan, 1999). Resistive strategies articulated toward the goals of social change and transformative politics are often constituted within the goals of the status quo. Neoliberal governance operates on the bodies of women through programs of development, often utilizing the language of development and empowerment to bring women under the purview and monitoring mechanisms of transnational corporations, IFIs, and nation states. Programs such as micro credit programs that position themselves under the framework of women-centered development serve as tools of control by placing women as individual agents responsible for their access to resources in the market economy, dependent upon their performance in the economy as producers. In the face of the unchanged gender relations within the dynamics of families, the responsibilities that women have to undertake further increase, adding to the burdens of women.

Neoliberalization and Gender

In the neoliberal configuration, women emerge as markers of the facade of the emancipatory politics of transnational expansion (Runyan, 1999; Spivak, 1996). It is on the symbol of the "woman" from the Third World that neoliberal politics plays out by framing neoliberal governance as favorable to the development of Third World women (Sharma, 2008). The economic agendas of TNCs are served through discourses and programs of woman-centered development, carried out under the premise of creating economic opportunities for women and promoting empowerment through self-help and entrepreneurial programs (Sharma, 2008). Development offers the rationale for economic and political penetrations of IFIs and TNCs through SAPs. IFIs create the openings for TNCs through their SAPs, many of which are imposed on Third World sites as rationales for development directed toward women. Neoliberal forms of women's empowerment are carried out through the promotion of the market; the empowerment of women is framed within the context of their capacity to participate in the market and to fulfill their needs through the market (Sharma, 2008).

Discourses of participation, democracy, empowerment, and dialogue are introduced into the discursive space precisely for the purposes of bringing subaltern women from the global South under the governance of neoliberalism (Runyan, 1999). The power of neoliberalism is exerted through its capacity to organize the symbolic representations of dialogue and emancipation to serve the capitalist logics of the free market. The market becomes synonymous with development, a marker of capitalist emancipation and freedom. The assumption that circulates in the neoliberal discourse is that women's freedom is achieved through the freedom of the market. The privatization of global resources, the minimization of state interventions, and the elimination of public spending on women's welfare are framed within the capitalist logic of the "free market" economy, tied to the notion that freeing the market would open up new emancipatory possibilities for women. As Runyan (1999) so eloquently notes, the principles of the free market are constructed as the tools to the emancipation of women.

Contrary to these emancipatory claims of the free market, though, worth noting in the neoliberal framework is the minimization of the opportunities for women's participation through the very calls to dialogue and participation that are issued in the mainstream (Dutta, 2007, 2008a, 2008b, 2008c, 2009; Dutta & Pal, 2010). Participation here is positioned as a strategic tool for scripting women as sources of knowledge, as data points to needs assessments done for the purposes of promoting neoliberal interventions, as labor to the transnational economy, and as markets for the goods and services produced by TNCs (see Dutta & Basnyat, 2008a, 2008b, 2008c). Dialogic platforms and spaces of participation are scripted within the neoliberal project as tools for diffusing the interventions planned out by program planners on the basis of neoliberal concepts of development (Dutta & Basnyat, 2010).

Critiquing the co-optive nature of dialogic forums at transnational sites such as the Fourth World Conference on Women held in Beijing, Spivak (1996) notes:

> The financialization of the globe must be represented as the North embracing the South. Women are being used for the representation of this unity—another name for the profound transnational disunity necessary for globalization. These conferences are global theatre . . . we are interested in *this* global theatre, staged to show participation between the North and the South, the latter constituted by Northern discursive mechanisms—a Platform of Action and certain power lines between the UN, the donor consortium, governments and the elite Non-Governmental Organisations (NGOs). In fact, the North organizes a South. People going to these conferences may be struck by the global radical aura. But if you hang out at the other end, participating day-to-day in the (largely imposed) politics of how delegations and NGO groups are put together—in Bangladesh, Sri Lanka or Central Asia, say, to name only the places this writer knows—you would attest that what is left out is the poorest women of the South as self-conscious critical agents, who might be able to speak through those very nongovernmental organizations of the South that are not favoured by these object-constitution policies.
>
> *(Spivak, 1996, p. 2)*

Although the language of empowerment provides the appearance of democratic inclusivity, the criteria for inclusion and participation of local voices are predicated through top-down policies of the governing structures that issue the calls for dialogue. The mechanics, processes, and content of dialogue within dialogic forums such as the UN are framed within the broader goals and strategies of neoliberalism. Worth noting here is the fundamental strategy of erasure of subaltern voices in order to justify the role of neoliberal dialogue as an intervention that is imposed on the global South. In forming the subaltern woman as the object of transnational policies, she is turned into a passive recipient, and is left out of the discursive spaces of representative politics and dialogue in the mainstream that are paraded as sites of emancipatory politics. Discussions in UN-based platforms of women's rights and issues of equality are framed within the logics of the market, foregrounding the role of the market as a panacea to women's underdevelopment in the global South.

The object-constitution politics of neoliberal hegemony operates on the basis of its privileging of the logics of privatization and minimum state involvement in the delivery of social welfare (Runyan, 1999). Therefore, as social welfare is depleted, the additional burden of work shifts onto women. Furthermore, as noted above, as traditional sectors such as agriculture become victims of transnational monopolies, women farmers find themselves at the margins, unable to provide food for their families. As heads of households and as providers of food within local contexts, women often bear the burden of economic marginalization in the subaltern sectors. Furthermore, as Runyan (1999) suggests, those civil society organizations are given access to the dominant spaces of policy-making that embody a market-oriented logic, and thus serve as strategic partners in the global diffusion of the "free market" logic. Civil society emerges as an ally of neoliberal hegemony, serving the interests of TNCs on the global arena, and co-opting the spaces of participation of subaltern women.

The political economy of neoliberalism is perpetuated globally through the power and control held by institutions such as the World Bank in the production of gendered knowledge about economics, progress, and development (Griffin, 2009; Peet, 2003). Griffin (2003) notes that World Bank discourse and policy-making operate on the basis of certain gendered dichotomies, with specific interpretations about the role of women in economies, which situate women across the globe as subjects of economic interventions that control the social and economic meanings of the work they participate in, and produce. It is on the basis of these dichotomies that the World Bank carries out the economic marginalization of women, reproducing certain gendered configurations within which women become the sites of oppression, framed within the realms of emancipatory politics of neoliberal institutions. As evident throughout this chapter, missing from the rhetoric of neoliberal governance are the stories of exploitations of women in sweat shops, oppressions in the SEZs, exploitations of women as migrant domestic workers in the neoliberal economy, trafficking of women, displacements of women under neoliberal policies, theft of women's knowledge bases, displacements of women from the agricultural sector, threats to women's health under privatization and deregulation, and the commoditization of women's love in new forms of neo-imperial transactions under neoliberal restructuring of global economies.

The rhetoric of free market that dominates the World Bank discourse operates on the basis of patriarchal assumptions about the nature of economic productivity and efficiency, while simultaneously continuing to perpetuate the marginalization of women's work. The goal of neoliberal governmentality is to create educational and training opportunities for women to enter into the productive workforce as sources of labor, and therefore, connected to the markets of neoliberalism. Therefore, the development and underdevelopment of women is measured in terms of their connection to neoliberal markets, and efforts of empowerment focus on creating spaces of participation for women in the neoliberal economy. What is absent from these assumptions in neoliberalism is the gendered nature of economic productivity under neoliberalism, and the taken-for-granted nature of the gendered exploitations that are carried out by capitalist structures operating at the intersections of patriarchy, transnational policies, and state participation.

Voices of Women

Because the achievement of neoliberal hegemony is strategically accomplished through the systematic erasure of women's ways of knowing from the dominant discursive spaces, the culture-centered approach offers the theoretical argument that the disruption of these global structures of domination is fundamentally achieved through the presence of the voices of women from the subaltern sectors of the globe in these dominant discursive spaces (Dutta, 2008c). The articulation of alternative rationalities in subaltern spaces ruptures the hegemonic narratives of the dominant structures, drawing attention to women's ways of knowing, economic organizing, sustenance, and living (Rose, 2001; Shiva, 1989).

Shiva's (1989) narrativization of the Chipko movement in the Garhwal Himalayan region of India offers one such alternate rationality by foregrounding the voices of women leaders and women activists who resisted government-supported deforestation projects on the basis of the feminine ecological principles of nurturing, sharing, conservation, producing and maintaining life, and living in harmony with nature. Here is the articulation of Sarala Behn, one of the key organizational leaders of the movement:

> From my childhood experience I have known that law is not just; that the principles that govern humanity are higher than those that govern the state; that a centralized government, indifferent to its peoples, is a cruel joke in governance; that the split between the private and public ethic is the source of misery, injustice and exploitation in society. Each child in India understands that bread (roti) is not just a right to the one who has money in his pocket. It is a more fundamental right of the one whose stomach is hungry. This concept of rights works within the family, but is

shed at the societal level. Then the ethic of the market reigns, and men get trapped in it.

(as cited in Shiva, 1989, pp. 71–72)

Worth noting here is the departure between the feminine principle of caring and nurturing, and the masculinist principle of market economics based on the ideas of competition and private property ownership. The demarcation of the private and the public carried out in patriarchal market economies is fundamental to the exploitation and deprivation of the poorer classes, as concepts of competition and economic growth drive social relationships and economic logics. The voices of the women of Chipko articulated against this backdrop share a different set of principles for organizing society and for conceptualizing the relationships of human beings with nature. The feminine principle, referred to as *Prakriti* in Sanskrit, is based on the core concept that nature is symbolized as the embodiment of the feminine, and is inherently an active, powerful force that lies at the essence of the dialectical struggles in the creation and maintenance of all life.

Similar articulations of alternative rationalities are heard in the voices of sex workers from Sonagachi, the largest red light area in Kolkata, who have come together in the form of the Durbar Mahila Swamanyaya Committee to organize against local, national, and global structures, and to create spaces of change both within the community as well as in the relationship of the community with outside stakeholders (Basu & Dutta, 2009). For example, as quoted earlier on p. 140, Gitadi notes: "We know what is best for us. We go around our community talking to people. They tell us what they need. Here we are in charge of things. We take care of the project that we run here" (as quoted in Basu & Dutta, 2009, p. 95). The rationality expressed here is precisely set in opposition to the dominant logic of passivity that establishes the sex workers as fixed categories to be targeted for social change campaigns run by experts situated in the West and North. Gitadi's voice in this narrative reclaims the ownership of the discursive space, and foregrounds the logic of the local voice as the impetus for the social change initiative. The alternative rationality shared here lies at the heart of a resistive articulation of social change processes that situates social change at the level of the local as opposed to the expert-based location of social change initiatives at an expert location elsewhere. The knowledge claim made by Gitadi privileges the community's knowledge of the local problems and corresponding solutions. It celebrates the local community's ownership of the change projects and the capacity of the local community to plan and implement the projects.

Listening to women's voices at the local level interrogates the stories of helplessness, low self-efficacy, and backwardness of Third World women that have historically been portrayed in dominant discourses in mainstream social change initiatives. Methodologically, the emphasis of the culture-centered approach on creating spaces and entry points for listening to subaltern voices challenges the erasure of subalterns in the mainstream by fundamentally noting the agency of subaltern communities to organize, to actively engage in problem definitions, and to come up with solutions that are responsive to the needs of the community. Here is another articulation by Lakshmi:

> We realized that to get sex workers to use condoms, go for regular check ups, the first thing we needed to do was determine the root of our problems and figure out ways we can address them. You have to live here to really know what's going on. You can't just come in, ask questions, and tell us what to do.
>
> *(Basu & Dutta, 2009, p. 95)*

Similar to what Gitadi had to say, Lakshmi notes the capacity of the community to determine its own problems. Discounting what experts are traditionally able to achieve through their minimal visits and sporadic contacts with the community, she emphasizes that one has to live in the community to really know what is going on. In this narrative, Lakshmi challenges the ontology and epistemology of social change campaigns by pointing out the limited capacity of experts in figuring out solutions because of their status as outsiders to the community. In challenging the ability of expert solutions that are imposed from outside to solve the local problems of the community, she establishes the claim of local forms of knowledge at the dominant discursive sites where knowledge is produced. In doing so, Lakshmi questions the very legitimacy and authenticity of these traditional sites of knowledge production because of their disconnection from local communities (see Figure 5.2).

Women Negotiating Agency

It is in the midst of the oppressive structures of neoliberalism that women seek out avenues to enact their agency, coming together as collectives, organizing legitimate spaces of collective support across borders, and laying claims to legitimacy by securing access to network structures and policy platforms where their voices can be heard (Ferree & Tripp, 2006; Moghadam, 2009). These claims to legitimacy articulated by women in the subaltern sectors of the globe challenge the principles of neoliberalism that exist at the foundations of the global flow of capitalism, and disrupt the homogeneous narratives of emancipatory politics that are articulated in the dominant structures of neoliberalism (Mohanty, 2006). The notion that the market offers freedom for the subaltern sectors is ruptured with the stories of oppression and exploitation that are carried out by the structural adjustment programs in perpetuating the agendas of transnational capitalism under neoliberalism. Situated amidst the tremendous inequities and oppressive forces of neoliberalism, women's voices and networks of solidarity share the stories of exploitation at local sites in global spaces, thus forever "making impure" the claims about women's emancipation and development that are continuously made by the dominant actors within these spaces.

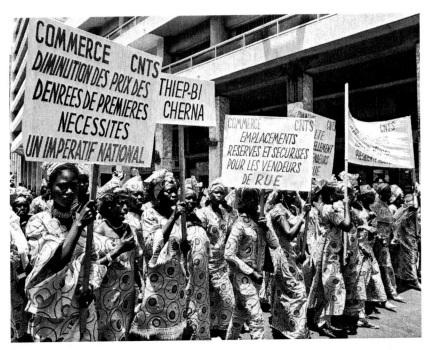

FIGURE 5.2 Women hold banners during a protest against the recent price rise for basic food-stuffs on May 1, 2008, in Dakar during the traditional workers' May Day march by the CNTS (National Confederation of Senegalese Workers) which brought together several thousand participants. (Georges Gobet/AFP/Getty Images)

Here is a narrative articulated by Irma, a Filipina worker in the Silicon Valley, California, cited by Mohanty (2006):

> We dream that when we work hard, we'll be able to clothe our children decently, and still have a little time and money left for ourselves. And we dream that when we do as good as other people, we get treated the same, and that nobody puts us down because we are not like them . . . Then we ask ourselves, "How could we make these things come true?" And so far we've come up with only two possible answers: win the lottery, or organize. What can I say, except I have never been lucky with numbers. So tell this in your book: tell them it may take time that people think they don't have, but they have to organize! Because the only way to get a little measure of power over your own life is to do it collectively, with the support of other people who share your needs.
>
> *(as quoted in Mohanty, 2006, p. 139)*

Irma shares with us her dreams of being able to offer the basic necessities for her children through her work, set at the heart of neoliberal hegemony. In Irma's voice, we hear the call for organizing as a way to have one's voice heard and to work toward addressing the local needs. In organizing, Irma finds power as she participates in a broader collective with other women who share her needs. Locally articulated stories of agency at global sites rupture the dominant narratives of subaltern agency in mainstream structures that erase subaltern agency in order to justify the acts of development and modernization, which in turn end up serving as mechanisms for carrying out the political economic agendas of transnational power. Agency therefore is constituted in the continually negotiated relationship between the individual and the collective.

Agency becomes evident in transnational feminist movements where women articulate oppressive structures that operate on the basis of gendered inequities, utilize gender as an entry point for mobilizing for change, create empowering spaces in which they challenge the inequities in gendered relations played out through the various roles and relationships in their lives, and build networks among women that operate on the basis of the identification of the oppressive nature of gendered relations (Ferree, 2006; Moghadam, 2009). Ferree (2006) further notes that successful feminist movements create spaces and places for the articulation of feminism within structures as well as within movements. Claims of gender equality are made within policy frameworks and structures locally, nationally, and globally; activist networks are mobilized for bringing groups of women together at various sites of organizing; and women organize to create knowledge through policy papers and research documents, which then offer the foundations for engaging in social change activities. The role of organizing serves as a fulcrum that connects women's voices locally and globally.

Global expressions of organized forms of women's agency are enabled through the creation of global political opportunity structures that are in turn constituted through globalization processes. Articulations of local forms of resistance are co-constructed at global sites, and in doing so, challenge the hegemony of global logics of neoliberalism. Simultaneously, local struggles offer theoretical, methodological, and practical models for resistance in the mainstream, thus forever disrupting the traditionally conceived one-way flow of communication under the neoliberal umbrella (Dutta, 2008c, 2009).

Conclusion

This chapter examined the intersections of structure, culture, and agency in the perpetuation of the hegemonic principles of the market across the globe. Critical interrogations of the project of development and the principles of scientific technical rationality embodied in development projects demonstrate the West-centric patriarchal agendas that are written into the articulations, processes, and strategies of development, which erase the voices of women, often paradoxically so through the perpetuation of the rhetoric of empowerment. This suggests the need for critical interrogations of dominant development institutions and the ways in which these institutions perpetuate the agendas of transnational patriarchy, operating at the intersections of the global and the local. Ultimately, the chapter wrapped up with a critique of neoliberalism and the ways in which neoliberal market economies marginalize women and constrain women's agency. The discussions of the structures of neoliberal market economics serves as a founding base for studying and working with women's movements of social change and redistributive justice that are situated amidst feminine principles of organizing from the global South. Because the marginalization of women has been perpetrated globally through the erasure of women's voices, the culture-centered approach begins with the emphasis on creating spaces of listening where women's voices from the marginalized sectors of the globe can be heard, creating entry points for solidarity building and transformative politics.

PART II

Communicating for Social Change

6

DIALOGUE AND SOCIAL CHANGE

At the core of the culture-centered approach is the privileging of the possibilities for listening to subaltern voices that have been historically erased from discursive spaces. This historical erasure is situated structurally, drawing upon the argument that inequities in distribution of resources play out communicatively. In other words, those with economic inaccess to resources are also disadvantaged in terms of their inaccess to communication platforms, spaces, processes, and resources (Dutta, 2008a, 2008b, 2008c). Therefore, dialogue offers a discursive opening for creating spaces of social change by transforming the structural inequities in the distribution of resources through the presence of subaltern voices in the discursive spaces. Stories of subalternity narrated through dialogues rupture the dominant ideological constructions that portray the subaltern as passive and without agency. Dialogic engagement with the margins seeks to disrupt the marginalizing processes that are carried out by the status quo by starting to listen to subaltern narratives. The goal of dialogue is not to operate within the structures to continue reifying the status quo, but to change the structures in order to address the inequities and injustices perpetuated by them.

In the culture-centered approach, voice is a key theoretical construct as it offers an opening for the possibilities of change. The very voices that have been systematically pathologized, scripted, and erased from the ontological and epistemological bases of knowledge production and praxis return to the discursive spaces of global politics through dialogue with the academic and the practitioner situated at the center of power. The politics of a dialogic approach to social change lies in the articulation of issues from subaltern standpoints, thus shifting the landscape of problem configuration and the development of solutions into the realm of subaltern agency. Rather than depicting the subaltern as bodies to be targeted in large-scale campaigns and interventions that focus on top-down logics of individual behavior change, the dialogic approach centers itself on the role of listening to subaltern voices, making note of problem configurations as seen through subaltern perspectives, and creating spaces of change through the voicing of subaltern agendas. For the academic or expert engaging in social change research and praxis, a dialogic engagement with the margins begins with humility, reflexivity, and openness to learning through engagement, thus shifting the traditional role of the expert from a producer of knowledge situated at the centers of power to a listener who works in solidarity with the subaltern sectors to create spaces of structural transformation.

In essence then, dialogue as a tool in the culture-centered approach offers a methodology for the academic and the practitioner to engage in the politics of social change. It creates an entry point for those at the centers to engage with the politics of subalternity, finding spaces for listening to subaltern voices in the ways in which policies are formulated and implemented locally, nationally, and globally. In this sense, dialogue becomes an epistemological tool for the subaltern politics of social change. It offers guidelines for communication scholars and practitioners participating in the politics of social change to envision communication processes and methods that engage with the marginalizing social structures and seek out avenues for changing them. A dialogic approach makes note of the dialectical tensions that emerge in the processes of social change. It also brings forth the tools of solidarity, commitment, and reflexivity into the communicative processes of social change, thus continuously renegotiating the role of the researcher and practitioner.

Simultaneously, the concept of dialogue also emerges as a tool that connects the politics of subaltern actors across the globe, therefore creating structural openings for social change by joining the local politics with the global. Through dialogue, the local gets foregrounded in the landscape of the global, thus taking up space in the global policy landscape, determining the agendas of global policy, and finding policy solutions in transforming structures that shape local outcomes. Simultaneously, the politics of the local dialogues with global networks of solidarity in creating spaces of change locally, thus bringing about transformations in local structural configurations. We begin this chapter by reviewing dialogue theories in communication scholarship, and by highlighting some of the key aspects of these dialogue theories. The review of dialogue theories in communication scholarship is followed by a discussion of the culture-centered approach to dialogue, engaging with the structural transformations of dialogue, the role of dialogue in structural transformations, reflexivity, solidarity, and the dialectical tensions that emerge in a culture-centered approach to dialogue. In reviewing the role of dialogue as a tool for social change, we will walk through the example of the United Nations Permanent Forum on Indigenous Issues (UNPFII) as a dialogic space for listening to the voices of the subaltern sectors.

Dialogue Theories in Communication Scholarship

Dialogue has strong disciplinary roots in communication, noting that dialogue is the prerequisite to an authentic relationship, therefore offering a space for co-construction of meanings through authenticity (Anderson & Cissna, 1996, 1997, 2008; Arnett, 1982, 1993, 2001; Baxter & Montgomery, 1996; Cissna & Anderson, 1996, 1998; Deetz, 1992, 1995; Eisenberg, 1990, 1994; Eisenberg & Goodall, 1997; Simpson, 2008). The works of Buber, Gadamer, Habermas, Bakhtin, and Freire have been pivotal in shaping the terrain of communication scholarship on dialogue, raising key debates as well as theoretical entry points about dialogue. In *I and Thou*, originally published in 1923, Buber (1958) presents the idea that human beings become persons through dialogue, and it is in this centering of dialogue as an entry point to embodiment that possibilities of change are constituted. Buber's *I-Thou* emphasizes that the *I* does not exist without the *Thou* or the other. Therefore, it is in relationship with the other that I finds meaning. For Buber (1958, 1965), listening or "turning toward the other" is an important aspect of dialogue, while for Gadamer (1982), the context is more important and he considers meanings as emergent through dialogue. Habermas (1989) takes the interpersonal concept of dialogue and connects it to a broader public domain; his philosophy envisions a public sphere where the speaker and listener engage with a common text that guides communicative action. Arnett (2001) notes that in Habermas' communicative action, dialogue becomes possible through a public domain involving common space, respect for the other and action in concert. Dialogue then connects the interpersonal context within which it is embodied to a more public context where public spheres offer opportunities for dialogue (see the special issue of *Communication Theory* by Anderson & Cissna, 2008). Given the emphasis of the culture-centered approach on the co-construction of meanings, dialogue offers the entry point through which meanings are co-created by the involved actors (Dutta, 2007, 2008a, 2008b; Dutta-Bergman, 2004a, 2004b). Relationships of authenticity are co-created through dialogic interactions, where the interaction between the participants opens up the space for mutual learning (Freire, 1970).

Bakhtin (1981) draws our attention to the concept of "heteroglossia" to articulate the diversity of voices in dialogue that offer the constitutive frame for the emergence of the self. Therefore, the self emerges through dialogue, through the imagination of what others see when they see us. The presence of multiple voices interrupts the totalizing effect of top-down discourse. It is precisely in this embracing of the multiple voices within dialogic encounters that Bakhtin's views on dialogue resonate with the culture-centered approach, foregrounding the possibilities for engaging with alternative utterances coexisting with, within, and in resistance to dominant discourse. So does Freire's (1970) argument to some extent, central to which is the recognition of the tension of human existence—a struggle between the oppressor and the oppressed that is articulated and negotiated through dialogic opportunities (Dutta & Pal, 2010). Freire (1970) suggests that only dialogic encounters entail the process of achieving freedom and alleviating this tension. In processes of social change, dialogic opportunities engage the tensions between the academic researcher and the community participants, continually creating spaces for reworking the identities, roles, and relationships of the researcher or expert with the community. In the culture-centered approach, dialogic interactions create opportunities for subaltern communities to articulate their viewpoints in a context that has traditionally silenced them. It is through these dialogic interactions that marginalized communities find access to dominant discursive spaces and articulate their voices in these spaces.

Early work on dialogue focused on the content of it, which in the 1970s moved toward the direction of humanistic psychology. While researchers and critics engaged with discussions on openness in dialogue and normative roles, a section of scholars, influenced by Gadamer, became interested in regarding dialogue as contextual, which is socially and historically situated. Ideas such as participation and collaboration in dialogue manifested in scholarship that suggested the intertextuality and multiplicity of dialogue. According to Anderson, Baxter, and Cissna (2004) a fresh intellectual intervention came in with the "Paradigm issues" volume of the *Rethinking communication* books in the late 1980s. The thrust on qualitative and interpretive research approaches gave momentum to the con-stitutive role of communication and rejected the unitary notion of reality. Along with it grew the consciousness of the central role of "listening to the other" in the realm of human experience. This consciousness about "listening to the other" connects dialogue theory with the subaltern studies project because of the commit-ment of the project to listening to the voices of the margins that have been erased from the dominant platforms of history making. The subaltern studies project suggests that the issue of "otherness" is ensconced within a larger politics of power and domination that concerns an engagement with the problematics of modernist epistemic structures that constitute the other through acts of erasure. What for instances are possibilities for engaging with the other where the "other" is created through a variety of material and symbolic resources put into motion in those very dominant public spheres of mainstream societies that have typically served as the spaces for privileged dialogue, simultaneously erasing the voices of the subaltern sectors (see for instance the critique of democracy promotion initiatives by Dutta–Bergman, 2005a)? As we see in the next section, dialogue for social change embodies the dynamic relationship with the tools and instruments of dominant structures in order to disrupt these structures. Methods such as photo voice and participatory video utilize the epistemological tools of mainstream spaces in order to disrupt dominant structures and meaningfully influence policy.

Inherent then in the conceptualization of dialogue for social change is the acknowledgement of the relationships of power that are negotiated at sites of dialogue. Hammond, Anderson, and Cissna (2003, p. 136) consider the problem-atics of dialogue in the realm of power by suggesting dialectical tensions that are permanent, "equivocal and difficult to pin down in dialogic moments" and are played out in the realms of identity, outcome, meaning, voice, and field. The issue of identity is constituted in the dialectical tension between the self and other where the participants in dialogue continuously negotiate between self-identity and group-identity. This negotiation of identities is critical to the role of dialogue in social change as experts and practitioners negotiate their own identities in the face of the dialogic interaction with the "other" that challenges the very foundations of mainstream knowledge. It is in making the self vulnerable to the "other" that opportunities are created for transformation, challenging the inequitable structures in the mainstream that perpetuate the erasures of subaltern voices based on the very assumptions of subaltern primitiveness and backwardness that inundate the mainstream (Basu & Dutta, 2008a, 2009; Dutta-Bergman, 2004a, 2004b).

The ways in which the outcomes of dialogues are negotiated play out in the realm of the dialectical tensions between content and process. Hammond et al. (2003) further indicate that cultural contexts determine the ways in which content and process are negotiated in dialogic outcomes. Tension over meaning resonates between coherence and incoherence; "coherence is affirming and temporary, and incoherence indispensable, drives a need for dialogue" (Hammond et al., 2003, p. 140). Questions of power in dialogue introduce an additional tension in the domain of voice that goes back and forth between monovocality and mutuality as dialogue struggles between the need for a collective voice in the realm of collective action, and simultaneously opens up the space for multiple voices and spaces for multiple contested meanings. Furthermore, Hammond et al. (2003) suggest that the dialogic field exists in a dialectical tension between emergence that contributes to change and creativity and convergence on outcomes and goals. The authors further go on to note that whereas convergent dialogue reifies and supports the dominant power structure by limiting the range of possibilities, divergent dialogue "challenges the processes and power bases of the status quo" (Hammond et al., 2003, p. 146). In contrast to the convergent self that draws its pre-established identity from traditional or juridical power, the emergent self comes to exist reflexively by engaging with the other through the process of dialogue. The subaltern studies project attends to this emergent dialogue by looking at the possibilities of engaging with subaltern voices that have otherwise been erased by convergent dialogue, supported by the dominant power structures. It also engages with and builds upon the possibilities of reflexivity as it foregrounds the privileged position of the scholar and the ways in which this position is intrinsically tied to silencing subaltern voices. The subaltern studies project further interrogates the discursive closures in dominant articulations and the spheres of emergent dialogue where the status quo nevertheless defines the discursive realm of possibilities that emerge from the dialogic process.

Deetz and Simpson (2004), Fernandez (2008), and McPhail and McCarthy (2004, 2005) grapple with some of these tensions by engaging with issues of power and race in dialogue. Deetz and Simpson note that power is pervasive across social structures that "routinely preclude otherness and block conversation . . . Systems of domination usually preclude genuine conversation." The authors caution that structural inequities are deeply embedded in human experiences, rendering them natural and invisible. Hence, traditional dialogic communication models supporting openness and acceptance advance a superficial treatment of equality without really addressing the underlying structural disparities; this is precisely the point where subaltern studies explores the linkages among the political economic functions of dominant discursive spaces that maintain hegemonic configurations and systematically erase opportunities for dialogue. McPhail and McCarthy (2004, 2005) argue that a broader discourse of color blindness limits dialogue by denying people of color their agency in defining their lived experiences of racism, thus suggesting the impossibilities that are constituted in the realm of dialogue in the discussions of race. Pointing out the ways in which mainstream dialogues in US society place issues of race as undiscussable (see for instance Ellinor & Gerard, 1998), McPhail and McCarthy (2004, 2005) note that dialogue is impossible when the materially constituted realities of African Americans are denied. Similarly, responding to the discursive closures that are brought about the dominant social structures, Deetz and Simpson (2004) articulate the transformative potential of dialogue in "radical encounters with otherness" (Simpson, 2008, p. 140) for meaningfully and profoundly engaging people across differences. The subaltern studies project provides an entry point for further interrogating the privileges in the dominant epistemic structures that silence the subaltern sectors and for exploring the conditions of silences that are historically produced through the communicative exercises of omission.

Culture-Centered Approach to Dialogue

The core components of the culture-centered approach, culture, structure, and agency, play out in the goals, configurations, and outcomes of the dialogic spaces. Culture, defined in terms of the continuously shifting local contexts and frameworks of meanings, defines the dialogic processes and the nature of dialogue. Dialogue, in turn, continuously shapes the local cultures of subaltern spaces, defining the meanings that circulate within these spaces, and the identities and relationships that define culture. Dialogue is situated against the backdrop of social structures, being defined by the social structures, the procedures, and processes set up by these structures, and the rules of participation in dialogue as defined by these structures. At the same time, as we see throughout this section of the chapter, dialogue creates an opportunity for redefining structures, for creating spaces of structural transformation that address issues of equity and social justice.

It is through dialogue that subaltern cultures enact their agency in challenging inequitable social structures. Dialogue shapes agency, both in terms of enabling agency and also in terms of constraining agency in policy platforms. Dialogue is also shaped by subaltern agency; it is through their participation that the subaltern sectors define the landscape of dialogue. It is in the midst of these interactions between culture, structure, and agency that the goals, processes, and outcomes of dialogue are determined. Let us look at the example of the United Nations Permanent Forum on Indigenous Issues created in May 2002 as a dialogic space for listening to the voices of indigenous peoples across the globe. The forum is created with the goal of opening up opportunities for listening to indigenous voices globally, where indigenous peoples can speak for themselves as members of a United Nations body. The forum, created by the United Nations Economic and Social Council, serves three important objectives: first, discuss indigenous issues within the broader agendas of the Council including economic and social development, culture, environment, education, health, and human rights; second, offer indigenous-based expert advice and recommendations to the Council and to other programs, funds, and agencies of the UN; and third, raise awareness about indigenous issues, and help to integrate and coordinate activities in the UN system.

Discursive Ruptures

In the culture-centered approach, dialogue is both an epistemological tool and a strategic marker of praxis. In other words, it is through dialogue that discourses are challenged, with opposing points of view being introduced into the discursive space. Resistance to globalization processes is fundamentally carried out through the articulation of alternative discourses embedded in alternative rationalities which question the individualistic, profit-driven logic of globalization that continuously seeks to take over the local discursive spaces across the globe. Possibilities of social change are primarily constituted over the ownership and construction of discursive spaces. Central to the change in dominant social structures is the articulation of discourse that challenges the existing ways of thinking, ruptures the taken-for-granted assumptions that constitute the seamless spaces of dominant public spheres, and entices the listener, viewer, or reader to consider alternative possibilities. This discursive shift lies at the heart of globally situated forms of resistance in local communities that seek to bring about shifts in structures of inequality and injustice.

Let us consider the example of China and the articulation of peasant resistance as a disruption of the hegemonic narrative of neoliberalism within which the images of China are constituted in contemporary global discourses. Since 1999, China has entered into the political economic spaces of globalization, played out in the form of economic reforms directed at modernizing China, restoring China's global citizenship, attaining possible world power status, and liberalizing the society. The narratives of Reform constituted in the global discursive spaces of and about China have celebrated the economic growth of the nation state, the substantial growth of a viable middle class whose values and lifestyles are increasingly congruent with Western modes of modern life, and the emergence of China into modernity. This economic story that predominates much of the discursive space is, however, accompanied by an equally absent narrative of the increasing polarization of Chinese society, with increasing deterioration and disenfranchisement in the rural sectors (Tiejun, 2001). Tiejun (2001) discusses the increasing presence of san-nong, "the three rural dimensions," referring to the emerging problems related to the rural population (peasants), rural production (agriculture), and the rural world (countryside).

It is against this backdrop of the hegemonic discourses of China that alternative rationalities are imagined through dialogic co-participation with rural communities. One such alternative discursive entry point is reflected in the work of the James Yen Institute for Rural Reconstruction (www.iirr.org/), focused on the tasks of training farmers and other learners in rural communities, and creating dialogic spaces for the voicing of alternative logics driven by relational harmony among people and with nature. The communicative construction of alternative discourses that challenge the hegemony of neoliberalism is complemented by structurally driven efforts of social change that seek to build capacities in rural communities such that farmers and rural residents can have a say in the stories of development that shape their lives. The basic commitment of the Institute is in reviving the traditions of the past in rural communities and enabling local communities to participate in self-management and self-governance at the local level based on traditional ways of knowing in contrast to the widespread logic of modernization based on principles of aping the West. Local communities organize in alternative discursive spaces that highlight the importance of collective community ownership of resources and decision-making processes.

Consider also the example of the Chipko Andolan in India as a space for articulating alternative rationalities to the economic rationality of neoliberalism. "Andolan" is the term that is often commonly used in the context of India to refer to a movement (Raina, 2004). The Chipko Andolan in Northern India originated from an incident in 1972 in Reni, a remote village in the Himalayan ranges, where the women of the village rushed into the forest and clasped the tree trunks to prevent a logging contractor from cutting the trees (Raina, 2004). Articulated around the question of ownership of the forest, the news of the protest spread rapidly through communities and media nationally and across the globe, thus putting tremendous pressure on the government who owned the land to negotiate with the local community, comprising mostly of women. The community began setting up committees to start addressing broader issues such as eco-friendly development in collaboration with the government. At the core of the movement was the tension over the definition of ownership of natural resources, and the ways in which the natural resources were put to use by the contractor in opposition to the local uses of the resources for the local community. For the women in the community, the defining question was one of the "right to use" the trees as a source of firewood for their hearths and the leaves for fodder as opposed to the cutting of the trees for timber to be used for manufacturing sporting goods. The branches of the trees were traditionally lopped off and the leaves were plucked by the community, allowing for the replenishing of the resource over time as opposed to the felling of the trees by the state-approved contractors. The kind of "use" offered a framework for entering the discursive space, situating the renewable use of the forest resources in opposition to the destruction of the trees. The dialectical tensions that emerge in the Chipko Andolan reflect the fundamental tensions over the question of ownership of common property resources, and the rights of the local community set in opposition to the rights of the state to define the uses of common property resources. In the contemporary global landscape where the economic agendas of neoliberal hegemony dictate the landscapes of development, movements such as the Chipko movement interrogate the discursive space with questions of ownership and rights, excavating the taken-for-granted assumptions underlying the agendas of development dictated by the State.

Similarly, Dutta-Bergman's (2004a, 2004b) culture-centered dialogues with the Santali communities in Eastern India disrupt the hegemonic narratives of health as situated in the realm of individual behaviors and individual lifestyles. Resisting the West-centric germ theory cosmology of biomedicine that takes a reductionist approach to health and illness, Santali narratives of health discuss health in its relationship to nature. Health is threatened when nature is disrupted by cutting trees and further urbanization. Therefore, the solution to illness is sought out in the realm of balancing the relationship with nature and in seeking to create spaces of harmonious coexistence. Along similar lines, indigenous movements such as the Land is Life movement (www.landislife.org/special/about) connects indigenous communities from across the globe to bring the subaltern sectors in dialogue with the dominant hegemonies, thus consistently challenging the reductionist thinking of the mainstream, its reliance on limited empiricism, and its politics of violence that has been carried out historically in the name of science and knowledge production. Here dialogue becomes a way of engaging the dominant structures; the Land is Life project brings indigenous leaders from twenty communities located in sixteen different countries in dialogue with international development institutions and leaders within the United Nations. It creates dialogic opportunities for indigenous communities, creating indigenous people's access to international policy-making structures, and working from within the UN to create global spaces of change in dominant structures and policy-making bodies. Dialogue here is situated in the realm of the agendas of the politics of structural transformation by creating opportunities for learning in dominant knowledge structures from ways of knowing that have been historically marginalized and silenced through the reductionist violence of science (see Figure 6.1).

Dialogue and Structural Transformation

In the culture-centered approach, calls for dialogue are not situated in the realms of apolitical interactions and relationships, but are at the core constituted in the domains of politics and access to power. Positions of power are crucial to the constitution of dialogic spaces, and these spaces become the sites for contesting power. Culture-centered dialogues ultimately do not stop at meaning making and

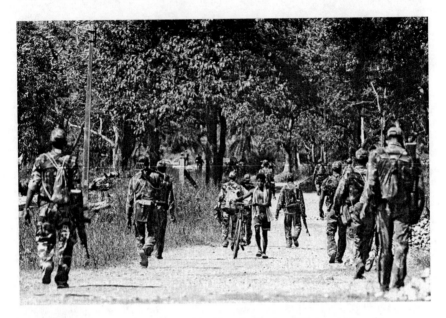

FIGURE 6.1 Paramilitary presence in Dantewada district of Orissa, India where indigenous communities are resisting their displacement. (Manpreet Romana/AFP/ Getty Images)

interpretation, but rather seek to mobilize the meanings created through dialogue in processes of social change. Power is central to dialogic processes, not only in terms of framing the terrains of dialogue, but also and more fundamentally in terms of challenging and changing structures that oppress the subaltern sectors. The dialectical tensions that emerge in dialogic moments also create entry points for social change, offering new avenues for challenging and changing those structures of inequality that continue to operate across the globe. Structural transformations are achieved through the incorporation of structures in discussions of problems and in the subsequent articulations of solutions through dialogic spaces. Dialogue creates opportunities for change by structurally engaging with the politics of change, and by continually seeking to bring about transformations in hegemonic structures of oppression.

Dialogue serves as a foundation for structural transformation by creating spaces for alternative rationalities, and by narrating alternative stories that bring forth the taken-for-granted assumptions of the status quo. The alternative narratives articulated through dialogue imagine possibilities that create the foundations for a different framework that departs from the mainstream and its conventions. Alternative rationalities articulated through dialogue lead us to alternative worldviews that interrogate the dominant narratives of development and modernity, and draw our attention to the spaces of violence that are carried out through these dominant narratives.

Consider, for instance, the following narrative articulated in the conversations of the Quechua community members of the Huancavelica community in Peru as a part of the "Conversations with Earth" participatory video project (www.conversationsearth.org/index.php?temp=media&id_story=21), depicting a ritual visit to Father Hyuaytapallana, referring to the mountain God, the snow from whose peaks have now melted, accompanied with the water shortages experienced in the plains of Peru:

> It hurts me to see the decay of Huaytapallana, he who gives us life and animates the entire world . . . All waters are contaminated. Here the water surfaces beautifully, but when it arrives to the river, it is full of garbage, contaminated by the fumes . . . I don't know what we can do about it. Pollution has started since the plastic factories came. It is obvious how things are getting worse. This is what I think, these are my thoughts, but who will listen?

Juxtaposed against the backdrop of visuals of dried out snow peaks and limited water flow, the narrative constructs the story of the decay of Huaytapallana. It ends with the following invocation:

> I invite you to get engaged in taking care of our Snow Mountains, to take care of our Mountains. I know if we take care, we can save what still exists and we can learn to live with what we have.

The articulation of the narrative of offering ritual homage to the mountains articulates the symbolic relationship of harmony between communities and nature, where nature holds the space of respect and veneration, being characterized as God to whom offerings ought to be made in order to ensure the sustenance of life forms. The story of learning to live with what we have and of taking care of the mountains is established in opposition to the stories of reductionist science and modernist development that construct development in terms of industrialization, deforestation, mining, and so on. Dialogue transforms structures through the entry of discourses of harmony and "respect for nature" that disrupt the hegemonic narratives of development, and create entry points for change by seeking to influence global policies through a wide range of platforms that engage in conversations with policy-makers, governments, and international organizations. Consider the following narrative articulated by a Marcos Terena, an indigenous tribal leader from Brazil in the video *Earth wisdom for a world in crisis*:

> The knowledge that we believe in is not just philosophical. Our knowledge derives from the nature and the environment. It is knowledge of the force that can be found in the wind, rain, rocks, rivers, and mountains. I am not talking about conservation or preservation but about utilizing this knowledge or what they call her "science" to improve everyone's life.

Ultimately, dialogues offer the openings for structural transformations in the neo-liberal political economy of the mainstream processes of globalization by bringing forth questions of social justice, and by reinterpreting the meanings of universal science and modernist development amidst global processes. The dialogic engagement with the local ruptures the political economic rationalities at global sites. Global is directly brought to question through dialogues with the subaltern sectors. The local-global sites of dialogue rupture the hegemony of mainstream knowledge and policy structures by co-constructing alternative rationalities with subaltern populations that draw attention to alternative modes of social, political, and economic organizing. In addition to the structural transformations in global rationalities through participations in dialogic processes, communication for social change operates on the basis of creation of platforms for participation by the subaltern sectors. The legitimacy of these platforms as well as their viability as dialogic sites is continually in question as such platforms for dialogues with the subaltern sectors struggle with mainstream platforms that serve the interests of the status quo.

Structural Transformations of Dialogic Spaces

The systematic erasure of subaltern voices from dominant discursive spaces that manufacture knowledge and then utilize this knowledge to create policies and interventions is resisted through structural transformations of public spheres and through the availability of dialogic spaces for participation by the subaltern sectors. Culture-centered projects of social change are constituted in the creation of dialogic spaces at local sites where local communities can come together and articulate their views (Basu & Dutta, 2009). The coming together at these common spaces of articulation is fundamental to the mobilizing of participants in processes of social change and structural transformations. The struggle for the creation of dialogic spaces therefore is a struggle for securing spaces where alternative rationalities are articulated, offering new and creative ways of organizing as opposed to the efficient mechanisms of free market economies. The legitimacy and existence of such spaces is always contingent upon the relationships of power and the continuous negotiations with dominant structures.

A subaltern studies reading of dialogue interrogates the very assumptions underlying dialogic spaces in mainstream public spheres, and instead suggests the relevance of engaging with subaltern public spheres where subaltern voices may be heard. The American Spanish *testimonio* (or testimonial narrative), as a genre, is one such communicative platform that disrupts the taken-for-granted assumptions about communication and dialogue in mainstream platforms where knowledge is circulated (Beverley, 2004a, 2004b). Beverley (2004b) describes the *testimonio* as a new form of communication:

> a novel of novella-length narrative in book, or pamphlet (that is, printed as opposed to acoustic) form, told in the first person by a narrator who is also

the real protagonist or witness of the events he or she recounts, and whose unit of narration is usually a life or a significant life experience.

(Beverley, 2004b, p. 31)

The *testimonio* serves as a site of social change by presenting the authority of the subaltern voice in its accounting of events and the narrative construction of these events; subaltern experiences strategically construct the narratives of testimony with an agenda, rupturing the dialogic expectations of the mainstream that construct the subaltern as the native informant and producing texts of "local history" that are concerned with elaborating hegemony (Beverley, 2004b). As a representation of those subjects who have traditionally been excluded from authorized representation, the *testimonio* operates as a resistive strategy, rupturing the dominant notion of "what is valued and understood as [culture] by dominant groups" (Beverley, 2004b, p. 19). Beverley adds:

> Almost by definition, the voice that speaks in testimonio is not, in its act of enunciation, part of what Hegel would have understood as civil society or what Habermas means by public sphere: if it were, it would address us instead in novels, essays, films, TV shows, letters to the editor, op-ed pieces. On the other hand, testimonio as an enonce—that is, as something materialized in the form of transcript of text—serves to bring subaltern voice into civil society and public sphere.
>
> *(Beverley, 2004b, p. 19)*

As a representation of the subaltern voice, the *testimonio* exists outside the traditional boundaries of civil society and dialogue, disrupting the articulations of dialogue as pure spaces, and offering dialogic hegemonies of the local by rupturing the modernist notions of what dialogue is and where it is made possible; simultaneously, by entering into conversations with civil society, the *testimonio* becomes the resistive site of the specific that challenges the hegemony of the universal. These dialogic hegemonies of the local, however, are politically directed at attending to the impurity of dialogue, and at transforming universal structures through the political co-optation of mainstream platforms of dialogue by rendering them impure (Beverley, 2004a, 2004b; Godalof, 1999). As a communicative form, the *testimonio* challenges our assumptions of both literary texts and ethnographies, rupturing these pure spaces with its boundary blurring impurities.

Dialogic spaces in subaltern contexts challenge hegemonic narratives when connected to the spaces in the mainstream. For example, the witnessing of exploitation and violence in the subaltern sectors carried out by SAPs brings forth the stories of structural and physical violence perpetrated on subaltern communities. Depicting the protest of an indigenous community in Mexico against military trucks and artillery armies invading their land, the following narrative in the video documentary *Earth wisdom for a world in crisis* seeks to disrupt the violence perpetrated by the status quo through the transformations of dialogic spaces in the mainstream by utilizing the technology of the video camera as a witnessing device that narrates the story of oppression and simultaneously resists the state–sponsored violence by documenting the protest:

> Difficulties can escalate into conflict when the issue involves ownership of land. In Chiapas Mexico, the confrontation evolves between native people and the government Native people all over the globe have decided that the fight for their land can no longer be fought in isolation.

The structural transformation of dialogic spaces facilitates the politics of social change by creating forums for the articulations of alternative rationalities and for the disruption of the seamless narratives of neoliberal hegemony. These politically connected and structurally vital dialogic spaces are essential to the mobilizing of communicative processes of change because they serve as sites for issue identification, identification of frames, and mobilization of resistance toward the goals of achieving social change.

Dialogue and Capacity Building

One of the assumptions in mainstream theories of dialogue and public participation is the assumption about the equality of participants engaging in the dialogic processes. Given the fundamental inequities that underlie access to communicative spaces and the avenues for participation in such spaces, the culture-centered approach to dialogue is critical of the celebratory rhetoric of dialogue that is unaware of the material inequalities underlying access to and participation in dialogic spaces.

The very requirements of certain skill sets and knowledge about dialogic procedures in dominant platforms keep these platforms inaccessible to the subaltern sectors, operating in a parallel sphere of domination and control. Dominant approaches promoting participation often operate within these spheres of inaccessibility because they do not engage with the structural capacities of subaltern communities.

Building dialogic capacities in subaltern communities involves the creation of structural resources and points of access within these communities. Such efforts at creating structural access have to happen both materially as well as communicatively. In the absence of developing material capacities in local communities, skills training for participation in dialogic spaces remain ineffective because of the lack of adequate material leverage in laying claims for social and structural transformation. The location of dialogic spaces within broader structures connect dialogic politics with the politics of structural transformations, working toward bringing about fundamental shifts in the inequalities and injustices constituted in neoliberalism.

Dialogue and Dialectical Tensions

In the culture-centered approach, dialogue in subaltern contexts exists amidst the tensions between the politics of change and the politics of co-optation, between the possibilities and impossibilities of listening to the subaltern sectors of the globe, and between representation and erasure. The interactions between culture, structure, and agency create a complex and dynamic web of dialogic possibilities, which are constituted in the midst of multiple and competing hegemonies. Even as scholars and practitioners working on issues of social change along with the participants of the subaltern sectors of the globe engage in dialogues with the dominant social structures locally, nationally, and globally, they continually operate within the possibilities of being co-opted within the broader hegemonic interests of these dominant structures. The very possibilities of representation created in dialogic interactions are set against the backdrop of the erasures of subaltern voices from these spaces. It is in the negotiation of these tensions that communication for social change engages with the tools of reflexivity and solidarity to create openings for structural transformation.

Politics of Change and Politics of Co-optation. Dialogue in the culture-centered approach is political in the sense that it interrogates and participates in the politics of the mainstream to seek out spaces of change. Therefore, one of the key criteria for evaluating the culture-centered approach to dialogue is on the basis of its ability to bring about structural transformation, to seek out changes in the status quo, and to challenge the practices of oppression and exploitation that are carried out by the mainstream. In this sense then, as noted earlier, social change becomes narrowly defined in terms of its ability to bring about changes in existing structural configurations, and not simply in terms of specific modifications within the structures that continue to reify the status quo. For instance, in the creation of the UNPFII, the UN opens up a space for dialogue with indigenous communities across the globe, particularly on projects of development, even as it co-opts the participatory agendas of these communities within the frameworks of the UN, thus threatening to minimize the resistive politics of the indigenous movements. Whereas on one hand, the participation of the indigenous actors at the table of the UN creates an opportunity structure for engagement with the dominant structures, on the other hand, it runs the risk of being co-opted within these structures.

Subaltern interpretations of dialogue suggest that the logic of dialogue within modern social systems is inherently tied to the interests of the capital and the ways in which this capital operates to create and sustain conditions of subalternity. The location of dialogic platforms within neoliberal spaces frames the agendas and strategies of dialogue with the interests of TNCs. For example, the indigenous-mining dialogue group set up by the Australian Uranium Association to bridge the gap between Aboriginal Australians and uranium mining industries is constituted within the agendas of the mining industry to usurp indigenous land to build mines

(Statham, 2009). Who gets to participate in dialogue is dictated by the interests of the system in sustaining itself as an economic enterprise. By turning our attention to the ways in which power shapes the nature, form, content, processes, and outcomes of dialogue, we become sensitized to the ways in which dialogue continues to sustain the imbalances and inequities within social systems. Along these lines, Dutta–Bergman (2005b) articulates that the subaltern is the subaltern precisely because she is located outside the realm of those discursive spaces that constitute the dominant notions of dialogue.

In modernist constructions of civil societies as avenues for dialoguing with the subaltern sector, the existence of civil society creates the condition of subalternity as the avenues of communicative exchange and the communication skills required to participate in civil society remain inaccessible to larger sectors of social systems. The basic requirements of civil society such as literacy, formal education, nuclear family units, and private property exclude significant sectors of the population from full citizenship and limit their access to communicative platforms. Subalterns, therefore, exist in the interstices of modern civil societies, rendered invisible through the lack of access to the discursive spaces of the mainstream public spheres where issues are debated and policies are formulated. They exist because of civil society, and because of the absence of discursive spaces that are accessible to them and responsive to their communicative needs.

Furthermore, the economic basis of civil society is built upon the creation of capital and the capital must continually create conditions of subalternity in order to sustain itself, finding markets for itself through colonialism (Dutta–Bergman, 2005a). What becomes evident here is the symbiotic relationship between civil society and colonialism as an economic enterprise that sustains it. The existence of civil society is dependent upon the creation and sustenance of markets, which in turn, suggests the necessity to continually manufacture positions of inferiority that would sustain the economic functions of such markets in the form of development interventions under the frameworks of neocolonialism and neo-imperialism.

On a similar note, discussing the politics of the transnational feminist movements, Desai (2005) notes that even as dialogic spaces have been created globally in the form of women's participation in the UN's International Decade for Women (1975–85), with a follow-up conference in Beijing in 1995, the strategic focus of movements has shifted from redistributive justice to discursive and policy changes. As a result, the dialogues at the UN have operated within a framework of empowerment without really addressing the structural injustices and material inequalities perpetuated by neoliberalism. She argues that the rights based framework that has emerged post-Beijing reifies the neoliberal configuration, because the rights discourse can coexist with neoliberalism, as demonstrated in the work of most UN agencies.

Possibilities and Impossibilities of Listening. Even as certain voices from subaltern contexts get privileged within dominant discursive spaces, other voices of subalternity get further erased from these discursive spaces. This notion of representation and erasures stems from the notion of multiple subalternities; the subaltern is not a homogeneous entity that can be counted as an aggregate, but rather a concept rooted in the negative, in loss, absence, and erasure. This makes subalternity complex and dynamic, constituted in competing and cooperating multiplicities hidden from dominant discursive spaces. Therefore, dialogues with the subaltern sectors operate on the basis of engaging with certain hegemonic configurations within subaltern spaces; these hegemonic configurations represent the dominant actors in the subaltern sectors. Simultaneously, those other voices from these subaltern sectors are further erased that do not have an opportunity to participate in the dialogic spaces, and exist at the margins of the margins. For instance, in dialogic interactions with subalternity, women's voices as the subaltern of the subaltern often remain erased from discursive spaces, written into a complex hierarchy of structural and discursive configurations (see Spivak, 1988).

For Spivak (1999), the subaltern sectors have historically been configured as subaltern precisely because they have been erased by the dominant dialogic plat-forms and the discursive logics of such platforms, being cut off from the processes of upward and outward mobility that would constitute them as colonized subjects. This erasure in contemporary neoliberal politics is not simply a product of the disconnection from the center, but also because of its linkages with the center as a source of profitable knowledge and as a subject of profit, at once linked to the contemporary political economic structures of neoliberalism and simultaneously erased from these structures (Dutta, 2009; Spivak, 1999). For example, the registration of the "TAM Mild Habanero Pepper" with the US plant variety protection (PVP) office database by the Texas Agricultural Experiment Station demonstrates the ways in which dominant sectors of knowledge production carry out their economic agendas through the silencing of the subaltern and through the erasure of dialogic opportunities for the subaltern (Robinson, 2009). The variety, *Capsicum chinense*, bred from a cross between an orange habanero pepper from the Yucatan peninsula and a mild habanero variety procured by a US Department of Agriculture official from a vendor in the Suarez province in Bolivia, promises to fetch a price of US$3 to US$4 per pound, as compared to the 50 cents per pound for comparable habaneros.

Ignored in the politico-legal discursive spaces of the PVP in the United States are the voices of indigenous communities in the Bolivian and Brazilian regions that have domesticated and bred mild varieties of habaneros for centuries, and therefore own the knowledge about breeding of the mild habaneros. Absent from the discursive space are the articulations of locally situated communicative pro-cesses that would determine issues of ownership and the extent of benefit sharing with the original breeders. The effectiveness of biopiracy under the neoliberal logic precisely works through the erasure of dialogic possibilities and through the absence of subaltern voices from the discursive spaces of bourgeoisie public spheres (legislative, judicial, as well as executive). Therefore, as noted by Dutta (2009), as the indigenous knowledge in the subaltern sectors continues to be stolen through the patenting of such knowledge by TNCs under the configurations of TRIPS in global spaces, subaltern voices are erased from these spaces as grounds for claims making.

Moreover, the erasure of subaltern bases of alternative knowledge claims is quintessential to the carrying out of the exploitative practices of the neoliberal project. In the case of the biopiracy of indigenous resources and knowledge bases, global spaces such as the Convention on Biological Diversity (CBD) and the International Treaty on Plant Genetic Resources for Food and Agriculture (ITPGRFA) remain inaccessible to the subaltern sectors through their impenetrable judicial-political frameworks, and basic requirements of language, literacy, communication skill sets, information seeking capacities, and legal knowledge, etc. The policies materially influencing the subaltern sectors are developed and implemented without the participation of the subaltern sectors of the globe in these platforms. Their effectiveness in usurping subaltern knowledge bases and turning them into exploitable resources fundamentally depends upon their ability to erase the subaltern from these discursive spaces at global sites of policy-making.

Therefore, culture-centered communication processes and strategies for social change ought to continually engage with the questions of representation and voice. Whose agendas are represented in dominant discursive spaces? Whose voices are privileged within such spaces, and whose voices are erased from these spaces? How to continually seek out dialogic opportunities that engage the subalterns of the subalterns? The theoretical understanding of the subalterns in terms of hetero-geneous identities and relationships, and constituted in the realm of competing hegemonies, offers the theoretical and practical tools for engaging in politics of social change that attends to the continual processes of marginalization and erasure that are intrinsic to acts of dialogue. For example, in Basu and Dutta's (2009) work on transformative organizing among sex workers, culture-centered dialogues with sex workers organized under the collective of the Sonagachi HIV/AIDS Intervention Programme (SHIP) engaged with the narratives of material resistance organized among the sex workers, and simultaneously erased the counter-hegemonies and counter-narratives in SHIP through its articulations of a collective narrative of resistance. However, this collective narrative of resistance and change articulated through dialogue is essential to the politics of transformative practice that organizes as a collective in order to challenge the material structures that create the conditions of subalternity. The materiality of the dominant structures that create the margins in their treatment of the margins as an aggregate can be disrupted by engaging in a politics of the margins at the level of the aggregate.

Furthermore, the dialogic commitment to listening exists within the competing tensions of what the academics and practitioners from the mainstream want to see, and the possibilities of learning that are created for them from such dialogues. The entry of subaltern voices within discursive spaces is often constrained within the rules of civility, communicative procedures, and guidelines for dialogue that are pre-established according to broader hegemonic agendas. The cultural processes in dominant social institutions and the methodologies of knowledge production typically determine the criteria for dialogue. In other words, what constitutes dialogue and what are the rules for dialogic engagement are determined by dominant social and cultural institutions across the globe. It may be argued that these very rules for communicative participation limit the discursive space and the realm of possibilities that are opened up by the discursive space, fundamentally shaping who can and who cannot participate in these discursive spaces. For instance, the transnational social movements continue to be largely represented by the North, and by participants from privileged middle-class backgrounds, with limited opportunities for participation from the subaltern sectors of the globe (Basu, 1995, 2004; Desai, 2005). This privileging of middle-class, educated women in TSMs therefore co-opts the participation of women under the agendas of West-centered patriarchal structures of neoliberalism and neo-imperialism, further limiting the space for the participation of women from the subaltern sectors of the globe.

Therefore, a culture-centered approach to dialogue calls for continually questioning the meaning of dialogue, the processes of dialogue, and the rules of dialogue that constitute the fundamental elements of the communicative practice of dialogue. Furthermore, the methods of knowledge production and the tools of praxis themselves need to be fundamentally questioned for the ways in which they represent the implicit interests of the status quo, and simultaneously limit the possibilities of real social change at the local level. Methodologies utilized by academics and practitioners at the center continually need to be interrogated for the values they represent, and for the assumptions they carry out. The rhetoric of mainstream dialogue needs to be evaluated against the backdrop of the actual practice, especially given the contemporary currency of terms such as dialogue. To what extent has a call for dialogue become a branding tool, a method to portray the image of democratic openness for the organization, institution, or structure as it fundamentally attempts to carry out the agendas of the status quo?

How do institutional processes and structures that have operated for decades on the logic of exploiting the subaltern become open to listening to the voices of subalterns, which in turn, might actually end up challenging those very processes and structures if we were to truly listen to the subalterns? The communicative procedures and practices of dominant social institutions at the local, national, and global levels need to be reconfigured such that they might become open to listening to the voices of the subalterns that they have historically erased. The sort of opening up of social structures and institutional processes demanded by the culture-centered approach so that we might start listening to the voices of subalterns calls for a profound change in the communicative practices of the status quo because these practices have operated systematically to silence the voices of subalterns.

Transformations in communicative processes and practices can begin with profound reflexivity that turns its critical gaze on the instruments of listening, continually asking the questions: to what extent are we really listening? What is our commitment to listening? How do we become listeners in the sense of listening so that we ourselves become open to change through the processes of listening? How do we become open to the challenges to our essentialist value systems if we were to truly listen to the subalterns? The emphasis of reflexivity is on investing the academic-practitioner team with the capacity to listen. Therefore, the culture-centered approach, as a starting point, turns the lens on those very academic structures and processes that have historically operated on the basis of turning the lens elsewhere. The academic practitioner becomes the subject of inquiry, interrogating his/her privileges, the ways in which these privileges are carried out in his/her ontologies and epistemologies, and thus seeking out ways to continually challenge the ontologies and epistemologies built into his/her engagement with the praxis of social change. The applications that develop through this sort of reflexivity are continually questioning the values they represent, the processes they undertake, and the possibilities of listening that they open up. The key evaluation criterion that these applications are measured against is their capacity to listen.

Representation and Erasure. Dialogue creates an entry point for structural transformations such as changes in policy, changes in how such policies are implemented, changes in the ways in which the policies are reported, by creating spaces in global, national, and local policy forums for listening to subaltern voices. The United Nations Permanent Forum on Indigenous Issues is an example of one such policy forum that brings forth the issues, ideas, and interests of indigenous actors across the globe in global policy discussions, in debates with local, national, as well as global policy-makers, and therefore creating opportunities for shaping policies on the basis of indigenous interests. The politics of representation through dialogue is not one of attempting to be in the shoes of the subaltern, but rather one of working with the subaltern sectors to represent subaltern issues in mainstream discursive spaces. Participation in dialogic forums offers subaltern groups opportunities for constructing alternative narratives that stand in resistance to the status quo. For example, resisting the patent of the Neem plant filed by the United States and the US-based multinational W. R. Grace in the European Patent Office (EPO), the grassroots group Navdanya organized a collective politics of change, creating participatory forums for discussing the biopiracy, mobilizing over 100,000 signatures in subaltern communities, and networked with international organizations to file an oppositional petition to the patent at the EPO in Munich, Germany (Shiva, 2007). The alternative narratives of biopiracy create symbolic and material openings for resisting the material exploitation of subaltern resources and knowledge bases by TNCs.

In its representative politics, dialogue remains a re-presentation of issues articulated in subaltern contexts within dominant discursive platforms. New stories are told that break the silences in the mainstream. Consider for instance the reflections of the American medical anthropologist Paul Farmer of his experiences working with the subaltern sectors of Haiti:

> Today, the world's poor are the chief victims of structural violence—a violence that has thus far defied the analysis of many who seek to understand the nature and distribution of extreme suffering. Why might this be so? One answer is that the poor are not only more likely to suffer; they are less likely to have their suffering noticed, as Chilean theologian Paolo Richard, noting the fall of the Berlin Wall, has warned: "We are aware that another gigantic wall is being constructed in the Third World, to hide the reality of the poor majorities. A wall between the rich and the poor is being built, so that poverty does not annoy the powerful and the poor are obliged to die in the silence of history."
>
> *(Farmer, 2003, p. 50)*

Farmer's engagement with subaltern communities across the globe as a doctor and as an anthropologist creates openings for listening to the voices of the poor that have been silenced by history. The observation that the poor are not only more likely to suffer but they are also more likely to have their suffering go unnoticed serves as the guideline for the praxis of social change. The role of the expert, rather than being one of changing the individual behaviors of community members based on interventions, becomes one of listening to the poorer communities to co-construct narratives that disrupt the status quo.

The paradox of the representative politics of dialogue in subalternity lies in the very impossibility of listening to the subaltern voices that is written into the politics of representation. Spivak (1988) notes that to the extent the subaltern could be visible, heard, and engaged with, she/he remains no longer a subaltern. The hope for culture-centered communication scholars is to continually participate in projects of dialogue so that the subaltern no longer remains a subaltern. Rather than romanticizing the subaltern space, the culture-centered project sees the imminent need for engaging in the politics of social change that works toward disrupting the structures that create subalternity, and continually interrupts the politics of the status quo. It utilizes the tool of dialogue to engage with the materiality of the dominant structures, simultaneously realizing that the very processes of categorizing, essentializing, and aggregating that must be done in order to create spaces of change also erase subaltern subjectivities, reifying these erasures. For example in Dutta-Bergman's (2004a, 2004b) dialogues with the Santali communities of West Bengal, the aggregation of Santalis as a category is essential for articulating the politics of change and for securing access to resources. Along these lines, in Farmer's (1992) work with the poorer sections of Haiti, the engagement with the material inequities and structural injustices experienced by the Haitian poor is necessary in order to find spaces of structural change.

Furthermore, as dialogue becomes a tool for representing subaltern issues and agendas in dominant discursive spaces, it also becomes a hegemonic tool for erasing authentic opportunities of dialogue. The rhetorical framing of a dialogic position can become just that, a strategic communication tool that delegitimizes the possibilities for authenticity. The very articulations of representative politics can turn dialogue into tokenism, as a replacement of the relationships of authenticity that seek to bring about structural change. Dialogue then simply becomes a way of bringing subaltern groups under the power and control of the status quo, serving as a hegemonic device that minimizes subaltern resistance by now creating a position at the table for a token subaltern voice. For instance, referring to the UNPFII, critical interrogations of the structures of dialogue draw attention to the specific rules, procedures, and processes for dialogue.

Solidarity

Solidarity refers to the participation in the journey of social change as collaborators, working toward the goal of challenging the inequitable structures that create the material margins of mainstream societies. Subaltern studies scholar John Beverley (1999) discusses the role of solidarity as an epistemological tool for the scholar who engages with the politics of structural transformation in the subaltern public spheres. Discussing the possibilities of a "concrete friendship with the poor," he notes:

> The desire for solidarity must begin, however, with a relation of what Gutierrez calls "concrete friendship with the poor": it cannot be simply a matter of taking thought or "conversation," or for that matter of romanticizing or idealizing the subaltern . . . in making the shift from "objectivity" to "solidarity," we cannot simply disavow representation under the pretext that we are allowing the subaltern to "speak for itself" . . . And there is a way in which the (necessarily?) liberal political slant Rorty gives the idea of solidarity may also be, as the 1960s slogan has it, part of the problem rather than part of the solution, because it assumes that "conversation" is possible across power/exploitation divides that radically differentiate the participants.
>
> *(Beverley, 1999, p. 39)*

Solidarity with the subaltern contexts turns the lens on scholarship, interrogating the hierarchies in scholarly projects of social change that engage with the subaltern sectors, exploring the privileges that get in the way of dialogic moments. Getting into dialogic moments of concrete friendships with subaltern communities calls for an openness to interrupting our own privileges as academics or experts, interrogating these privileges, and seeking to unlearn them.

The postcolonial theorist Gayatri Spivak (1999) discusses this sense of willingness to unlearn our privileges as academics/experts as a primary epistemological tool for the postcolonial scholar who desires to participate in the politics of social change. For Spivak (1999), the possibility of engaging in emancipatory politics begins with unlearning one's privilege through the deployment of similar kinds of strategies based upon which we learn our privileges. Unlearning one's privilege means critiquing and challenging the history that has closed the opportunities for alternative knowledge, other options, and other possibilities; therefore, unlearning one's privilege is coming face-to-face with one's loss. It is this notion of unlearning one's privilege as one's loss in Spivak's writing that is eloquently articulated by Landry and MacLean (1996):

> Unlearning one's privilege by considering it as one's loss constitutes a double recognition. Other privileges, whatever they may be in terms of race, class, nationality, gender, and the like, may have prevented us from gaining a certain kind of Other knowledge; not simply information that we have not yet received, but the knowledge that we are not equipped to understand by reason of our social positions. To unlearn our privileges means, on the one hand, to do our homework, to work hard at gaining some knowledge of the others who occupy spaces most closed to our privileged view. On the other hand, it means attempting to speak to those others in such a way that they might take us seriously and, most important of all, be able to answer back.
>
> *(Landry & MacLean, 1996, p. 5)*

Unlearning one's privilege as a scholar and practitioner is fundamental to the creation of communicative spaces that allow opportunities for dialogue with marginalized voices that have otherwise been erased. In this sense, power cannot be wished away, and yet it is the reflexive awareness of the power attached to one's positionality that creates opportunities for dialogue (see Figure 6.2).

Reflexivity and Performance

As noted in the depiction of solidarity, reflexivity lies at the heart of the dialogic interactions with the subaltern sectors, continually questioning the credibility and meaningfulness of the theoretical categories and interrogating the viability of the methodological tools that constitute the domains of expertise of the researcher, scholar, or expert (Basu, 2005, 2009; Basu & Dutta, 2009; Dutta-Bergman, 2004a, 2004b; Ellis & Bochner, 2000). Culture-centered narratives of social change processes bring into question the very legitimacy of the knowledge structures that become the sites of neoliberal governance. Therefore, reflexivity in the study of communication for social change interrogates the privilege embodied in the assumptions of academic participation in spheres of knowledge production and knowledge circulation. Addressing such forms of privilege as barriers to engaging dialogically with the subaltern sectors that have been continually erased by the structures of knowledge production that constitute the scholar-researcher, Spivak

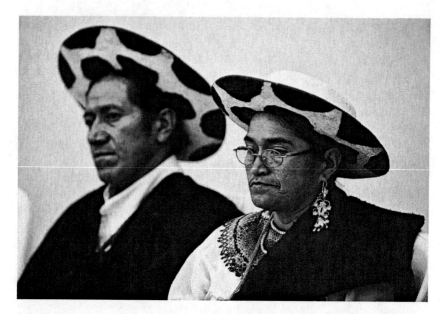

FIGURE 6.2 Ecuadorean natives take part in a working session regarding the Climate Justice Tribunal, during the "People's World Conference on Climate Change and Mother Earth Rights," in Tiquipaya, 12 km from Cochabamba, Bolivia, on April 21, 2010. (Aizar Raldes/AFP/Getty Images)

(1999) notes the notion of "privilege as loss" as a theoretical entry point for engaging with the politics of social change through a dialogic sensibility.

The dialogic element of the culture-centered approach notes that the encounter with the "other" is a moment for turning the gaze toward the self, of critically engaging with the taken-for-granted assumptions and privileges that constitute the self, and of interrogating the foundations of the Eurocentric knowledge structures that freeze the other as passive subjects of studies (Ellis & Bochner, 2000; Holman Jones, 2005; Tomaselli, Dyll, & Francis, 2008). Through a dialogic method immersed in reflexivity, participants become equal co-constructors of narratives. Knowledge from elsewhere interrogates the identities of scholars and destabilizes the knowledge categories in mainstream neoliberal structures, thus offering new openings for co-constructions of knowledge. The essence of knowledge categories are fundamentally rendered fragmented and incomplete through the dialogue with subaltern communities. Methodologically, the process of reflexive dialogue creates openings for social change through its engagement with theories from elsewhere which create impure spaces of theorizing.

In this instance, the dialogic sensibility turns toward the subject of the researcher, making him/her the subject of interrogation, and leading to the continual interrogations of the interpenetrations of class, gender, caste, race, nationality, etc. that constitute the identity of the researcher. When the scholar, researcher, or activist embedded within the dominant structure come to understand the profound implications of privilege as loss, their participation in processes of social change is evaluated in terms of their commitment to work with subaltern communities through the spaces of privilege, and simultaneously to unlearn it, to examine the margins constituted by it, and to critically examine it.

Culture-centered dialogues with subaltern contexts depend upon the ability to open up to the other in ways that would challenge the very bases of expert identities protected through the safety of methodological jargons. The performative elements of dialogue attend to the embodiment of the whole person in the dialogic space, the presence of the whole being that engages dialogically with the other through the complexities of all the senses put together at the dialogic moment, in the engagement between participants.

Authenticity and Commitment

Most importantly, dialogue is embodied in the quest for authenticity in the relational space, and a commitment to the dialogic process as a gateway to social change. The authenticity of the relationship in subaltern contexts is fragile, contingent upon the terrains that the scholar must negotiate as she/he participates in the journeys of social change in subaltern contexts. On one hand, a critical engagement with subaltern studies theory deconstructs the very roots of the processes of knowledge creation through which paths are carved out for the politics of representation; on the other hand, a positive co-constructive framework has to be continuously developed for creating discursive shifts in dominant platforms.

In the development of this positive co-constructive framework, scholars are continually brought face-to-face with the limits of the epistemological foundations that constitute their methodological toolkits as they enter the field, confronted by questions such as: What is truth? What are the entry points to social justice and structural transformations through the stories being shared? What are the political entry points for action? What are the ways in which communicative processes of social change are dialogically engaged by scholars and practitioners at the hegemonic sites of transnational knowledge production?

Take for example the transformative politics of resistance to the neoliberal processes of industrialization and development that have threatened to displace indigenous communities from their spaces of livelihood in the Eastern Indian states of Bihar, West Bengal, Chattisgarh, and Orissa (Bhattacharya, 2009; Navlakha, 2010). As indigenous groups are collectively engaged in protesting these oppressive neoliberal policies of the state using a variety of non-violent and violent strategies, the resistance of indigenous participation has been complexly constituted at the intersections of community-based participatory processes, processes of mobilizing catalyzed by the Naxalite groups in the region, and the local, state-level, and national political actors at the grassroots (Navlakha, 2010).

Social researchers interjecting themselves into this political space of social change are situated amidst the impossibilities of reconstructing adequate narratives of the local processes of social change even as they work toward piecing together the narratives through fragmented articulations, disjunctures, and gaps in the stories that are circulated, and work toward a journey of solidarity with the indigenous collectives in their resistance, narrating stories amidst the state-sponsored structures of violence. The impossibilities of co-constructing authentic narratives of social change (at such sites where the sheer volume and intensity of terror has disrupted narrative possibilities) are articulated amidst a commitment to co-creating stories that offer the foundations of a humane practice of dialogue amidst such violent forms of oppression and marginalization meted out by neoliberal governance. The sharing of stories, however fragmented, unfinished, contingent, and complex, is situated amidst a commitment to act and to challenge the material realities of oppression written into state-sponsored mechanisms of neoliberal governance.

Conclusion

In this chapter, we examined the role of dialogue in the politics of social change. Dialogue emerges at the heart of social change processes through the creation of spaces that interrupt the hegemonic frames of economic progress, efficiency, and free market economy under neoliberalism. The theories at the center are rendered impure as the lens is turned inward, the gaze is fixed on the structures of knowledge production, and embodied performances in dialogue imagine alternative visions of social, political, and economic organizing through the articulations of alternative rationalities co-constructed in dialogues with the subaltern sectors. Dialogic spaces and processes are quintessential to the politics of social change, when contextually situated in relationship with the structures at local, national, and global sites. It is ultimately through the epistemological tool of dialogue that scholars engage in co-constructive processes of knowledge production through which they participate in rendering a global imagination founded on the values of harmony, peace, collaboration, humility, respect, and social justice.

7
PERFORMING SOCIAL CHANGE

do you hear the police sirens? Beautiful, eh?
Ammmeeeeeeerica, what a beautifully scary place to be
But then living in fear is normal to us
We are all scared shitless of the immediate future
By the way, are you scared of me?
("On Fear of the Other," Performance Poem, Gómez-Peña, 2000, p. 61)

Narrating his experiences of being the "other" within the neoliberal landscape of migration politics, the performing artist Gómez-Peña disrupts the hegemonic narrative of globalization by foregrounding the everyday experience of living in fear. Performance for social change embodies the politics of representing issues of social injustice, oppression, power, control, and resistance in public spaces through the use of aesthetic forms of representations. In discussing the performance of social change, this chapter draws our attention to the gamut of micro and macro practices of communication that disrupt the status quo through their embodiment of alternatives to dominant configurations. These alternatives open up new possibilities for imagining states of being, feeling, and living, and thus bring about shifts in consciousness in how social realities are approached, lived in, reaffirmed, and challenged. It is through these shifts that possibilities are opened up for material transformations.

Performance disrupts the status quo not only through the articulation of content that resists the dominant narratives that circulate in mainstream structures, but also through the fundamental presence of communicative avenues and communication channels that exist outside the realms of the status quo (Conquergood, 1986; Harter, Dutta, Ellingson, & Norander, 2009; Singhal, 2001, 2004). Performative avenues express an alternative rationality that exists outside the world of rational deliberations in mainstream public spheres (Denzin, 2003). Through their narrating of stories embodied in a multisensory field, performances draw upon sensibilities that exist outside the realms of objectivist and instrumental rationalities of mainstream public spheres. They draw upon aesthetic sensibilities that are deeply connected to the perceptive faculties of sight, hearing, touch, smell, and taste, and engage with the human capacity for aesthetic judgment (Gagliardi, 2006; Harter et al., 2009; Strati, 1999, 2007). These avenues and channels reiterate the alternative rationalities of subaltern organizing that consistently challenge the status quo (see Figure 7.1).

Sites such as streets and public spaces become places for enacting social change, thus disrupting the aesthetic representations that circulate within these sites and the expectations that are typically attached to them. As opposed to the mainstream mass-mediated forms and channels of communication that are conceptualized in dominant approaches to communication scholarship, performance-based communication avenues bring about messages of social change through the presence of community participants at the sites of articulation, narrating alternative stories and introducing alternative rationalities. Further, this chapter explores the intersections of storytelling, art, and social change, demonstrating how alternative conceptualizations of aesthetics direct us toward social transformations. In order to substantiate

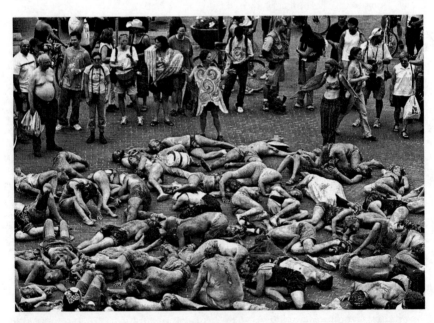

FIGURE 7.1 Anti-globalization protesters participate in the "mud dance," June 27, 2002 in Calgary, Canada. Mud-smeared protesters, some cavorting topless, cartwheeled and twirled their way through the streets of Calgary in a pagan-inspired "dirty" protest against the Group of Eight summit. (Paul J. Richards/AFP/Getty Images)

the key points made in this chapter, examples are drawn from around the globe to demonstrate how performance has been utilized in efforts of social change.

Performative Tactics

The political capacity of performance to constitute social change lies in its ability to disrupt the dominant structures and the assumptions built into these structures through the use of cultural symbols. The conservative elements of the culture embodied in the symbols that are circulated widely are pieced together at performative sites to bring to crisis the status quo. As noted by the performance artist Gómez-Peña (2000):

> Performance as an artistic "genre" is in a constant state of crisis, and is therefore an ideal medium for articulating a time of permanent crisis such as ours. Performance is a disnarrative and symbolic chronicle of the "now" and the "here." Performance is about presence, not representation; it is not (as classical theories of theatre would suggest) a mirror, but the actual moment in which the mirror is shattered. The act of creating and presenting a performance carries a sense of urgency and immediacy that does not exist in other artistic fields.
>
> *(Gómez-Peña, 2000, p. 9)*

Performances mobilize change through the embodiment of the performers in collaboration with the participants at the performance site. The presence of the actors in the performative space attaches a sense of urgency and action to performances. In this section, we explore various tactics of performance that often act together to communicate the message of transformation.

Street Protests

Streets protests are performances on streets that challenge mainstream hegemony by seeking to reclaim the streets as public sites of dialogue and debate (Ferrel, 2001; Harvey, 2001). They are typically expressed in the form of planned marches, rallies, and walks that are organized on the streets on specific issues, policies, and social injustices (Cockburn, St. Clair, & Sekula, 2000). The goal of these protests is to challenge structures and social institutions, and to voice alternative rationalities publicly, although contemporary theorists studying street protests articulate the wide divergence of these projects in their capacity to challenge the neoliberal hegemony (Ferrel, 2001; Harvey, 2001). The politicization of urban spaces seeks to recapture these spaces to narrate alternative stories that resist the mainstream narratives of consumption, commodification, and privatization.

The meanings of streets as public spaces are reappropriated and reinterpreted as streets become sites for struggle and contestation, articulating the vision of streets as sites of public dialogue and debate as opposed to the highly corporatized, privatized vision of streets (C. Smith, 2004). Street protests seek to draw public attention and attention of policy-makers by taking over the signifiers attached to the streets and by utilizing these signifiers to articulate the politics of change. In contemporary neoliberal politics, as more and more communicative spaces have been taken over by neoliberal hegemony, excluding the poorer sectors from participating in these spaces, global social movements foreground the vitality of resisting the taking over of the streets by private corporations and participating in the streets as sites for articulation of resistance and alternative rationalities into the discursive spaces of knowledge production (Bogad, 2003; Ferrel, 2001; C. Smith, 2004).

As streets have largely become privatized sites of merchandizing products of TNCs, an increasing number of social change projects have emerged to contest this appropriation of the streets, and to lay claims of legitimacy to streets as public sites and spaces (C. Smith, 2004). Based on the notion that streets are community and social spaces that facilitate communal and collective action, these movements have sought out to reclaim the streets so that they can offer alternative spaces for resisting neoliberalism. In responding to the privatization of urban spaces across the globe, contemporary urban social movements have emerged to legitimize these spaces as sites of public participation, dialogue, and political engagement. For example, the Reclaim the Streets (RTS) movement emerged in London in the early 1990s in order to resist the explosion in car culture and highway capitalism. Noting its vision, the London Reclaim the Streets (http://rts.gn.apc.org/prop 05.htm) movement explains:

> The privatisation of public space in the form of the car continues the erosion of neighbourhood and community that defines the metropolis. Road schemes, business "parks", shopping developments—all add to the disintegration of community and the flattening of a locality. Everywhere becomes the same as everywhere else. Community becomes commodity—a shopping village, sedated and under constant surveillance. The desire for community is then fulfilled elsewhere, through spectacle, sold to us in simulated form. A TV soap "street" or "square" mimicking the arena that concrete and capitalism are destroying. The real street, in this scenario, is sterile. A place to move through not to be in. It exists only as an aid to somewhere else—through a shop window, billboard or petrol tank.

The movement to reclaim the streets is situated within the politics of resituating the politics of change within the community, as a counter-narrative to hypercapitalist development projects that have taken over urban planning. It is not only an articulation of change in terms of bringing to the fore alternative issues that lie outside the mainstream hegemony of the shopping malls and billboards that have taken over public spaces, but also fundamentally a resistive strategy for laying claims over the very spaces that have been taken over by capitalism. Therefore, the calls to social change made by Reclaim the Streets (http://rts.gn.apc.org/prop07.htm) are also situated as contemporary critiques of capitalism:

> The struggle for car-free space must not be separated from the struggle against global capitalism—for in truth the former is encapsulated in the latter. The streets are as full of capitalism as of cars and the pollution of capitalism is much more insidious.

What is articulated in the propaganda documents of the RTS is the politicization of its project of reappropriating the streets. The cannibalizing of the streets to serve the merchandizing and marketing interests of global business needs to be resisted through a broader resistance offered to capitalism, and therefore, RTS movements throughout the globe have been channeled toward resisting transnational hegemony and the logic of neoliberalism. For instance, in Toronto, RTS organizers challenged the city's "public space" initiative at the Yonge-Dundas Square as a marker of the "public-private partnership" between the City of Toronto and downtown private sector interests represented by the Yonge Street Business Improvement Association (BIA) to turn the square into a merchandizing showplace for commercial interests, subjecting the public space to the "privatizing, militarizing and sanitizing forces of capitalist urban development" (C. Smith, 2004, p. 159).

> If the Board of Management declares that riding a bike in the Square is prohibited, we need to begin arriving on our bicycles *en masse*, in a critical mass; if they continue to restrict economically marginalized people such as panhandlers and the homeless from accessing the square, we need to invite our friends to begin physically occupying the site with tents and sleeping bags; if they want to turn Dundas Square into a venue for corporations to showcase their products, we have to set up our own socially-organic marketplace of competing ideas and alternative lifestyles.
>
> *(C. Smith, 2004, p. 160)*

The cultural articulations of the RTS are also materially situated. The material inequities reiterated in the contemporary urban development projects in the neoliberal era are challenged through cultural representations and symbolic markers, reiterating the linkage between the material and the symbolic. Symbolic acts such as arriving on bicycles in a critical mass, setting up tents and sleeping bags at the Square disrupt the sanitized image of the square as a de-politicized merchandizing space.

The streets remain alternative sites for disrupting the neoliberal logics propagated by the dominant global structures, and therefore street protests organized at specific sites of neoliberal hegemony disrupt the seamless logic underlying this hegemony, and draw attention to the taken-for-granted assumptions that constitute it. The very problematization of the streets as sites of enunciation and collective action remains at the heart of the struggles of legitimacy that seek to organize in the streets to disrupt the status quo. For instance, during the World Trade Organization meetings in Seattle, protesters from across the globe took to performing on the streets to draw attention to the oppressive political economy of power and control carried out by the WTO (Cockburn et al., 2000). The protests were performed at the sites of the WTO convention, and thus disrupted the symbolic markers of WTO with alternative narratives. In this instance, the street protests were performed through symbolic markers of resistance such as sea turtle costumes for the marchers to wear to protest the WTO's ruling of the Endangered Species Act, which requires shrimp to be caught with turtle excluder devices, to be an unfair trade barrier. The environmentalists were joined by the labour union members from the Steelworkers and Longshoremen, filling the streets with the chant that symbolized the Seattle protests, "The people united will never be divided" (Cockburn et al., 2000, p. 17). Marchers carried posters and slogans that symbolically articulated the politics of the movement, constructing alternative stories to neoliberalism. Human-size effigies of major political and business leaders were taken through the streets and burned. The "truth" claims of the global corporations, policy-making bodies and nation states were ruptured with alternative truth claims narrated on the streets.

In performing the stories of change, street protests take on a carnival-like character, imbued with banners, posters, songs, dances, speeches, poetry slams, graffiti writing, chanting of slogans, and so on. The celebratory performances on the streets become symbolic markers of the protest, mapping out a space in public memory and public discourse that challenges the neoliberal narrative. Depicting the creative nature of urban protest practices symbolically constituted by the street protests, Christopher Smith (2004) uses the metaphors of "playfulness" and "carnivalesque." Graffiti and property destruction are used strategically to mark up public sites, and to interrupt the narrative of neoliberalism with multiple counter-narratives. For instance, the slogan "Trade, making life better," displayed on a McDonald's window, is altered into "Trade, making life bitter." Furthermore, both symbolically and materially, the Seattle protest intended to disrupt the WTO meetings, seeking to stop the meetings from taking place. The hegemonic control of the state in carrying out the agendas of neoliberalism became explicitly evident in the deployment of police, National Guard, and federal agents on the streets; it is also at these very junctures that in response to police violence, protesters chanted "The whole world is watching, the whole world is watching" (C. Smith, 2004, p. 25). The sites of state control also became the very sites of resistance, disrupting the hegemonic narrative of the street by making explicit the function of the state in protecting the interests of neoliberal hegemony. Street protests as forms of performance interrupt hegemonic narratives through the circulation of symbolic markers and messages that explicitly question the status quo and the public relations messages of the status quo that inundate mainstream media.

Gheraos and Barricades

Gheraos refer to the encircling of public spaces that are perceived by community participants as spaces for achieving social justice. Gheraos draw their performative capacity from the ability to disrupt and challenge the status quo through the public performance of resistance, demanding justice, equity, and structural transformation. The taken-for-granted inequities that are often built into dominant structures become visible through the presence of the collective in the geographic spaces of the power structure. The presence of the collective encircling the public site stands as a representation of disruption, attempting to stop the day-to-day activities of the dominant structural configuration and drawing attention to the issue at hand. For example, commercial sex workers organized under the Durbar Mahila Samanwaya Committee in Kolkata, India, used gheraos to interrogate the role of the local police in perpetuating their oppression, and in demanding action against pimps, clients, local criminals as well as members of the police that harassed them (Basu & Dutta, 2008a).

Resistance is also communicated in the disruption of public spaces by taking over these spaces. For example in the case of the EZLN, on January 1, 1994, when the North American Free Trade Agreement took effect, rebel farmers from the local jungle communities moved into several cities in Chiapas, briefly occupying these cities, and thus drawing attention to the oppression of the indigenous peoples and rural poor in the mainstream discursive spaces of Mexican and global politics (Gollnick, 2008). The taking over of the cities marked off the public sites in these cities, and therefore the broader discursive spaces, with messages of resistance that challenged the hegemony of neoliberalism, drawing attention to the oppressive forces of neoliberalism that operated in carrying out the marginalization of the subaltern sectors.

Similarly, in their protests against the privatization of water in Cochabamba, Bolivia, the people of Bolivia took to the streets, battling the police and indefinitely blockading the regional highways and roads (Olivera, 2004). The privatization of water resources in Cochabamba, Bolivia, played out against the backdrop of water shortages faced by the people, World Bank directives of water privatization in the region, the passing of Law 2029 that declared the privatization of the water and the confiscation of wells and alternate forms of water use, and the signing of a forty year contract with a consortium of enterprises named Aguas del Tunari. With the majority of the interests in Aguas del Tenari held by US-based Bechtel Corporation, and including Bolivian companies with political linkages, it became clear that the privatization of water served the interests of the global and transnational elites, simultaneously putting large price tags for water for the poor, who could not afford the price of the water. The Coordinadora (Coalition in Defense of Water and Life) emerged in response to the inability of local community members to pay the rising price of water; the privatization of water, which Cochabambinos believed was a natural gift and a public service; the nature of government decision-making; and the erasure of the local community from decision-making structures that contracted out resources that belonged to the community without involving the community. In their protest, on January 12, 2000, the Coordinadora members blockaded traffic, smashing car windows and forcing shops to close; this was followed by a town meeting in the plaza that demanded that the government send a commission. Subsequently, resistance was expressed in the form of planning a peaceful demonstration that was publicized as the "takeover of Cochabamba," constituting the taking over physically of the main plaza, symbolically representing the coming together of the workers to make their own decisions. On February 4 and 5, 2000, marchers took over the streets of Cochabamba, setting up barricades and blockading the entire city. Subsequently, between April 4 and April 12, 2000, the Coordinadoras organized protest marches in Cochabamba, with blockades cutting off the main highways and masses of protestors occupying the city centers in Cochabamba.

Speeches

Messages of social change are often communicated by the leaders and members of communities participating in the processes of change; social movements narrate their identities and goals through speeches given by the key actors of the movements (Browne & Morris, 2006). Speeches articulate the key issues of the social change process, frame these issues, and persuade audience members to join the movement and participate in the processes of social change. The narrative element of speeches is tied to their ability to weave together stories of change that challenge dominant structures, by questioning the dominant taken-for-granted assumptions that circulate in these structures and by disrupting the mainstream rationalities within dominant structures. These speeches are delivered at the public sites of protest that are explicitly resistive such as rallies, marches, street protests, or at public sites that fall within the realms of the status quo. Public speeches play vital roles in the politics of social change, articulating the identity of the movement, defining the organizational agendas, and mobilizing public participation in social change efforts. Whereas on one hand, public speeches participate in the democratic politics of neoliberal structures by working to change policy agendas, policy frames, specific policies, as well as the implementation of these policies, they also participate in articulating a disruptive politics of change that operates through exhortations to disruptive actions as ways of challenging dominant structures.

Poetry

Poetry is one of the most powerful and quintessentially utilized forms of performance through which social change activists seek to raise public consciousness about issues (Reed, 2005). Consciousness raising through poetry involves the juxtaposition of ideas and narratives in order to communicate the message of the movement and to inspire action. Drawing from the everyday lived experiences of audience members, performances of poetry expose the underlying ideologies of dominant structures and the inequities embedded within the structures we inhabit. Poetry as a symbolic expression inspires social change through the reinterpretation of cultural rules and roles as it simultaneously draws upon cultural symbols to make its arguments (Reed, 2005). Broader cultural narratives are continually disrupted and reinterpreted in order to create spaces for change.

Reed (2005) analyzes the powerful role of poetry in the politics of social change specifically in the context of the feminist movement, noting that the feminist movement critically shifted broader cultural perceptions about issues of women's equality by juxtaposing the private against the backdrop of the public through poetry. Poetry emerged as a vital tool to identify, name, formulate, and disseminate issues, spread through leaflets, performance in small groups, public performances at large events, and performed as songs. The false dichotomy between the private and public spheres is communicated through poetic rationality, as the realms of the public and private are superimposed on each other. In doing so, feminist poetry communicates the injustices and oppressions that are carried out in the separation of the private and the public, thus raising awareness, changing belief structures, and creating openings for broader cultural transformations (Montefiore, 1995; Whitehead, 1996). For new recruits into the movement, poetry served the function of communicating the movement ideology (Reed, 2005).

Poetry also became a key site for the theorization and contestations of feminisms. These "art theoretical" discourses were central to the production of feminist identities, feminist politics, and feminist cultures (King, 1994). Movement identity and the broader theoretical issues in feminist organizing were constituted, negotiated, and expressed through poems. For example the book *This bridge called my back: Radical writing by women of color* published much of its content in the form of poetry, contesting the limits of the "whiteness" of the normative identity that was being circulated in the women's movement culture, thus creating an entry point for engaging feminist theory through the articulations of women of color (Moraga & Anzaldua, 1981). Poetry here emerged as a form of practicing, mediating, and doing feminist theory. To stretch this linkage between poetry and the political further, poetry became a form of feminist theory. Reed (2005) notes:

> the point is that poetry does not simply "reflect" ideas already in the air, but rather in giving "form" brings the ideas into public existence, and helps to invent identities, not merely to express them. Movements in general are highly productive places, sites of a great deal of "cultural poetics"—the bringing into visibility and audibility of new thoughts and feelings. In this case, the cultural poetics occurs through actual poetry. But the line across genres in this respect are constantly transgressed; Rich, Lorde, and Anzaldua are as well known for their essays as for their poems, and each reinforces and adds nuance to the other.
>
> *(Reed, 2005, p. 94)*

Cultural poetics represents an alternative rationality through which dominant cultural institutions and practices are engaged, cop-opted within movement politics, and transformed (Harter et al., 2009; Reed, 2005). Aesthetic renderings challenge dominant representations, mainstream ideologies, institutional structures, and dominant structures of knowledge production by creating new emancipatory possibilities (Johnston, 2009). The value of cultural poetics to processes of social change lies in the transformative capacity of aesthetic representations and embodiments by generating new thoughts and feelings, new ideas, new ways of being and seeing, new belief structures as well as new structures of feeling (Harter et al., 2009).

Discussing the intersections of structure and culture in the enactment of agency through cultural poetics, communication scholars Harter et al. (2009) suggest that the poetic is political. Symbolic expressions of art and aesthetic cultural forms create possibilities for challenging and reconfiguring dominant structures through the new meaning structures, thoughts, feelings, and thinking-feeling associations that they bring about in dominant discursive spaces.

Visual Art

The expression of social change politics in aesthetic platforms challenges dominant structures through the creation of cultural forms and circulation of expressions that stand in resistance to the status quo (Gómez-Peña, 1993, 1996, 2000; Teune, 2005). Juxtaposing the political against the backdrop of the aesthetic fundamentally challenges the rationalist logic to discourses of social change that emphasize the written word as the means of communicating change (Harter et al., 2009). The identity of a movement as well as its resource mobilization and impact on society are rooted in the symbolic representations that circulate around it. Art can, therefore, serve as a site of change both in terms of its illustrative potential as well as its conceptual basis (Teune, 2005).

As illustration, art aesthetically represents the political economy of contemporary issues, drawing audiences to the consequences of these issues and the complex web of meanings constituting these issues. For instance, posters and banners serve as important spaces for demonstrating the value of a message, offering visually constituted narratives to audiences, and appealing to audiences through the images and symbols they introduce into the cultural spaces. Art installations perform the resistive politics of change through the symbolic representations of meanings that disrupt the dominant cultural spaces and their taken-for-granted assumptions.

At a conceptual level, visual arts offer the interpretive framework for reorientation of collective action, interrupting and questioning the interpretive frames that circulate in the mainstream (Harter et al., 2009; Teune, 2005). The taken-for-granted constructions of meanings are disrupted, and these disruptions create new possibilities by opening up the interpretive frames that circulate in the culture.

The Border Arts Workshop/El Taller de Arte Fronterizo (BAW/TAF) created in the 1980s conducted art installations and performances that disrupted the hegemonic narratives of state-sponsored violence, racist media depictions, and US policies toward the South (Gómez-Peña, 1993, 1996, 2000). Visual representations such as make-up, dressing up, and spatial set-ups are utilized to disrupt dominant symbolic markers. In one of the early performances of the BAW/TAF in 1986 titled *End of the line*, Mexican, Chicano, and Anglo group members dressed up as "border stereotypes," sat at a large bi-national table that was bisected by the borderline between the United States and Mexico, "illegally" holding hands and exchanging foods across the borderline, "illegally" entering into each other's countries by turning the table 360 degrees, and setting fire to the three carabelas of Columbus.

The agendas of movements of social change are often carried out through the circulation of visual markers that denote the movement. For example, the iconic photograph of Che Guevera taken by Alberto Korda in 1960 became a marker of socialist students' movements and movements of the Left across the globe in the 1950s and 1960s. Similarly, the symbols of the raised fist and the colour red emerged as markers of revolutionary politics that sought to take down the status quo. Art also serves as a site for revolutionizing the fundamental conceptualization of society, thus offering a basic framework for reimagining the ways in which material and symbolic relations are constituted. For instance, in the 1950s, the concept of art as an object presented to the audience started being questioned, thus bringing a paradigm shift in worldviews of human interaction, and constituting the bases of new forms of protest that interrogated the divisions between the subject and the object. Robert Rauschenberg created his "White Paintings," which was a projection screen for the shadows of the audiences that were looking at them. Audiences, therefore, were no longer passive observers, but were active participants in the creation of the art. This move toward participatory art emerged as an important marker in projects of social change, particularly in terms of engaging with concepts of participatory opportunities for the margins. This philosophy is well articulated in George Maciunas' (1965) *Manifesto on art/fluxus art amusement*, "to establish artist's non-professional status in society, he must demonstrate artist's dispensability and inclusiveness, he must demonstrate the self-sufficiency of the audience, he must demonstrate that anything can be art and anyone can do it" (as cited in Teune, 2005, p. 7).

Songs

Songs of protest draw deeply from cultural resources and turn these cultural resources against dominant structures (Reed, 2005; Routledge, 1993; Sanger, 1995). Through songs, cultural articulations and narratives enter into the discursive space to create avenues for structural transformations. The universal politics of neoliberalism is resisted through the articulation of local narratives weaved through songs that are culturally reproduced and distributed across subaltern communities. Songs narrate stories of oppression and exploitation, and in the midst of these narratives of marginalization of the poor, create openings for change by narrating resistance and stories of subaltern participation in processes of change. The song "We shall overcome" stands globally as a symbol of resistance to oppressions and exploitations by dominant structures, drawing upon locally situated cultural symbols tied to the US civil rights movement and diffusing globally to articulate meanings of resistance in local spaces across the globe (Carawan & Carawan, 1963; Reagon, 1975; Reed, 2005). Similar roles played by songs are observed in the global labor movement, drawing upon labor songs to craft local as well as transnational movement identities and strategies.

On one hand, songs offer the identities of social change processes by communicating the message of the collective, by noting the stories of exploitation and oppression; on the other hand, songs mobilize solidarity, communicate points of action, and communicate specific tactics and strategies in processes of social change. Songs connect collectives of resistance across local sites dispersed throughout the globe. At sites of protest, through songs, local collectives resist the universalizing narratives of development and modernization, by drawing out the hypocrisies and paradoxes in development policies.

In peasant mobilizations in the subaltern sectors of India, religion offers the moral justification for resistance, serving as the foundation of the epistemology, ontology, and the practical code of ethics, including political ethics, in the local community (Chatterjee, 1982). Responding to the decision of the government to build a missile test base called the National Testing Range in the Baliapal area of Orissa, the community responded as a collective to resist the taking away of their land, livelihood, and way of life. The cultural markers of the movement, referred to as the Baliapal movement, were expressed through songs that referred to the local cultural articulations of land as mother, associated with the Hindu deity Laxmi, goddess of good fortune, prosperity, and abundance. Here's an excerpt:

> We feel this is Laxmi's storehouse
> This is our land
> By strength of which virtue
> Have we been born into this land?
> Blessed are our lives . . .
> Soil 'tis not—Our Mother
>
> *(Purushottam Behera, as cited in Routledge, 1993, p. 61)*

Land becomes imbued with meaning, not only as a source of prosperity, but also as a blessing, as the mother who protects her children. Songs frame key issues within the broader agendas of the processes of social change, mobilizing public support and public participation in challenging the dominant structures of oppression and exploitation.

Reed (2005) notes that for the Black civil rights movement, music was the primary medium for creating, framing, diffusing, and sustaining the movement's culture and through its culture and its politics. One of the key elements of the movement was its mobilization through the churches; the liberation theology of the movement was accompanied by liberation musicology. Old gospel songs that drew upon the Christian tradition and connected to the history of slavery offered the connection that linked the movement with the past. The traditional hymns that got built into the movement were recontextualized to fit the politics of civil rights. Movement activists also reworked traditional songs into new ones, with the lyrics being recontextualized to connect the narratives of the new movement with the stories of struggles against slavery. Referred to as freedom songs, these songs of emancipation became organizing and mobilizing tools, giving an identity to the movement, recruiting public into the movement, and continuing the struggles against structures. Freedom songs opened public meetings and were sung at mass protests; they became the center stage of many public performances, articulating the stories of oppression, and situating these stories amidst narratives of resistance and hope. Music groups such as the Nashville Quartet and the Freedom Singers connected the various networks of the movement ideologically, created persuasive entry points for recruiting activists, conveying the key values of the movement, and emerging as sites for communicating strategies and tactics. Singing also became a movement strategy as participatory singing enlisted audience commitment, engagement, and participation in processes of change.

Dances

The body is a performative site that enacts resistance through its presence as disruption amidst dominant structures. It is through the presence of the body at the sites of protest that social change activists communicate the messages of social change to outside actors and to dominant actors. Dances represent ways of aesthetically constituting the body in opposition to the ideologies and hegemonic configurations of dominant structures, writing scripts of resistance through the body, punctuated between its moves and ruptures, between stops and starts (Martin, 1998). Choreography becomes a way for reorganizing the spatial logic of power and control with the goal of narrating stories that challenge the oppressions and exploitations embedded in the status quo (Lepecki, 2006). Through movements, the body writes new stories, and introduces new imaginations into the cultural space, inviting entry points into the politics of change (Thomas, 2003).

Dances organize movement identity and mobilize participation at sites of challenge. Through the embodiment of emotions, feelings, thoughts, and counternarratives at the sites of protest, dances communicate messages of social change by restructuring belief structures and disrupting the dominant cultural narratives. Dance tells the stories of colonial erasures precisely through its representations of postcolonial silences, erasures, and absences at the very sites of cultural production.

Dances narrate stories of violence through the embodiment of movement brought to crisis, questioning the legitimacy of the dominant structures that write over the body as a subject of intervention. Through choreography, new openings are imagined, and these imaginations constituted the beginnings of social change in the cultural and political landscape (Foster, 1996; Martin, 1998).

Dances at sites of protest communicate resistance through the presence of bodies, through choreographies that challenge the mainstream, and through joyous celebrations that invite participants to stand in opposition to structures. At anti-globalization forums and the various social forums across the globe, dances of resistance bring about the intersections between culture and structure. It is through performances of cultural symbols embodied through the movements of body and perceived through the complexity of multiple senses that messages of social change are articulated.

Theatre

Theatre has historically been conceptualized as an aesthetic product for consumption by audiences; challenging this conceptualization of the subject-object dichotomy in theatre, theatre activists involved in projects of social change articulate the political role of theatre as a communicative space for enacting collective identities, building solidarity, and mobilizing people for collective actions of change (Cohen-Cruz & Schutzman, 2006; Freire, 1970, 1973). The theoretical development of the concept of theatre for social change is perhaps most widely recognized in the work of the Brazilian theatre activist Augusto Boal, conceptualized under the framework of the Theatre of the Oppressed. Referring to the concept of *conscientization* developed by the educator Paulo Freire (1970, 1973), where the poor and the oppressed people learn to analyze the oppressions that constitute their own social, political, and economic realities, Boal developed Forum Theater as a participatory model of political performance, where spect-actors are invited to actively participate in constructing the drama, articulating their own solutions to the problems presented in the plays, and thus rehearsing resistive strategies for revolution through the experiences of everyday life (Boal, 1979, 1992, 1995, 1998). Later in his work, Boal (1998) developed the legislative theatre to work with health practitioners, legal participants, educators, policy-makers, civil servants, as well as other professional citizenries to identify potential areas for new legislation that would address social oppressions. Working through specific problems, spect-actors engaged in developing solutions, in the process, identifying situations where solutions could not be found using existing laws. These problems were then brought to the city council with the goal of developing new policies (Boal, 1998). Theatre here emerges as a site of social change by directly putting communities, experts, and policy-makers in contact, within discursive sites that create openings for legal transformations.

Emphasizing this articulation of theatre as situated in the active meaning-making and creativity of the local community, radical black aestheticians refer to the term "methexis," meaning the communal "helping out" action of all those who have assembled for a performance (Benston, 1980). Theatre here becomes a site for collective ritualistic participation in creative meaning-making and as a site for solidarity building rather than the consumed spectacle, as traditionally conceptualized in the mainstream interpretations of theatre. For Boal (1995), methexis is the state of being in between, the state of belonging to two different worlds, "the image of reality, and the reality of the image." It is in this interplay of the real and imaginary that the possibilities of change are constituted, serving as the "rehearsal space for real life" that disrupt the taken-for-granted assumptions (Boal, 1995, pp. 43, 44).

The Theatre for Development (TFD) movement in Nigeria was started in the 1970s with the goal of creating spaces for communities at the margins to resist neocolonialism by sharing their stories of oppression and by mobilizing for social action (Amkpa, 2003). TFD trained facilitators conducted community workshops, created performances, and organized communities to stage performances as sites of meaning-making that drew attention to the neocolonial oppressions and created openings for transcending the oppressive neocolonial articulations in the mainstream. Social change is conceptualized in the form of creating spaces of change in self-concept, attitudes, skill sets, and behaviours against the backdrop of neocolonialism. Communities are organized to participate in decolonizing discourses and to create open spaces for community involvement through the use of theatre in determining the agendas for the community. Theatre here is a communicative process for organizing communities to come together to create community-driven articulations of development programs, and to articulate projects of change as envisioned by community members through their active engagement in these projects from identification to problematization to planning to implementation.

In India, street theatre has had a history of serving as a site for social change and revolutionary politics (Deshpande, 2007). The Indian people's theatre movement, Badal Sircar's Third Theatre, and Jana Natya Manch (JANAM) emerged as some of the main political actors in the early years of participatory people's theatre. JANAM came to occupy a key place as a leader of the activist street theatre movement in India, staging over 8,000 performances in over 140 towns, cities, and villages of India. Explaining the street theatre movement in the Indian context, Safdar Hashmi (2007), one of the co-founders of JANAM and the leader of the organization until he was killed in 1989 at a street performance, notes: "It is basically a militant political theatre of protest. Its function is to agitate the people and to mobilize them behind fighting organizations" (Hashmi, 2007, p. 13). Worth noting here is the emphasis of street theatre on politically organizing with the subaltern sectors, and seeking out spaces of collective organizing based on the narration of stories.

In South Korea, protest theatre, categorized as a separate genre called *madang guk*, incorporated folk culture to narrate counter-hegemonic narratives that challenged neocolonial multinational capitalism (Choi, 1995). *Madang* refers to an idealized space where agricultural communities collectively produced and shared goods before the advent of the capitalist market economy and, therefore, the symbolic articulation of *madang guk* in and of itself becomes an anti-capitalist site of resistance. Incorporating folk art forms such as the mask-dance drama, protest theatre disrupted the narrative of transnational domination with counter-narratives of subaltern solidarity, articulating the voices of peasants and workers, and sharing stories of marginalization. Theatre was essential to activism, involving activists alongside workers and farmers, serving as a subaltern discursive forum as well as a means of resistance to global hegemony. *Madang guk* performances such as *Sorigut Agu* (*Agu* is a shamanic ritual of cry) and *Unification Rice* become collective sites of articulating the alternative discourse of *minjung* that symbolically represents the collective resistance of the people.

In resisting the political economy of migration in the neoliberal landscape, the performer Guillermo Gómez-Peña uses a combination of props, costumes, make-up, song, drama, and poetry to narrate the oppressive forces of violence that play out in border crossings, in US immigration policies and in racialized portrayals of Mexico and Mexicans. Through his disruptions of the dominant narratives attached to specific spaces and sites, Gómez-Peña questions the hegemonic assumptions about immigration. For instance, in his protests against the xenophobic immigration politics of California's governor Pete Wilson, Gómez-Peña, along with his collaborator Roberto Sifuentes, created the Cruci-fiction project in 1994. The artists crucified themselves on sixteen-foot high crosses, symbolically narrating the crucifixion in the hands of the Immigration and Naturalization Services (INS) and the Los Angeles Police Department. The audiences were given a handout that read, "free us from our martyrdom as a gesture of political commitment" (Gómez-Peña, 1996, p. 102). The project received international media attention and disrupted the hegemonic narrative of immigration that circulates in mainstream media. The political and cultural dimensions of what he calls "border art" are noted by Gómez-Peña (1996) as entry points for material transformations.

Self-Sacrifice: Hunger Strikes and Suicides

Self-sacrifice has historically operated as a powerful frame for social change movements. The self is subjected into the space of political action; the body becomes the site of enunciation, and symbolically creates a discursive space for resistance as it disrupts the taken-for-granted assumptions about politics and citizenship (Sweeney, 1993). Hunger strikes, for instance, depriving the body of food, have remained a powerful act of resistance in movements of civil disobedience across the globe.

In protesting against the oppressive policies of globalization that have placed them at the margins of contemporary economies, and sharing the stories of deprivation and material inaccess faced in their own lives, farmers, miners, and indigenous people across the globe have committed suicides as the ultimate expressions of resistance to the state-sponsored neoliberal violence carried out in the form of globalization (Majid, 2000, 2008). Majid narrates the story of the suicide committed by a South Korean farmer, Kyung Hae, president of the Korean Advanced Farmers Federation, in the Mexican resort of Cancun in 2003 when he was attending the Fifth WTO Ministerial Conference:

> On the day the WTO conference opened (coinciding with the Korean Thanksgiving holiday of Chusok and around the second anniversary of 9/11), Kyung Hae climbed the steel barricades separating protesters from officials and stabbed himself to death, thus concluding a long attempt (including a self-stabbing in Geneva a decade earlier) to bring the world's attention to the destructive impact of globalization on South Korea's rural communities: "I am crying out the words to you that have so long time inside my body," he wrote.
>
> *(Mahid, 2008, p. 137)*

Kyung Hae's suicide at the very site of neoliberal hegemony became a media spectacle, thus disrupting the representations of the WTO with the stories of violence perpetrated by global policies that reify the power and control of TNCs in the global South.

Suicide, as a performance, ultimately disrupts the status quo through its narration of the structural violence that remains hidden underneath the marketing strategies, advertising campaigns, and public relations initiatives of global corporations. It breaks past the controlled and strategic use of symbolic markers by TNCs, articulating stories that are altogether different. These are stories of deprivation, of structural violence and desperation, and of loss in the face of the neoliberal project and its instruments of power and control played out through global policies. As a symbolic marker of violence, suicide enters into the discursive space to draw attention to the much more deep-seated, hidden forms of structural violence that are perpetrated by the agendas of neoliberalism in the global landscape.

Strikes

Workers' strikes across the globe have historically served as critical symbolic and material markers as avenues of protest, demonstrating the "collective, instrumental, material, and occasionally revolutionary politics of labor" (Cloud, 2001, p. 270; see also Cheney & Cloud, 2006; Cloud, 2005, 2007). The disruption of the means of production has traditionally been the predominant symbolic and material marker through which the capitalist hegemony has been disrupted, by directly attacking the economic base of capitalism. Interrupting the systems of production has been effective in creating a discursive space for engaging with the dominant power structures by undermining their profitability. In recent years, workers' strikes such as the strikes of the United Parcel Service (UPS) workers demonstrated the collective bargaining power of labor and securing workers' rights by fundamentally disrupting the processes of production and, therefore, by bringing direct interruption to the economic profitability of capitalism.

Strikes are performative as they symbolically narrate the voices of the labor in securing material improvements in the lives of workers by taking over the sites of narration in mainstream platforms. In neoliberal economies, industrial labor remains one of the predominant elements in the production cycle although workers remain erased from dominant discursive platforms. Therefore, strikes symbolically perform narratives of resistance as they disrupt the hegemonic stories of consumption and commodification by drawing attention to the oppressions of the working classes, and by foregrounding the class antagonisms that lie at the heart of the neoliberal project. Also, through various forms of aesthetic representations such as posters, banners, placards, art, songs, and slogans that they simultaneously use, strikes disrupt the hegemonic constructions in mainstream discourses, replacing them with otherwise untold stories.

Communicative Processes in Performance: Culture-Centered Notes

Based on our review of the specific tactics of social change processes, in this section we examine the broader theoretical tenets underlying these communicative practices. In doing so, we utilize the culture-centered approach to communication as the overarching framework for theorizing the use of communicative processes and practices to serve the goals of transformative politics in the realm of neoliberalism (Dutta, 2006, 2007, 2008a, 2008b, 2008c, 2009; Dutta–Bergman, 2004a, 2004b). We have noted throughout the book the three key elements of culture, structure, and agency; the interplay among these elements defines the theoretical framework of a culture-centered approach to performance. Performance is both a cultural artifact as it draws upon existing cultural practices, and an expression of agency at both the individual and collective levels. The expression of culture and agency, however, is constrained and enabled by the social structures that constitute performances. Even as performance operates within the realm of the structures that define the range of resources and interpretive frames to be mobilized, it also becomes a site for creating new frames and constituting resources creatively, thus pushing the boundaries of the cultural resources available within a community (see Figure 7.2).

Disrupting Structures

The performance of social change is fundamentally directed at articulating change through the disruption of structures (Kershaw, 1992). It serves as a communicative framework for challenging the structures of inequity and injustice that make up

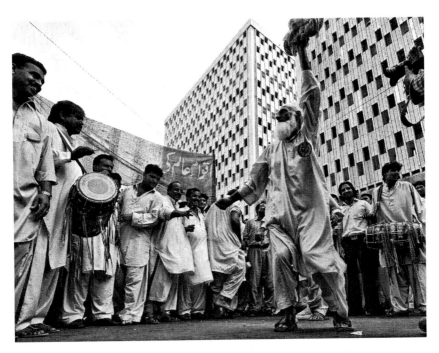

FIGURE 7.2 Members of Pakistani trade union dance against the increase of food prices during a demonstration in Karachi on May 18, 2008. (Rizwan Tabassum/ AFP/Getty Images)

the status quo. It does so by disrupting the narratives that constitute the mainstream discourses; those structures of neoliberal hegemony that perpetuate global violence in the form of the oppression of the subaltern sectors are foregrounded. For instance, the performance of suicides disrupts the stories of progress and development constructed by the World Bank, International Monetary Fund, and WTO, juxtaposing these stories with stories of hunger, poverty, and inequality. In the stories of the farmers committing suicide, the rhetoric of "progress" is countered by the rhetoric of "poverty." In this instance, performance disrupts the status quo symbolically by situating the dominant rhetoric of progress beside the lived experiences of hunger, pain, and poverty among the subaltern sectors of the globe. By opening up avenues for participation of the subaltern classes in sites of representation and enactment, performance creates an opening for social transformation.

Performances not only disrupt structures through the participation of the subaltern sectors, but also create openings for change by serving as collective sites at which new narratives and meaning structures are co-constructed by participants, and by issuing direct calls to action motivated toward disrupting structures (Basu & Dutta, 2009; Johnston, 2009; Reed, 2005). Culturally, performances issue calls for change by drawing attention to the structural injustices, and articulating calls for participation of the subaltern sectors in efforts of disrupting the structures of oppression. Consider the following excerpt from the poem "Revolution," written by the poet Langston Hughes and published in 1934:

> Great Mob that knows no fear—
> Come here!
> And raise your hand
> Against this man
> Of iron and steel and gold
> Who's bought and sold
> You—
> Each one—
> For the last thousand years.

Evident here is the narrativizing of oppression situated amidst a call for collective action in challenging these forms of oppression. The cultural narrativizing of the oppressive structures serves as the backdrop for articulating the disruptive politics of structural transformation. Participants come together at performance sites to weave together stories of change. These stories that are co-created by the performers and the members of the audience move toward active involvement in crafting a collective identity on the basis of the identification of fundamentally material inequities.

Collective identities that are created through performances weave new stories of change and structural transformation, bringing together the dreams of social justice and access to resources and juxtaposing them onto the spaces of performance. In doing so, performances open up avenues for imagining specific solutions to the oppressive conditions of marginalization among subaltern groups, and imagine alternative ways of thinking, feeling, and being that challenge these structures of oppression. As a marker of culture, performances demonstrate the material possibilities of dynamic cultural expressions that deconstruct old meanings and create new ones, participating in a "ceaseless process of unmaking old meanings and making new ones, unmasking old ways of being, thinking, and acting, and making newer ones" (Reed, 2005, p. 79). As demonstrated by the feminist movement, cultural politics opens up spaces for change in consciousness, which in turn forms the basis for legislative and other forms of political change with material ramifications.

At a material level, the performance of strikes, blockades, and barricades extend the symbolic sites of resistance to the realm of the economic by fundamentally disrupting the economic modes of production in dominant capitalist systems that extract profit through the exploitation of workers. In other words, performances disrupt the material structures of exploitation and oppression by physically interrupting the hegemonic spaces of oppression and by directly targeting the processes of production. Direct interruptions of the economic processes of capital generation continue to remain one of the most powerful strategies utilized in performances. In addition, the threats of violence narrated and presented through performances complement the symbolic articulations of resistance.

Reinterpreting Structures

Along similar lines, performance takes up the institutional structures of communication to redefine them, and to create new avenues for expression that question the hegemony of the existing institutional structures of communication, and suggest entry points for changes in existing policies. For example, the strategy of misappropriation that extracted symbols of neoliberal hegemony in everyday life and rearranged them to create new meanings demonstrates the role of performance in creating new interpretive frameworks based upon existing resources within the dominant structure (Vienet, 1967).

In the instance of misappropriation, performances become sites for articulating changes in policies by offering new meaning and thought structures, and new bases for putting forth arguments in the public sphere. Here, the aesthetic rationalities of performances perform their transformative roles by engaging with the objectivist and rationalist spaces of policy-making by creating, presenting, and re-presenting new meaning structures. Performances create openings for reforming structures by shaping public opinion and, through public opinion, influencing public agendas, public policies, and the implementation of these policies (Giugni, 2004; Tarrow, 1993; Tilly, 1978). In reinterpreting structures, performances demonstrate the ways in which the dynamic interactions between culture and agency create avenues for structural transformations. Cultural artifacts and symbols are constituted within new meaning structures to suggest entry points for policy changes.

Constituting Identities and Mobilizing Resources

The construction of identities in processes of social change is pivotal to the collective organizing, differentiating the movement or organization from other movements or organizations. It is through the articulation of a collective identity that participants are recruited into a social change organization. Identities also create entry points for mobilizing action against dominant structures. Performances serve as identity-building tools in processes of social change through the narration of the politics of change through cultural symbols, practices, and rituals (della Porta & Diani, 2006). Even as performances change within shifting cultural and structural forces, collective identities continually metamorphose, serving specific strategic purposes directed toward achieving social change (Reed, 2005).

Performances are pivotal to the telling of stories through the alignment and realignment of cultural symbols, artifacts, and myths. In processes of social change, performances connect historical narratives and culturally circulated symbols with the structures of inequities and injustice. Through performances, oppressive structures are interrupted in the narrativizing of specific problems inherent in these structures. Performances therefore work toward the identification of specific problems, placing these problems on public agendas, and disseminating the agendas and frames among broader collectives, with the goals of recruiting participants and sustaining the processes of social change. The very act of witnessing constituted in performance is a mobilizing strategy that connects the viewer, listener, or reader to the performer and the narratives of oppression. The presence of evidence embodied in the materiality of the performative site communicates the story (Pezzulo, 2004). Toxic tours through areas polluted by toxins invite the viewer, tourist, or observer into the narrative, persuading people to understand the effects of toxins in the environment and participate in active decision-making to protect the environment. The witnessing of the materiality of toxic poisoning first hand invites the audience as participants into the story, placing the responsibility on them to act.

Performances enact the identity of the movement and in doing so create internal spaces of solidarity and support within the movement, drawing upon collective participation to mobilize resources and work with institutional structures to bring about transformations in structures. Performances mobilize resources by communicating the material needs of the processes of social change, and by connecting local communities with other community networks and organizations. Furthermore, the development of community identities through performances creates a base for persuading members, leaders as well as the members of the public, to contribute resources toward the processes of social change.

Stories of Change: Culture and Agency

Performances create openings for social change through the enactment of agency at individual and collective levels (Johnston, 2009). As noted in the resistive performance works of Gómez-Peña (1993, 1996, 2000), individual performances draw upon cultural resources to challenge structures, articulating the agency of cultural participants in utilizing the cultural resources creatively and simultaneously reinterpreting these cultural resources to articulate the messages of change. For example the "Cruci-Fiction Project" drew upon the religious story of the crucifixion of Christ that circulated in the broader culture to reinterpret the violence carried out by US immigration policies. Situating the immigration policies against the backdrop of the biblical narrative of violence brought forth the hidden spaces of violence that often underlie policies on migration. Individual artists, working both individually and in collectives, participate in imagining spaces of change by creatively narrating cultural stories against the backdrop of contemporary issues of neoliberal oppression and global development.

Narratives perform social change through the circulation, adoption, and reconstitution of cultural symbols in order to draw attention to unequal structures (Polletta, 2006). Stories mobilize participants through narrative structures, utilizing metaphor, synecdoche, and metonymy. Framing of events, problems, and solutions in performances draw upon cultural resources to articulate certain frames around issues and to mobilize these frames in addressing structural inequalities. For mobilizations to be successful, studies demonstrate that the frames in performances need to be consistent with the cultural values and interpretive structures (Diani, 1996).

Social change is also enacted collectively through the mobilization of cultural symbols to narrate stories of structural violence and injustices. For instance, in the example of the Baliapal movement in the state of Orissa, India, noted above, the cultural markers such as religious stories and metanarratives were utilized in the context of the movement to refer to the fight for justice. Cultural rituals such as the blowing of the conch shells (these are to be found in every Hindu home in the area and are used to offer prayer to the Hindu deities) and *thalis* (metal plates that are used to serve food) to warn the villagers of approaching government vehicles, thereby immediately drawing villagers to the barricades, where they would lie down to create a human roadblocks that would prevent further entry into the village. Here, the cultural artifacts of conches and *thalis* enter into the symbolic space of the movement, as mobilizers for gathering people at the sites of protest. In the songs of the movement, religio-cultural narratives appear in the calls issued to the youth and women in the community:

> Blow upon your conches
> Mothers, aunts and sisters
> To shake the parliament with your sound
> Destroy the evildoers and their descendants
> In mother Durga's form . . .
> Says Purushottam, O youth
> Cower not your sorrows today
> Bear not silently but rise
> To create Baliapal
> From a second Kalinga war.
> *(Purushottam Behera, as cited in Routledge, 1993, p. 62)*

In this instance, the role of the women in the movement is articulated in the domain of the shakti (power, energy, and action) of the Hindu goddess Durga, who is a warrior goddess and was called upon to destroy evil. The sounds of the conches are called upon to shake the parliament. Similarly, the youth are urged to join the resistance against oppression through references to the war of Kalinga. Religious narratives serve the purpose of articulating the agendas of social change and for mobilizing participation. Cultural symbols offer the framework for the enactment of collective agency, thus offering the cosmological space and the repertoire of resources within which agency gets played out.

Dialectical Tensions in Performing Social Change

Culture-centered theorizing of social change posits that communication of social change is situated in a dynamic field where structure and agency are continually negotiated amidst the strategic uses of cultural symbols, tropes, and stories. Because these stories are drawn from the toolkit of the broader culture, communicative processes of social change continually negotiate the relationship between the conservationist and creative functions of culture. Culture in its conservationist elements passes down the shared values, meanings, and belief structures from one generation to the next through stories, communicative practices, relationships, and community ties. In its creative elements, culture creates new meanings, novel forms of art and performance, and new stories that open up windows to processes of change. Performances as culturally situated communicative enactments, continually negotiate between these static and dynamic elements of culture, at once picking up on the stories circulated in the dominant culture, and simultaneously opening up spaces of change.

Social Change versus Co-optation

One of the essential dialectical tensions in the mobilization of performance-based avenues is situated in the purpose served by the performance. Whereas performances have historically been and continue to be enacted as sites of articulating resistive narratives that challenge the exploitative and oppressive elements of dominant structures, performances have also been co-opted within the dominant structures in order to serve the goals and objectives of these dominant structures. For example, the widespread use of performances in entertainment education (E-E) programs is constituted within the goals of objectives of international funding agencies, campaign planners, program developers, and program evaluators, where performances become tools for optimizing the effectiveness of the behavior change messages sent out by the status quo.

For example, as Dutta (2006) demonstrates in his critical analysis of performance strategies in E-E programs, street theatres are often used by program planners to increase the reach and effectiveness of programs of family planning and population control, which in turn are situated within the status quo politics of national and international actors in framing problems of poverty and inaccess as products of population growth rather than as outcomes of large-scale inequalities and injustices perpetrated by global structures of neoliberal governance. The solutions articulated through E-E-based performances place responsibility on individual behavior change (promoting the adoption of contraceptives) whereas the solutions in resistive performances are tied to pointing out the structural inequities and issuing calls for transformative social justice and redistribution of wealth. The fundamentally resistive capacity of performances as sites of change is co-opted by the broader umbrella of E-E to carry out the overt and covert agendas of dominant global actors such as USAID, UN, and WHO, simultaneously serving the goals of the national elite. Participatory elements of performances are co-opted within the agendas of transnational hegemony to effectively diffuse messages of individual behavior change, and simultaneously reinforce the neoliberal ideology of individual responsibility among participating audiences.

The vitality of performances as sites of social change is not only tied to the strategic use of performance by social change processes toward the articulation of transformative goals, but also critical for social change theorists and practitioners to continually engage in discussions about the nature of performances and the role of performative sites in the politics of social change. In so doing, theoretical engagements need to explore the ways in which performance is shaped by the goals and agendas of the dominant institutions that mobilize performance. How are performances constituted by the goals of the change agents creating and participating in them? Whom do performances serve? What are the messages narrated through performances? What are the agendas of performances? How are these agendas carried out? Realizing the participatory capacity of performances as sites of change is intrinsically tied to the delineation and operationalization of performance, especially as it ties to the politics of performance.

Also worth noting in the articulations of social change in performance is the relationship between the symbolic and material elements of performance (Reed, 2005). In their expressions of narratives, performances create material avenues for structural transformations by drawing attention to the material bases of oppressions and inequities and by articulating transformative imaginations that are founded on the bases of material transformations.

Open versus Closed Fields

Performances of social change move along a broad continuum in the context of the degree of openness of the field of performance. On one end of the continuum, open fields of performances are highly participatory and operate on the basis of emerging scripts and narratives that arise out of the performative field. In these instances, the agendas of performance as well as the problems and solutions to be constituted through performance are left wide open. The performers and audience members come together to brainstorm about problems, corresponding solutions, and the ways in which they would enact the solutions. Members of the audience become the storyteller as they participate in the telling of the story, and the boundary between the audience and the performers disappears as audience members turn into performers of stories based on their lived experiences, dreams, aspirations, and understandings of problems or solutions of subaltern life situated at the margins of the mainstream. More fundamentally, communities become the narrators of stories through performances as open fields, drawing upon local cultural processes and symbols to share stories.

Performances as closed fields occupy the other end of the continuum, serving as sites for sending out the messages of change agents through forms of art. In these instances, the agendas of the performance are predetermined, and the message to be communicated is already dictated by the goals and objectives of the program planners. Communication in these cases is top-down and is determined within specific goals of behavior change and persuasion. The treatment of participation as a functional tool positions participation as a tactical toolkit within the broader objectives and goals of the campaign in achieving success in bringing about behavior change in the target population. The nature of performance is framed within the broader goals of campaign planners. Although local involvement may be enlisted to achieve institutional goals, the objectives of such involvement are to put together effective and efficient performance-based campaigns.

Performances navigate the broad field between these poles. Particularly worth noting are those forms of performances that are closed in the sense of being constituted by top-down agendas and are open in the appearance of their strategies and tactics of incorporating audiences in the creation of scripts and narratives to achieve the objectives of dominant social, political, and economic structures. Audience involvement in these forms of performances is directed toward enlisting the participation of local communities toward achieving the goals and objectives of transnational hegemony. The appearance of participation and local involvement is rhetorically positioned against the backdrop of the actual politics of co-optation that is achieved through such forms of participatory forums and spaces.

Furthermore, even in closed sites of performance, the continual flow of interpretive frames creates openings for multiple meanings and interpretive strategies used by members of the audience, thus leaving performances as fragmented and continually constituted texts. These elements of openness create avenues for change and transformation by creating possibilities for resistive practices. In spite of the possibilities of the enactment of subaltern agency at status quo–driven performances, it is worth emphasizing that the intent and the messages coded into these performances are situated amidst the interests of the dominant social actors. Furthermore, even as we acknowledge the fragmented sites of performances, it is worth noting that the agendas of performances are very much situated within the material elements of access and power over performative spaces.

Tied in with the notion of performances as open versus closed fields, it is also worth noting that performances of social change are on one hand strategic in the sense that they are often predetermined by social change activists and movement actors. In these instances, issues such as core objectives of the performances, the broader scripts and the roles to be enacted, etc. are already strategically determined by the performers. On the other hand, performances often emerge collectively at sites of resistance and protest, spontaneously responding to the structure and mobilizing cultural symbols in order to enact agency. In these instances, performers put together cultural symbols and artifacts and continually recreate them within new frames in order to respond to the structural inequities and oppressions, and convey messages of change. The carnivalesque feel of performances at sites such as G8 summits and WTO meetings is tied to the spontaneity that erupts at these sites, as activists come together to express their views through art, building on each other, and creating together a narrative of change. Similarly, Reed (2005) describes the scenario at Highland Folk School in Tennessee in 1960 where a group of activists, gathered together to discuss the civil rights movement, were confronted by the police. As police charged in, forcing the activists to sit in the dark, harassing them by searching through their things, a girl spontaneously started singing a new lyric of the then popular civil rights song "We shall overcome." She sang "We are not afraid. We are not afraid today." Describing this spontaneous moment of performance that stood in resistance to the oppressive structures of racism both at the moment as well as across the United States, Reed (2005) observed:

> Of course, she was afraid in that moment. Anyone would be. But in singing the fear is both indirectly acknowledged and directly challenged. Singing away a bit of her fear, she asserts the rights she and countless others are prepared to fight and die for—the right to freedom and justice in their own land.
>
> *(Reed, 2005, p. 1)*

Unity and Diversity

As noted in the performance of poetry in the feminist movement (Reed, 2005), performances of social change shuffle between their representations of collective movement identities and the negotiations of multiple competing issues, agendas, and frames within the broader questions of feminisms and the ways in which feminisms are constituted at the intersections of race, class, and gender. Performances articulate new imaginations by weaving in narratives that connect cultural symbols in sharing a collective story of social change; as they work through these new imaginations and emancipatory possibilities, they negotiate the fragmented sites and terrains of resistance that come together in articulating a resistive hegemonic presence. Furthermore, performances become the very sites of theorizing social change, engaging differences, and counter-hegemonies in processes of social change, working through differences to create entry points for social change and structural transformation. With the aesthetic openings in the terrains of art and the tools of creative sensemaking in performative expressions, they emerge as the spaces for negotiating the dynamic processes and tensions within the processes of social change.

Conclusion

Performances connect the symbolic and expressive elements of culture to the politics of structures that constitute the margins of the globe. In order to challenge and bring about transformations in political, economic, and social structures, performances connect the spaces of culture with the broader agendas of transformative politics.

Collective identities co-created through performances create openings for change, and mobilize local, national, and global public to challenge dominant structures. The aesthetic rationality of performances disrupts the objectivist rationality of public discursive spaces, thus creating new openings for stories put together at performative sites that challenge the hegemony of the dominant structures. Through their emphasis on alternative rationalities, performances fundamentally create openings for listening to the voices of the subaltern sectors and creating bridges for the expression of these voices in dominant platforms of policy-making and policy discussion.

8
ORGANIZING FOR SOCIAL CHANGE

Processes of social change are founded on the capacity of local communities to come together as a collective. It is in its identity as a collective that the community becomes a key stakeholder in decision-making processes, developing the capacities to identify the absence of resources, developing community-based understandings of problems, and putting together solutions that are directed at addressing these problems. The community becomes the locus for enacting agency, and organizing processes offer a framework for the collective agency of the community that draws upon the cultural resources to seek out spaces of structural transformation. The communicative processes involved in the formation of the collective, the crafting of a collective identity, and the development of infrastructures, capacities, and resources to meet the needs of the collective constitute organizing for social change. In this chapter, we examine the processes of organizing in the culture-centered approach that seek to bring about transformations in social structures, and rupture the silences that are perpetuated in the dominant structures of global hegemony. Particular attention will be paid to examining the specific communicative processes and practices that seek to bring about changes in social structures that perpetuate global inequities.

The margins in subaltern contexts are marked by their erasure from the sites of the mainstream. They are considered "subaltern" precisely because their stories have been erased from the dominant discursive spaces. As noted earlier in this book, the communicative erasure of the margins typically goes hand in hand with the deprivation of structural resources. Not having access to communicative spaces further reifies this structural marginalization by not offering avenues for articulating the absence of resources and finding solutions to such absences. Organizing becomes a gateway for the articulation of community-specific needs and agendas by bringing together the collective under an umbrella and therefore creating spaces of legitimacy within local, national, and global sites. It is a focal point of social change initiatives because it offers the very base on which processes of social change are constituted. To bring about changes in social structures and to secure access to resources, local communities need to be organized so that they can have a voice in policy-making platforms.

What then are the ways in which subaltern communities come together to resist the marginalizing structures that constrain their lived experiences? What are the communicative processes through which local communities work with academics and practitioners to organize for social change? What are the communicative processes and practices that are utilized by development communication scholars and practitioners in order to foster local community organizing? Although these three questions presented above are driven by fundamentally different epistemological and ontological assumptions, they share a common thread in their emphasis on community organizing as a channel for social change (see Figure 8.1).

This chapter explores the organizing function of communication as an entry point for mobilizing marginalized communities. Members of marginalized communities come together by deploying a variety of communication processes and strategies, and utilize these processes and strategies to constitute themselves into a collective. It reviews these communication processes and strategies through use of empirical evidence, case studies, and large-scale analyses of activist projects. Ultimately, the goal of this chapter is to demonstrate how communication serves as a fulcrum for the subaltern sectors to organize themselves in resisting the dominant structures. We begin by examining the communicative processes of

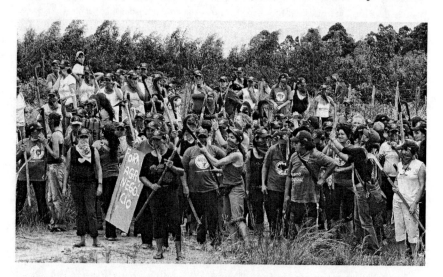

FIGURE 8.1 Members of the "Via Campesina" peasant movement shout slogans during the occupation of lands belonging to multinational firm Stora-Enso on March 4, 2008, in Rosario do Sul, 400 km south of Porto Alegre. (Duda Pinto/AFP/Getty Images)

organizing that are enacted in local communities in projects of social change, followed by a discussion of the tensions and contradictions experienced in organizing for social change.

Processes of Organizing: Culture, Structure, and Agency

Papa et al. (2008, p. 31) describe organizing for social change as "the process through which groups of individuals orchestrate their skills, resources and human potential to gain control of their future." Organizing therefore connects individuals into a collective, creating a shared space of action among them. Essential to the processes of organizing is the emergence of the collective that connects individuals and pools together their skills, resources, and human potential in order to achieve some desired objectives and agendas.

Collectives not only are organized locally in the contemporary global landscape, but also reach out beyond national boundaries, being organized across borders (Brecher, Costello, & Smith, 2000; della Porta & Diani, 1999; Tarrow, 2005). These global social movements are organized as sustainable and durable networks that identify themselves as global social movements around the "countersymbol of globalization" (Tarrow, 2005, p. 7). Acting as a collective requires organizing for the mobilization of resources, becoming aware of opportunities and seizing them, framing demands in ways that create opportunities for aligning with other activist groups and joining forces with them, and identifying common targets to act upon (Tarrow, 2005). Furthermore, della Porta and Diani (1999) note the importance of a collective identity and a durable network structure to movements of social change.

Information Sharing

Marginalization is achieved and reified through the limited access to information resources among the subaltern sectors of the globe. These global inequities in spaces of information get carried out in terms of the absence of subaltern voices from the discursive spaces of knowledge production as well as the absence of adequate communication infrastructures for sharing information about important policies with subaltern communities. Spatially, the subaltern sectors remain hidden from dominant discursive spaces precisely because of their location at the margins of mainstream information resources. In other words, to a large extent, the global margins are constituted in the inequities in information infrastructures and the limited accessibility to such structures in the mainstream. Processes of social change, therefore, fundamentally work toward addressing these inequities, so that communities at the margins have access to information resources, and to spaces of policy-making where they can share their voices.

Furthermore, information sharing is also pivotal to the organizing processes of the movement. The infrastructure of the movement is built upon information, as individuals in the collective share information to create common foundations and agendas for the collective. Similarly, information sharing is crucial to the identification of resources and to the mobilization of the collective for the purposes of securing access to these resources in the processes of change. It is also through information sharing that specific strategies and tactics are evaluated and decisions are made collectively about the next steps of the social change process.

Information is a key resource in processes of social change, offering access to resources for local communities, developing community-wide platforms for discussions of issues, communicating about strategies, tactics, and events, as well as offering process-based knowledge that is necessary for structural transformation. Collectives are organized through the sharing of information, and community knowledge of critical community issues, local and global policies, as well as the implementation of these policies is essential to organizing. Therefore, information seeking, information gathering, and information sharing are vital functions in organizing that are carried out in local communities participating in processes of change. One of the essential elements of community solidarity building is the sharing of information about the situation, the problem specific to the local community, vital resources, avenues of change, and strategies and tactics of communication to be utilized by the community. Therefore, most social change projects focus on creating awareness initiatives in the preliminary stages, with the goal of developing community networks around relevant issues.

Identifying Issues

Collectives of social change are typically organized around community-specific issues that need change (Giugni, 2002). In other words, change becomes a key element in organizing processes, and it is constituted around issues that are seen as problems by community members. The articulation of a common problem becomes the central point of organizing, the reason behind the coming together of individuals and groups into a broader collective. Therefore, a core component of the organizing process is to identify an issue that threatens the community and to articulate the ways in which the issue relates to the members of the community. Issue relevance is pivotal in the early stages of the collective organizing processes. It is in situations when a community perceives an issue to be present, sees it as relevant to itself, and interprets it as a threat that the seeds of social change processes are sown. For instance, the interests of those directly affected by the building of dams in southern Brazil led to the formation of the Comissao Regional de Atingidos por Barragens (CRAB), constituted around the issue of land struggle (Rothman & Oliver, 2002). Similarly, the Narmada Bachao Andolan in India was organized around the issue of the land rights of communities threatened to be displaced by the building of a dam over the river Narmada (Dutta & Pal, 2007).

Although the issues identified are locally situated within the experiences of local communities, they often embody globally positioned arguments. The identification of the issue of class struggle lies at the heart of the revolutionary project of Marxism, played out in projects of resistance across various local communities of the globe. In other words, in Marxist processes of social change, class antagonisms fundamentally underlie social change initiatives. Here, social change processes are constituted on the basis of the identification of the oppressive elements of capitalist social systems, including the exploitation of labor that results in the profit margins for capitalists. The inherent conflict in the interests of the proletariat against the backdrop of the interests of the capitalist classes serves as the framework for the organizing of social change. For instance, several Marxist and Marxist-Leninist movements across the globe are constituted on the framework of class struggle, calling for transformative practices that would overthrow the neoliberal systems of oppression and exploitation of the poorer classes (Giugni, 2002). Poverty and exploitation of the poor emerge as the key organizing concepts that constitute such movements. Along these lines, the organizing of global movements against neoliberalism is founded on the issue of the negative economic effects of neoliberalization on the world's poor and the increasing chasm between the world's rich and the poor brought about by the large-scale adoption of neoliberal policies (Reed, 2005; Starr, 2005).

Similarly, the global movements against dams connect various local and transnational actors on the issues of the negative economic, political, environmental, and displacement effects of dams (Blaser, Feit, & McRae, 2004; Burt & Mauceri, 2004; Chatterjee, 1983; Chaturvedi, 2000; Pal & Dutta, 2008a, 2008b; Rothman & Oliver, 1999). The global base for collective organizing connects the local actors on globally situated issues that are constituted within global structures. Therefore, issues that are situated amidst structures take on local meanings in the cultural contexts of the lived experiences of marginalized communities, and simultaneously draw upon a global framework to create spaces of resistance the cut across geographic and cultural boundaries. The global social change network International Rivers connects several communities, movements, NGOs, and other partners across sixty countries to protect rivers by protesting the building of dams and promoting alternative development frameworks for meeting water, energy, and flood management needs (www.internationalrivers.org/). These alternative development frameworks are situated locally even as they are constituted within a broader global agenda of resisting the development projects funded by the World Bank and other financial institutions.

As noted in the examples presented here, resistive organizing around issues exists in a dialectical relationship with the structures of power and control through which the issues arise. Subaltern organizing often emerges in response to issues raised in the mainstream that are directed toward further carrying out the agendas of power and control in the hands of the status quo. The issue becomes the site of the collective organizing, bringing together the collective in networks of solidarity. For instance, with the large-scale funding of the Human Genome Diversity Project with the goal of mapping genetic variations in indigenous samples across the globe, indigenous collectives and activists responded by questioning the fundamental violation of the indigenous worldview, the continued colonization of indigenous spaces, and the political economy of exploitation of indigenous spaces to create knowledge resources that could then be used by TNCs (Wood, Hall, & Hasian, 2008). Indigenous communities organized around the issue, came together at a collective meeting of several interested indigenous organizations, and put forth "The Declaration of Indigenous Peoples of the Western Hemisphere Regarding the Human Genome Diversity Project" (www.ipcb.org/resolutions/htmls/dec_phx.html) stating:

> In the long history of destruction which has accompanied western colonization we have come to realize that the agenda of the non-indigenous forces has been to appropriate and manipulate the natural order for the purposes of profit, power and control. To negate the complexity of any life form by isolating and reducing it to its minute parts, western science and technologies diminishes its identity as a precious and unique life form, and alters its relationship to the natural order. Genetic technologies which manipulate and change the fundamental core and identity of any life form is an absolute violation of these principles, and creates the potential for unpredictable and therefore dangerous consequences. Therefore, we the Indigenous Peoples and Organizations participating in this meeting from North, Central and South America reject all programs involving genetic technology. We particularly oppose the Human Genome Diversity Project which intends to collect, and make available our genetic materials which may be used for commercial, scientific and military purposes. We oppose the patenting of all natural genetic materials. We hold that life cannot be bought, owned, sold, discovered or patented, even in its smallest form.

Here indigenous resistance is constituted around the perception of the Human Genome Diversity Project as a violation of the indigenous worldview. The principles of gene mapping are juxtaposed in the backdrop of the indigenous worldview of harmony and balance with nature. The issue is identified within the realm of Western colonialism and destruction of nature, thus drawing upon grand narratives that are pertinent to the lived experiences of indigenous communities across the globe. It is on the basis of the identification of the issue that the collective articulates its site of struggle, creating an entry point for the mobilization of resistance. Resistive politics of social change works around the interrogation of issues within social structures that perpetuate the marginalization of communities. As noted earlier, issue identification processes involve information gathering, information dissemination, and creation of knowledge bases among collectives. Collectives continually come together to actively enact their agency in the interpretation of information, and in the processes of organizing around issues. Furthermore, in their organizing as collectives, the subaltern sectors create frames around issues that offer alternative entry points for processes of social change.

Framing Issues

The ways in which issues are framed are critical to the organizing of social change processes (Benford & Snow, 2000; della Porta, 2009; Johnston & Noakes, 2005; McAdam, McCarthy, & Zald, 1996a,1996b). Frames are interpretive lenses for constructing issues, and serve as sites of resistive practice by offering alternative and/or competing interpretive frameworks for understanding issues, thus challenging the dominant interpretations and modes of political and economic organizing (Meyer & Staggenborg, 1996; Noakes & Johnston, 2005; Staggenborg, 1986, 1988, 1989, 1991). They focus our attention on what is relevant and draw attention away from extraneous items in the field of view, persuading a wider collective to participate in processes of change. The term *collective action frames* or *framing processes* refers to the dynamic processes of defining what is going on to create a collective site of action. Snow and Benford (1988, 1992; see also Snow, Rochford, Worden, & Benford, 1986) categorize three basic framing tasks as diagnostic (focusing on the detection of problems and pointing out what is wrong and why), prognostic (presenting a solution to the problem identified in the diagnostic framing process), and motivational (giving potential recruits a reason for joining the collective action).

For social movements to work, they have to break the accepted frames that operate within the status quo, in dominant institutions of society, and in the media, working to serve the dominant interests and discouraging collective action (Noakes & Johnston, 2005). Frames, in summary, create resistive entry points into policy-making, implementation, and evaluation by challenging the taken-for-granted assumptions in the dominant systems of knowledge production (Desmarais, 2007). For example, the Via Campesina movement (http://viacampesina.org/en/index. php) is a transnational movement made up of several local organizations of peasants, farmers, farm workers, indigenous agrarian communities, and rural women spread across the globe that seek to offer alternative meanings of development and agriculture, challenging the neoliberal framework of agricultural development (Desmarais, 2007; Via Campesina, 1996, 1999). The alternative framing of development emerges at the core of the collective organizing processes of Via Campesina.

The roots of the movement are situated in the Managua Declarations that emerged out of the discussions among representatives of eight farm organizations from Central America, the Caribbean, Europe, Canada, and the United States:

> Neoliberal policies represent a dramatic constraint on farmers throughout the world, bringing us to the brink of irredeemable extinction and further aggravating the irreparable damage which has been caused to our rural environs . . . We note that GATT affects farmers in poor countries and as

well impoverishes farmers in rich countries to the benefit of monopolies and transnational corporations. Trade and international exchange should have as their fundamental goal, justice, and cooperation rather than competition and the survival of the fittest. We as producers need to be guaranteed sufficient income to cover as a minimum our costs of production. This, to date, has not been a concern of the negotiators of the GATT. We reject policies which promote low prices, liberalized markets, the export of surpluses, dumping and other export subsidies. Sustainable agricultural production is fundamental and strategic to social life and cannot be reduced to a simple question of trade.

(Managua declaration, 1992, as cited in Desmarais, 2007, p. 76)

The foundations of the social change process in the Via Campesina movement are based upon the critique of neoliberal hegemony and the widespread narrative of neoliberalism that promises uncontrolled development through privatization, allocation of land for large-scale development projects, displacement of farming communities, and liberalization. The grand narrative of neoliberalism that promises economic growth and a trickle-down effect is challenged through the articulation of an alternative frame that reinterprets the goals of trade and international exchange in the realm of social justice and cooperation. The competition-based framework of neoliberalism is challenged by an alternative framework of co-operation and sustainability. Trade is juxtaposed against the backdrop of social life in driving the criteria for the measurement of the effectiveness of a development model, thus disrupting the taken-for-granted ideologies underlying the articulations of development in mainstream globalization processes.

Frames are particularly important as communicative mechanisms for connecting resistive movements that seek transformations in neoliberal policies that operate on the basis of their global reach and penetration. On a global scale, the global social justice movement (GJM) emerges on the discursive and material spaces of social change through the framing of global concerns and by targeting global enemies within a global field of action (della Porta, 2009). One of the key frames that emerges in the GJM is the framing of alternative mechanisms for regulating markets, trade, and development on the basis of issues of human dignity, economic justice, social and political justice, equality, and access among the marginalized to basic resources. Connecting the various groups from across the globe that come together to organize for global change under the GJM network of networks are the frames of rights, social justice, another democracy through participation from below, and the global nature of action. Frames here serve the symbolic function of connecting actors within organizing processes, connecting various organizing processes together into networks, and furthermore, connecting these networks into "networks of networks" in the global arena.

Movement frames draw upon the existing symbols, interpretive resources, and artifacts from the cultural stock, putting together these symbols in the context of resistive strategies, articulating new frames for looking at issues, problematizing existing structures, suggesting alternative solutions, and seeking to recruit participants into the movement (Snow, Rochford, Worden, & Benford, 1986; Swidler, 1986). The relationship between the symbols circulated in resistive processes of social change and the broader domains of popular culture is dynamic because even as communicative processes of social change draw upon existing cultural symbols in order to create spaces of change, they do so in negotiation with the status quo that is embedded within the popular culture. Frames advocating social change continually negotiate the divergent needs of aligning with broader cultural rationalities and simultaneously utilizing these symbols to create a mobilizing frame that motivates participation in processes of social change.

As Valocchi (2005) notes, the effectiveness of resistive frames depends upon the extent to which the cultural symbols in these frames resonate with the potential constituents of the social change process, mobilizing these constituents into action. The concept of *frame resonance* taps into the congruence between the collective action frame, the interpretive frameworks of the targeted community, and the broader culture (Gamson, 1992). Snow and Benford (1992) note that frame resonance is influenced by frame consistency (frames are logically consistent in their core values, beliefs, strategies, and tactics), empirical credibility (frames make sense with the ways in which the target audience sees the world), experiential commensurability (the congruency of the frames with the everyday experiences of the target audience), centrality (the importance of the core values and beliefs articulated by the frame to the lives of the targets), and credibility of the frame's promoters (the perceived expertise and trust of the sources of the social change messages). To increase the resonance of frames, four frame alignment strategies are often put to use: frame bridging (linking two or more previously unconnected frames that have an affinity, such as indigenous rights and environment), frame amplification (communicating the essence of the movement in a catchy phrase or slogan), frame extension (extending specific aspects of a frame to new areas that are considered to be important to the target audience), and frame transformation (generating new meanings and changing old interpretations and meanings) (Snow et al., 1986).

Frames are communicated to the audiences of social movements through the communicative processes of articulation and amplification (Benford & Snow, 2000; Snow & Benford, 1998; Tarrow, 1998). The process of articulation involves the connections among and aligning of events, the selection and packaging of cultural symbols, and the representation of particular narratives such that dominant structures may be challenged. Articulation involves the selective "punctuating and encoding of objects, situations, events, experiences and sequences of action" in order to create a meaningful interpretive framework for the audiences of the message. Particular symbols are picked from the cultural framework and are positioned in specific alignments to craft particular narratives around a specific set of selected events in order to mobilize public participation in the processes of social change.

The processes of articulation are complemented by the processes of amplification that select and highlight various issues, events, or beliefs from the broader cultural universe and interpretive frameworks of the movement. Amplification strategies are evident in the use of slogans and bumper stickers that communicate the salient points about the movement. Similarly, catchphrases crystallize some key ingredients of the movement in an easily memorable message. Noakes and Johnston (2005) note that powerful tactical choices highlighting the messages of a movement include historical examples, metaphors, visual images, and cultural stories. Frames can also be communicated through art, songs, dances, and other forms of performances. Along similar lines, non-verbal signifiers such as dress, gestures, and facial expressions are also strategically used to amplify the core messages of processes of social change.

Empowerment, Local Representations, and Voices

Empowerment refers to the creation of relational spaces within local communities that situate positions of power within these local spaces. Empowerment processes are critical to organizing for social change as they bring about the collective recognition of the community of its ability to participate in processes of social change. Unless communities and collectives believe in their ability to bring about change, they would not be activated to participate in processes of change. In the participatory development approach, local communities are empowered through the interventions by outside experts that impart the skills of empowerment in these local sites.

The culture-centered approach notes the agency of the subaltern sectors to participate in processes of change as the starting point for its politics of change. In doing so, it departs from highly deterministic conceptual frameworks that construct subaltern communities as passive and without agency. Instead, it makes the fundamental argument that communities and collectives that live at the margins of dominant societal configurations have the inherent capacity to resist such configurations. Empowerment, therefore, is understood as the understanding of the relational processes of power dynamics that operate at the intersection of the local and the global. Empowerment in the culture-centered approach is concerned with the acknowledgement of the capacity of local communities to make their own decisions that are aligned with their lived experiences.

One of the key elements in processes of social change is the representation of diverse local stakeholders in the social change collective. The organizing of social change draws its legitimacy from the grassroots organizing of local actors with specific geographic ties within local communities. The representation at the grassroots level creates a channel for the articulation of issues, and for the participation in identification of solutions, and development of strategies and tactics. Local representations at global sites are quintessential to social change processes that disrupt globally situated structures through the presence of locally situated narratives. The inequities in representation between the various sectors of the globe are addressed through the creation of spaces for presenting the voices of the poor and historically oppressed sectors of the globe.

Processes of social change are organized on the basis of identifying the erasure of the subaltern sectors from the mainstream spaces of policy-making. For example, as noted earlier, global movements against neoliberalism are constituted on the issue of the absence of subaltern voices from policy-making circles. The undemocratic decision-making structures of global financial institutions such as the World Bank and the WTO become the sites of organizing for global activist groups, seeking to create spaces for the enactment of subaltern agency, where the voices of marginalized groups may be heard. The undemocratic communicative processes embodied in the global structures emerge as the site of social change organizing that seeks to address this inequity by creating spaces where the voices of marginalized groups may be heard. Therefore, a key element in organizing for social change is the creation of spaces and spheres of listening to voices of the marginalized sectors.

Along similar lines, the global anti-dam movement seeks to disrupt the hegemonic spaces of development policy-making and World Bank policy-making by seeking to create opportunities for listening to the narratives of the poor who are affected by the building of the dams (www.internationalrivers.org/). Noting the absence of the poor from the dominant spaces of knowledge production and policy-making, the transnational movement notes the importance of creating spaces where the voices of the poor can be heard in policy circles and alternative narratives of development can be created. The emphasis on creation of spaces is seen in the policy reports and correspondences that the organization engages in with funders in order to hold them accountable and to interrogate the hegemony of the dam discourse that circulates in dominant structures of development.

Similarly, the Via Campesina movement that developed in response to the agricultural policies of GATT that excluded the world's poor engaged in the agricultural sector, sought to create spaces of change by creating entry points for listening to the alternative narratives presented by the farming and peasant communities across the globe (Via Campesina, 1996). Noting that the exploitation of the peasant communities in the hands of neoliberal structures is fundamentally tied to the absence of the local voices from the discursive space, Via Campesina sought to open up discursive spaces for articulating the voices of the peasant sectors:

> To date, in all the global debates on agrarian policy, the peasant movement has been absent; we have not had a voice. The main reason for the very existence of the Via Campesina is to be that voice and to speak out for the creation of a more just society . . . What is involved here is [a threat to] our regional identity and our traditions around food and our own regional economy . . . As those responsible for taking care of nature and life, we have

a fundamental role to play . . . The Via Campesina must defend the "peasant way" of rural people.

(Via Campesina, 1996, pp. 10–11, as cited in Desmarais, 2007, p. 77)

Worth noting here is the work of the collective toward the creation of spaces such that the voices of the peasants may be heard in those very policy circles that make decisions about their lives. Situating the oppression of the agrarian sectors in the absence of these sectors from policy circles, Via Campesina works toward creating spaces and serving as a voice of the peasant movement. The creation of spaces such that local voices may be heard within such spaces is a key element in the organizing of social change processes. Neoliberal structures are disrupted through the enactment of agency; simultaneously, the enactment of agency is facilitated through the availability of certain structural configurations within dominant spheres that leave openings for resistance. The culture-centered approach makes note of this cyclical relationship between structure and agency; on one hand, structure is disrupted through the enactment of agency; on the other hand, structures offer opportunities for the enactment of agency even as they constrain agency in a wide variety of ways.

Negotiating Identity

Processes of social change are organized around specific identities that drive the ability of collectives to recruit and retain members, and to participate in communicative processes of social change. Therefore, critical to the organizing of social change is the creation of specific identities for the social change processes (Klandermans & de Weerd, 2000; Melucci, 1996). Identities of movements are central to the existence of the movement, to its articulations of problems and solutions and to the mobilization of frames for the purposes of recruiting participants. These identities are expressed in the actions of the collective, therefore offering the broader template for symbolic and material actions (Touraine, 1985). Simultaneously, identities offer the defining framework for collective action, determining the range of strategies and the ways in which these strategies are negotiated and expressed in order to bring about social change.

For instance, transnational feminist networks are globally organized across disparate local spaces on issues of women's rights and participation, and follow similar sets of strategies and tactics in critically engaging with policy and legal issues at the local, national, international, and global levels (Moghadam, 2009). The identity of these transnational feminist networks is founded on the principles of women's rights, and is broadly constituted around the issues of neoliberal economic policies, religious fundamentalism, and peace. The three strands of transnational feminist networks of protests are constituted against global neoliberal policies that economically exploit women, religious fundamentalism that oppresses women, and the military-industrial complex that wages war and threatens women through various forms of state-sanctioned violence.

The framing of maternal identity foregrounds the collective solidarity that binds together the organizing of the Mothers of Heroes and Martyrs of Matagalpa, a political organization controlled by the Sandinista National Liberation Front (FSLN), and comprising mostly very poor women in Nicaragua who had lost at least one child in the war or revolution in Nicaragua (Volo, 2000). The communicative efforts of the mothers was directed at an international audience, particularly against the backdrop of US involvement in the Contra war, the international solidarity movements against it, and the resulting economic and political crises that were tied to the war. The Mothers of Matagalpa drew upon their roles as mothers of the fallen Sandinistas to mobilize the identity of Las Continuadoras (the continuers) to carry on the struggles of their children. In subsequent years, after the end of the war, the group continued to build on the frame of continuation to mobilize against the structural adjustment programs triggered by neoliberal policies. As Dona Maria, a participant in the mothers' movement, narrated:

> As long as we participate . . . [in] our revolution, our children haven't died. Our children continue to live because they fought so that we would know our culture, so that the poor would have land, so that the poor would have a house . . . And so we can't stop struggling for land for the *campesino*, for housing, for health because for all this our children died . . . The important thing is to keep alive the memory of the heroes who loved us . . . It's that as long as we struggle, they haven't died—nor are they going to die.
>
> *(Volo, 2000, pp. 142–143)*

The identity of motherhood is negotiated by the Mothers of Heroes and Martyrs through the framing of continuation, built around the theme of continuing the struggles that were once carried out by the now-dead children of the mothers. The obligation to continue the struggles of the children emerges as a mobilizing frame, constituting the commitment of the mothers to the struggles for social justice and equality.

Resource Identification and Mobilization

The capacity to effectively form a collective organization that comes together to articulate the politics of change is tied to the access to structural resources, and to the ability to put together these resources in order to meet the needs of the collective as it participates in the processes of social change (Lofland, 1996). Therefore, communicative processes of social change emphasize the identification of resource needs, and the further mobilization of the collective to create basic resource capacities in order to establish the foundations of the social change processes (della Porta & Diani, 2006). The symbolic becomes the realm of organizing the material, issuing persuasive messages seeking material support, and communicating with key stakeholders to develop economic resources for the processes of social change.

This element of community organizing for processes of social change draws attention to the intersections of the symbolic and the material; the symbolic is continually projected onto the spaces of the social change process in order to maintain the material necessities of organizing for social change (Giugni, McAdam, & Tilly, 1998, 1999). Social change processes depend upon their economic bases and access to material structures in order to bring about changes in these structures. Therefore, activists working on change engage in a wide variety of steps in order to attract material resources, working with stakeholders within the processes of social change as well as with outside stakeholders. The deployment of strategic communication attains the goal of securing funds for the movement organizing, working through institutional mechanisms as well as a wide variety of community networks and ties. The formation of ties outside the local has increasingly become relevant in the global formations of resistive politics, organizing in collaboration with global support structures to bring about change locally, nationally, and globally.

The framing of the issues, their problematization, and the appeal of the possible solutions being proposed are tied to the ability of the social change processes to generate an economic base of support. The effectiveness of the processes of social change are tied to the effectiveness of the networks built, and the ability to communicate clearly with these networks to articulate common points of praxis. The organizing of networks is also critical to the optimization of resources, developing movement alliances across a wide range of issues in order to create a powerful resource network. For instance, the linkages between the indigenous land rights movements and the movements of the environment optimize the resources of multiple organizations to articulate a clear and powerful message against neoliberal policies of industrialization that have displaced subaltern communities and simultaneously threatened the environment. A large number of material resources such as grants, local fund collection, government aid, private funds, dues, direct mail, phone banks, fundraising events, sales revenue, canvasing, and public place solicitation and selling are explored in order to develop supportive infrastructures and create spaces of change (Lofland, 1996).

Elite Relationships with Institutional Political Actors

As processes of social change seek out opportunities for structural transformation, they engage with institutional political processes and political actors to bring about changes in global, national, and local policies (Moghadam, 2009). Noakes and Johnston (2005) describe political opportunities as structural factors that are external to social movements and affect the actions and results of social change processes by creating linkages to positions of power. Tarrow (1992) notes that political opportunities include channels of access to political institutions of decision-making, the availability of political allies to resistive groups, the stability of political alignments and institutions, and divisions among political elites. These political opportunities are dynamic and continually negotiated amidst relationships of power; they create openings for the articulations of the politics of social change within dominant political and economic spaces (McAdam, McCarthy, & Zald, 1996a, 1996b). Political opportunity structures on one hand shape the communicative frames in social change processes, and on the other hand, are shaped by the frames of protest in processes of social change.

The political networking with dominant institutional structures is crucial to the success of social change processes. For instance, the implementation of the Biodiversity Law in Costa Rica that protects the rights of indigenous people and peasant communities to the local knowledge that has been developed in these communities was made possible through the development of linkages with resource-based allies (Miller, 2006). In the face of the neoliberal agendas that seek to bring knowledge under the control of TNCs, the Biodiversity Law in Costa Rica sought to protect the intellectual property rights of the rural communities for the uses they have developed for the natural resources and the plants and animals they have bred (Miller, 2006). In organizing to create the spaces for the discussion and creation of the policy in response to the growing threats of bioprospecting, a coalition of legislators, lawyers and scientists came together to work with the National Indigenous and Peasant Boards. The experts in the coalition were organized under the broader framework of the Office for Mesoamerica of the World Conservation Union (IUCN) and the National University of Costa Rica.

The National Indigenous and Peasant Boards received outside support in the form of legislative involvement from among the political elite, legal and scientific advising from IUCN, and the support of the National University of Costa Rica through the CAMBIOS program that sought to train indigenous and peasant leaders about the biodiversity law debates and how to protect their indigenous forms of knowledge. Furthermore, international linkages were fairly crucial in developing the support structures for the processes of social change among the indigenous and peasant communities, with resources, information, training, as well as funding resulting from transnational linkages. Similarly, in the Philippines, the networks of scientific communities have worked collaboratively with legal experts and civil society to develop the biodiversity laws (Swiderska, Dano, & Dubois, 2001) and in India, NGOs working with indigenous communities have been actively involved in attempting to shape the biodiversity policies (Anuradha, Taneja, & Kothari, 2001).

International Networks of Solidarity

As noted earlier in this book, globalization processes have produced severe structural inequalities and poverty through the SAPs imposed by the IFIs such as the IMF and the World Bank, creating similar threats and opportunity structures across nation states throughout the globe (Johnston, 2009; Johnston & Noakes, 2005; Walton & Seldon, 1994). Against the backdrop of globalization and internationalization, social change collectives are increasingly organized in transnational activist groups that seek transformations in global policies because these policies create similar types of threats and opportunity structures (McAdam & Rucht, 1993; J. Smith & Johnston, 2002). Collective transnational networks become increasingly relevant globally as they address grievances of a global character and work simultaneously to address state-level organizations (J. Smith & Johnston, 2002). They do so by engaging with international opportunity structures that offer an entry point for articulating their voices at the international level, articulating resistance against issues of global character (Reimann, 2002).

Social movement organizations work collectively by building cooperative networks with other social movement organizations across borders that resemble their own, sharing a common base of experiences, identities, and organizational forms. Local-global connections become vital to the organization of resistance. For example, local church-based and labor-led mobilizations in the anti-dam movement in Brazil connected with international environmental challenges to World Bank lending policies, thus offering a new political ecology frame that offered novel and globally informed ideas about local grievances and their solutions (Rothman & Oliver, 2002). Powerful frames for addressing local problems emerge when activists get together across borders and generate frames and strategies of protest (J. Smith & Johnston, 2002). The linking of environmental movements and movements of indigenous rights, for example, creates new frames and strategies for collective global organizing against transnational targets such as the IFIs, UN organizations, and TNCs.

These international opportunity structures have been facilitated by, first, the increasing availability and use of the Internet as a communicative platform; second, the UN conferences of the 1990s that created global political opportunity structures for non-governmental organizations, activist groups, and transnational advocacy networks to interact with each other, disseminate their publications, and lobby delegates and policy-makers; and third, the election of the left-wing Worker's Party (PT) in Brazil, which sought to facilitate global networking among activists through the support for the World Social Forum (WSF). The rising importance of international organizing among resistive solidarity networks across the globe is also a response to the increasingly global control of neoliberal policies articulated at the centers of global power, the effects of these technologies of power and control felt across the various sectors of the globe, and an increasing acknowledgement of the necessity and urgency to act as a global collective to resist the hegemony of neoliberalism.

Inherent in the international networks of solidarity are the interconnections between the local and the global that are communicatively constituted. Local network actors connect globally through their articulation of issues and the framing of these issues within resistive paradigms. The overarching frame offers a platform for the international networks that connect the local movements, putting points of pressure both locally and globally, and thus creating and sustaining sites of change. For example, the international network of movement against dams connects multiple locally situated anti-dam movements across the globe. The international network here offers an overarching global framework for organizing against global policy-making and funding bodies such as the World Bank, thus creating sites of collective power at the global level. Similarly, Via Campesina operates at the global level as a transnational solidarity network of peasants, farmers, and land workers who resist the oppressive elements of neoliberal policies that deal with agriculture (Desmarais, 2007). The global collective becomes an organizing site for drawing resources for local processes of resistance as well as for constituting global processes of resistance at the sites of global power. For example, Via Campesina exerts its presence at the major meetings of IFIs, articulating the relevance of listening to the voices of the peasant communities in forming agriculture-related global policies.

International networks are often created, nurtured, and further strengthened through international meetings that bring together activists from around the globe in transnational forums that seek to resist the dominant economic forums of neoliberalism (Moghadam, 2009). For example, the World Social Forum was created as an alternative to the World Economic Forum that brings together transnational elites to discuss policies, develop goals, and strategize about global economic policies. The WSF was conceptualized as a space that would bring together grassroots activists from around the globe on a common platform, both in the form of institutional structures necessary for concerted organizing and also in the form of open spaces for activists from around the globe to meet, exchange ideas, develop strategies, and mobilize collectively against global neoliberal policies. Groups that identify themselves as part of the GJM participate in transnational events such as the World Social Forum and/or European Social Forum, taking part in Global Days of Action as well as specific counter-summits that are organized at the meetings of International Governmental Organizations. In addition, these social justice groups participate in national and local social forums, coordinating with dispersed local and national social forums across the globe (della Porta, 2009) (see Figure 8.2).

Tensions in Organizing Processes

The organizing of social change is a dynamic process that exists at the intersections of culture, structure, and agency. In this section, we examine the interplays among culture, structure, and agency that constitute the paradoxes in organizing for social change, thus offering insights about the theory and practice of organizing for social change. The two key tensions discussed here negotiate the politics of resistive transformation within the increasing global presence of neoliberal ideology amidst global, national, and local structures.

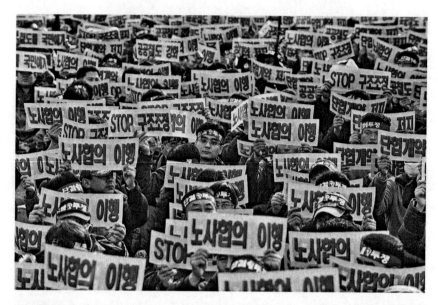

FIGURE 8.2 Railway workers wave banners reading "Stop Restructure" during a rally in front of Seoul station on November 26, 2009. South Korean railway workers went on strike to cripple the nation's cargo train service after talks with management over working conditions failed. (Jung Yeon-Je/AFP/Getty Images)

Conflict versus Solidarity

Organizing processes in social change initiatives continually negotiate the tensions between conflict and solidarity. Whereas much of the emphasis in organizing is placed on solidarity, the coming together of a collective around issues and frames also involves the discussion of opposing viewpoints and the negotiations of conflict. Conflict is integral to processes of solidarity building as collectives negotiate opposing viewpoints, stances on issues, frames to be adopted, strategies, and tactics. Collectives also typically draw upon various stakeholders with competing interests and agendas, thus creating a complex web of multiple competing hegemonies. These conflicts within organizing efforts exist side by side with solidarity networks that hold the collectives together, and drive the core identity of the collective. Solidarity refers to the feelings of trust, camaraderie, and commitment that exist in efforts of social change. It is on the basis of the principles of solidarity that collectives come to challenge and transform unequal social structures, operating as a singular entity organized around a certain set of issues, and working to challenge the social structures around these issues.

In organizing the processes of social change, conflict is capable of producing solidarity within a democratic framework. The goals to align community actions with specific community demands generate conflicts over specific issues among the various organizations and organizational practices, thus also creating a space for dialogue and trust, and producing social cohesion and solidarity. In other words, creating spaces for disagreement and conflict also brings about opportunities for open dialogue in local community contexts, thus increasing the opportunities for the community to come together to articulate its visions, objective, and strategies through dialogue.

Resistance versus Co-optation

The effectiveness of resistive organizing depends upon its ability to work through the structures of neoliberal governance, bring about shifts in global policies, and offer alternatives to neoliberal forms of global economic and political organizing. In constituting a politics of resistance, processes of social change continually negotiate the tensions between resistance and co-optation, particularly as they network with political institutions, structures, and resources in order to build viable sites of resistive politics. For example, communicative practices carried out by organizations such as community relations (CR) and corporate social responsibility (CSR) can create spaces for resistive organizations to seek out and articulate the politics of resistance in dialogue with organizational stakeholders. Simultaneously, these very sites of CR and CSR also emerge as sites of co-opting community resistance through manipulative practices that give the appearance of dialogue. For example, the indigenous–mining dialogue group set up by the Australian Uranium Association to bridge the gap between Aboriginal Australians and uranium mining industries is constituted within the agendas of the mining industry to usurp indigenous land to build mines (Statham, 2009). Who gets to participate in dialogue is dictated by the interests of the system in sustaining itself as an economic enterprise and in carrying out its exploitations through minimization of resistance.

Similarly, large environmental movements have emerged as important sites of negotiation of power, playing into the hands of TNCs in order to negotiate spaces of legitimacy and economic support for their operations (Switzer, 2001). For instance, major environmental organizations such as Green Peace receive large sums of donations from major petrochemical TNCs. The material support received from the TNCs that lies at the heart of the practices that threaten the environment then raises questions about the legitimacy of such processes of social change.

The agendas of social change here get situated within the broader agendas of the dominant power structures that are also the sources of exploitation and oppression. This fundamental paradox in resistive politics and the co-option of resistance within dominant platforms is intrinsic to organizing for social change, as processes of change negotiate their relationships with key stakeholders on dominant platforms, seeking to co-opt these platforms for the goals of social change and simultaneously being threatened to be co-opted by the goals and agendas of these platforms (Dutta, 2009; Dutta & Pal, 2010; Pal & Dutta, 2008a, 2008b).

Conclusion

Organizing is a key element in communication for social change. It is through organizing that social change collectives are formed, identities are developed, and resources are mobilized toward achieving collective goals. Processes of organizing are symbolic as well as material. In the realm of the symbolic, organizing processes express the values of the culture and simultaneously create new meaning structures and thought-feeling combinations in order to bring about transformations in global structures of exploitation and inequalities. Simultaneously, the material is embedded in the performative in its calls for bringing about changes in material structures. Organizing processes against the backdrop of globalization operate through the building of networks among multiple organizations, and the continual negotiations of relationships through transnational solidarity networks. In the face of the global control of neoliberal hegemony and the expanding power of neoliberal governance not only to work through coercion but also to work much more effectively through consensus building, dialogue, and participation, organizing for social change continually negotiates the tension between co-optation and resistance. Reflexivity in organizing practices creates entry points for continually engaging critically with the practices of organizing, and exploring the co-optive moments and processes through which resistive practices are threatened by the increasing power and control of transnational hegemony.

9

PARTICIPATION, SOCIAL CAPITAL, COMMUNITY NETWORKS, AND SOCIAL CHANGE

As discussed so far in this book, social change in the culture-centered approach is achieved through the participation of local actors in the processes of change, with local participation offering ontological entry points for transforming global knowledge configurations and concept structures (Basu & Dutta, 2009; Dutta-Bergman, 2004a, 2004b). It is through the commitment and active involvement of locally situated actors that agendas of social change are articulated, and actions are taken to bring about transformations in the structures constituting the lived experiences of community members (Basu & Dutta, 2008a, 2009; Dutta, 2007, 2008c, 2009). In other words, participation in the culture-centered approach offers the avenue through which local agendas are shaped and articulated, thus creating entry points of social change. In this chapter we examine the processes of participation, complexities in participation, and the tensions negotiated in participatory processes in the realm of social change. We will also engage with the concept of social capital,[1] as this concept offers insights into community-based spaces of social change and the possibilities of structural transformation that are written into these processes.

Participation serves as a key element in the processes of social change by introducing locally situated issues as well as the framing of these issues into the dominant discursive spaces of neoliberal governance. It is through participation in local community forums that community members articulate their agendas of change, identifying the key issues and objectives of social change processes, as well as outlining the strategies and tactics for change. Transformations in structures are achieved through the involvement of local communities, bringing forth local community voices in participatory platforms. Simultaneously, it is through their participation in a variety of platforms both inside and outside the mainstream that community members open up possibilities for challenging and changing social structures.

Communication with stakeholders outside the community, such as policy-makers, agencies, academic partners, practitioners, and juridical systems, happens through participatory platforms that open up the opportunities to communicate the agendas of the grassroots to mainstream social actors. The community not only communicates within itself as a foundation for organizing, but also networks, affiliates with, and collaborates with actors dispersed across the globe to create entry points for transformative politics that has a global network, and that is able to draw upon this global network to mobilize for social change. In essence then, participation is integral to the communicative processes not only within the local community, but also in the engagement of the local community with outside actors at the local, national, and global levels. This inside-outside negotiation is also reflective of the broader politics of negotiating the local and the global in processes of social change communication.

Although participation can offer an avenue for creating locally driven structural transformations, the concept often gets utilized as a tool to serve the agendas of mainstream actors at the center. Increasingly, participation has become a tool in the hands of hegemonic global institutions to carry out the economic and political agendas of dominant social actors. The language of participation, in such instances, serves as a cover for the hidden agendas of dominance and control played out by the status quo. Local participatory spaces and platforms get co-opted within the neoliberal agendas of the global actors in order to create spaces of market opportunity for these actors. In the face of such co-optation, local communities also engage with these hegemonic participatory spaces to negotiate their agendas and goals, thus rescripting the global agendas in locally situated narratives and creating a complex web of participatory tensions.

Acknowledging these complexities and tensions, this chapter argues for the continued necessity for critically interrogating the usage of participation in the contemporary neoliberal landscape and the agendas served by such participation in co-optive politics, situated against the backdrop of discussions of power and the ways in which power gets constituted in the logics of participation that are carried out to exploit local communities in order to serve the agendas of neoliberal hegemony. Even as we engage with postcolonial theory as an entry point to the praxis of social change, our critical reading of participation will interrogate the value of postcolonial concepts such as hybridity in the politics of interrupting the agendas of the status quo. We examine the role of theory in guiding the praxis of change, evaluating the applicability of theory on the basis of the rubric of change. Here once again we refer back to the differentiation between social change and status quo as defined in the Introduction and Chapter 1.

The organizing framework presented in Chapter 8 is further built upon in this chapter, where attention is drawn to the role of communication in the realm of social capital and community networks. Here, the emphasis is on the role of communication as participation, particularly in the realm of community infrastructures and community networks that can be mobilized for social change. What are the ways in which the scholarship and practice of communication engages with participatory avenues in subaltern spaces? What are the possibilities of structural transformation that are brought about by these partnerships? What are the tensions negotiated in such partnerships? In this chapter, we examine the participatory processes through which community networks are mobilized, reinforced, and utilized for purposes of social change, simultaneously attending to the many tensions that are imbued in these participatory processes. Furthermore, the chapter specifically explores the theoretical tensions that emerge in participatory processes, attending to the connections between theory and praxis. Ultimately, the goal of the chapter is to engage with the praxis of participation that is directed toward social transformation (see Figure 9.1).

Participation and Social Change

In response to the vertical development campaigns of early communication social change projects that conceptualized communication as a vehicle for carrying out the messages of development to target communities in the Third World, communication scholars suggested the role of participatory processes in social change communication. Scholars such as Chambers (1983, 1994a, 1994b, 1994c) noted the fundamental inequities in the expert-driven model of social change communication within the development framework that fundamentally operated on the basis of assumptions of backwardness of the rural sectors of the globe, and the

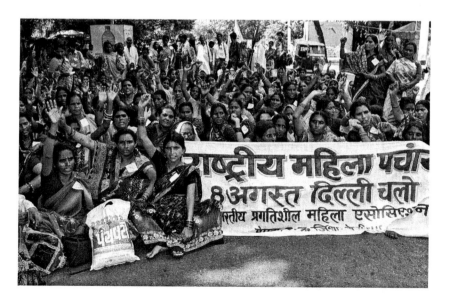

FIGURE 9.1 All India Progressive Women's Association (AIPWA) protesting against the United Progressive Alliance (UPA) Government in New Delhi, India. (Yasbant Negi/The India Today Group/Getty Images)

solutions were generated by outside experts. Here is what Chambers (1994a) articulates in discussing the underdevelopment of the rural sectors in development discourse:

> Much of the mystery disappears if explanation is sought not in local people, but in outsider professionals. For the beliefs, behavior and attitudes of most outsiders have been similar all over the world. Agricultural scientists, medical staff, teachers, officials, extension agents and others have believed that their knowledge was superior and that the knowledge of farmers and other local people was inferior; and that they could appraise and analyze but poor people could not. Many outsiders then either lectured, holding sticks and wagging fingers, or interviewed impatiently, shooting rapid fire questions, interrupting, and not listening to more than immediate replies, if that. Outsiders' reality blanketed that of local people. They "put down" the poor. Outsiders' beliefs, demeanor, behavior and attitudes were then self-validating. Treated as incapable, poor people behaved as incapable, reflecting the beliefs of the powerful, and hiding their capabilities even from themselves. Nor did many outsider professionals know how to enable local people to express, share and extend their knowledge. The ignorance and inabilities of rural people were then not just an illusion; they were an artifact of outsiders' behavior and attitudes, of their arrogant and ignorant manner of interacting with local people.
>
> *(Chambers, 1994a, p. 963)*

Chambers notes that the "backwardness" of rural populations is epistemologically and ontologically manufactured through the inherent biases built into the theory and practice of development campaigns. The very assumptions of the superiority of expert knowledge bases and the inherent inferiority of rural knowledge script the rural sectors in terms of ignorance and inability. It is this very scripting and fixing of the inability of the rural actors that then defines the parameters of development, without listening to the voices of rural participants.

Along similar lines, the writing of Paulo Freire (1970, 1973) served as one of the most influential lines of work on the role of participation in educational processes, articulating the idea that community member involvement is quintessential to challenging and transforming the oppressive nature of top–down educational systems which use a "banking" model of education, transferring information to the passive recipients. At the heart of Freire's work is the idea of dialogical communication that respects the personhood of each human being and attends to the active meaning-making capacity of community members. Furthermore, participation is quintessential to the collective capacity of communities to address structural deprivations such as poverty and cultural subjugation.

Based upon examples of grassroots-based participatory processes of social change utilized by NGOs in South Asia, the work of Robert Chambers (1983, 1994a,

1994b, 1994c) further added to the emphasis on participation in development, proposing the idea that local communities need to be actively engaged in developing understandings of key problems facing the communities and in the prioritization of these problems in terms of what is relevant to the collective community and its local needs. Acknowledging the capacity of rural communities to actively analyze information and develop solutions, Chambers (1997) proposed participatory research appraisal (PRA), focusing on the development of participatory methodologies for facilitating the active involvement of local communities. It is on the basis of the community involvement in prioritizing problems to be addressed that community members then participate in developing solutions that would address the problems as identified by the community.

> The essence of PRA is changes and reversals—of role, behaviour, relationship, and learning. Outsiders do not dominate and lecture; they facilitate, sit down, listen, and learn . . . they do not transfer technology; they share methods which local people can use for their own appraisal, analysis, planning action, monitoring, and evaluation.
>
> *(Chambers, 1997, p. 103)*

Worth noting in PRA is the reversal of the traditional roles of experts and recipients of interventions. The role is defined in terms of working with local people to enable their participation in their own processes of analysis, action planning, and evaluation. The community becomes the locus of problem definition and solution development.

Responding to the critique of the early top-down development campaigns, an increasing number of international organizations, funding agencies, academic institutions, campaign planners, and non-governmental organizations have started incorporating participation in their communication for social change processes. Large-scale bureaucracies such as the World Bank have incorporated participation in their conceptualization and application of development principles and interventions (Francis, 2001). Empowerment of local communities has emerged as a key principle in several World Bank projects, as well as government and public-private partnerships. In addition, a large number of activist projects, projects of resistance, and social movements involve local communities in processes of social change. How communication is being conceptualized in social change processes is intertwined with the ways in which communicative processes are deployed to achieve social change, and the different contexts in which communication is utilized in the realm of achieving the social change agendas of the involved actors.

Definitions of Participation

At a foundational level, participation is defined in terms of the involvement of the local community in decision-making processes. Essential to the idea of participation is the conceptualization of a discursive space or site that brings together participants, and where the views of the participants are articulated. Participation is operationalized in a wide spectrum of roles that includes participation in information gathering, participation in information dissemination, participation in consultation, and participation in decision-making (Dutta, 2007, 2008a, 2008b, 2008c; Dutta & Basnyat, 2008a, 2008b; Dutta & Basu, 2007a, 2007b). The degree of decision-making located in the realm of the local community varies immensely among these different approaches to participation. At one end of the spectrum, processes of participation as information gathering use participatory channels for the purposes of gathering data in order to create more effective social marketing messages. The emphasis is on creating the strongest social change communication effort with the highest reach, effectiveness, and efficiency. Participation as information dissemination conceptualizes participatory processes and spaces as channels for carrying out information. Therefore, participation is configured in the form of radio listener groups, support groups, community meetings, folk performances, and community art in order to be developed as a strategic component of the channel mix for the social change campaign.

In participation as consultation, the role of the local community emerges into one of offering guidelines to the dominant structures, with the goal of ensuring that local voices are considered in the development of the program planning. The greatest level of community-centeredness is seen in the participation in the decision-making framework, where the local community participates in developing the problem configuration and subsequently in the consideration of possible solutions to the problem. In this framework, the locus of decision-making is situated in the local community. Not only do grassroots communication processes of social change often emerge from the communication as decision-making framework, but also they have to negotiate the other functions of participation as consultation, dissemination, and information gathering.

How participation is defined in the context of a social change initiative is framed within the broader goals of the initiative, and in turn, frames the strategies, tools, and tactics that are deployed in the participatory processes. For example, in recent years, responding to the criticism of the top-down economic restructuring programs and the limited success of structural adjustment programs (SAPs), the 1999 G7 Summit proposed the Heavily Indebted Poor Country (HIPC) initiative, making debt relief contingent upon the creation of a national poverty reduction framework and suggesting a shift in the organizational cultures and attitudes of the World Bank and IMF. It is in this climate that the World Bank started emphasizing the role of participation in the newly formulated poverty reduction strategies, highlighting the relevance of country ownership of poverty reduction strategies as well as the role of public participation in deciding the strategies to be worked on in the country-specific poverty reduction strategy papers (PRSP) process (Bradshaw & Linneker, 2003; World Bank, 2002). In spite of the widespread rhetoric of participation, World Bank policies continue to define poverty reduction in terms of the existing strategies of economic growth, with striking similarities between the PRSP guidelines and the SAPs (Bradshaw & Linneker, 2003; Verheul & Cooper, 2001).

Furthermore, World Bank documents reveal the conceptualization of participation primarily as a consultative process; here the role of the local community becomes one of offering some tentative guidelines and suggestions for the World Bank. These guidelines rarely figure into the social change processes determined by the World Bank as the poverty policies are formulated and implemented through top-down economic agendas. In this case, examining the definition of participation within the broader context of the institutional processes, goals, and frameworks creates not only a theoretical but also an empirical space for delineating among the various types of participation in social change processes.

Theoretical Conceptualizations

A key theory that has often been referred to in the realm of participatory communication for social change is Habermas' (1989) theory of the public sphere. For Habermas, the public sphere is an autonomous space in which citizens participate and act through reasoned debate and dialogue. Free speech creates and broadens the foundations of democratic processes, and the public sphere is established on the basis of specific deliberative processes. Habermas (1996a, 1996b) establishes a set of procedural guidelines and communicative presuppositions through which arguments arise and are negotiated, and fair bargaining processes are established. For Habermas (1996b), the "ideal free speech situation" serves as a normative goal for establishing the procedures for dialogue, setting up formal institutional structures through legal and constitutional mechanisms. He notes that the ideal speech situation promotes uncoerced rational dialogue among equal and rational participants. It is, therefore, inclusive, coercion free, and open. Inclusivity refers to the idea that no one is left out of the discursive space in participating in discussing topics and ideas that are relevant to him or her. Freedom from coercion refers to the ability to engage in arguments and counter-arguments freely without feeling intimidated by others or being dominated by others. Openness refers to a situation where each participant can raise and continue discussions on a relevant topic, including the very procedures governing the discussion.

Coming from an altogether different lens, postcolonial theory deconstructs the binaries that have been constituted in the terrains of development knowledge production, noting the absences within Eurocentric structures that constitute the knowledge about the Orient. The Orient emerges as a subject of study, as a category to be known, measured, and evaluated in dominant articulations of development. Postcolonial theory argues that these binaries of the primitive/modern, underdeveloped/developed, and colonized/colonizer have fundamentally operated to reify the differentials in access to positions of power, further producing the Third World savage on whom disciplinary bodies of development knowledge and praxis have been situated (Escobar, 1995). Therefore, inherent in postcolonial thought is the notion of access to communicative spaces and the creation of postcolonial spaces that challenge the dichotomy inherent in the universal narratives of development. Postcolonial theorists such as Homi Bhabha have noted the hybrid nature of postcolonial spaces that operate at the intersections of control and resistance, creating opportunities for participation.

The subaltern studies project further builds on the postcolonial agenda by interrogating the erasure of subaltern voices from the dominant discursive spaces of knowledge production, and seeking to co-create spaces for listening to subaltern voices by interrogating that which is missing. The underlying assumptions constituting the ontological and epistemological foundations of dominant systems of knowledge production are interrogated, attending to the ways in which they have participated in the production of elitist narratives of knowledge, simultaneously devaluing and making irrelevant other ways of knowing. The subaltern is constituted in her/his erasure from the discursive spaces. Therefore, listening to subaltern voices offers an avenue for challenging the politics of power and control played out in the dominant spheres where knowledge is produced and circulated. Subaltern studies theorists articulate the existence of subaltern spheres of participation in parallel with the mainstream public spheres. Participation of the subaltern sectors of the globe in subaltern public spheres creates opportunities for disrupting the dominant discursive spaces in the mainstream.

The culture-centered approach builds on both postcolonial and subaltern studies theories to theorize about local participation as an entry point to social change through its engagement with the interpenetrations of local and global structures. Making note of the agency of individuals, relationships, and communities to make sense of oppressive structural configurations, the approach attends to the processes of change through which these structures are challenged locally as well as globally. Theoretically, the dominant structures of neoliberalism are interrogated structurally through the participation of local communities in processes of change locally, nationally, as well as globally. Global activist networks and networks of solidarity create connections through which the local emerges on the global arena, and it is precisely at these sites of subaltern participation that oppressive structures are interrogated. Also, these solidarity networks connecting disparate and distant local communities across the globe participate in processes of structural transformations within communities as well as across communities affiliations.

Agendas of Participation

Participation then broadly can be categorized on the basis of the purpose that it seeks to serve. The theoretical conceptualization of participation is tied to the practical goals, objectives, strategies, and tactics that are tied to it (more on this in the section on participatory tensions later in this chapter). For example, participatory development communication efforts utilize participatory channels for the purposes of information gathering and information dissemination. The information-gathering function is primarily put to use in the form of formative research in strategy development, message design, and tactical execution. The inputs of the local community are sought for the purposes of fine-tuning the message so that it can be effective in achieving the proposed behavior change in the target population. Multiple social marketing campaigns utilize participation as part of their strategic marketing goals.

Dutta (2007) discusses the cultural sensitivity health campaigns that utilize participatory tools to gather data about local cultures in order to create more effective health messages that are fine-tuned to the characteristics of the culture. Tools such as focus groups and group discussions are utilized here for the purposes of message development and message testing, in order to create effective safe sex, cancer screening, and fruit and vegetable promotion messages in target communities. The goals of participation therefore constrain and define the nature and usage of the participatory channel as a tool for information gathering.

The information dissemination function of participation is conceptualized within the capacity of participation as an effective message dissemination tool, creating large-scale exposure to campaign messages through trustworthy interpersonal channels and networks that are more intimate with the local community than mass-mediated channels. The immediacy of participatory networks serves as an effective tool in changing beliefs, attitudes, and behaviors (Dutta & Basnyat, 2008a, 2008b). For example, the Avahan campaign run by the Bill and Melinda Gates Foundation uses peer-led participatory forums such as group discussions as channels for diffusing the message of safe sex:

> The Avahan trucker project is the first Indian national program to successfully use active truckers along with former truckers as peers to reach their fellow truckers. This dialogue-based interpersonal communication approach now employs 348 truckers and ex-truckers (50 percent of whom are active truckers) across the major transshipment locations where the program operates. They have been fully trained and conduct approximately 5,000 group discussions with fellow truckers every month. These peer workers use nine participatory tools and visual aids to facilitate discussions among groups of 10–12 fellow truckers about HIV, STIs, common misconceptions, and the importance of condom use.
>
> (Gates Foundation, 2008, p. 17)

Here the participatory channel of group discussions is utilized to bring truckers together to create dialogues around the issue of safe sex. The participatory spaces of the group discussions are utilized for framing the goals, complexities, and textures of communication within the broader objectives of the Avahan campaign in diffusing safer sexual practices among the long-distance truckers of India.

Therefore the participatory tools and visual aids that are utilized to facilitate the discussions serve as framing devices that define and construct the nature of participation. The agendas of participation here then are defined within the broader goals of campaign agencies, funders, and program planners to create greater reach, penetration, and effectiveness of individual behavior change messages that are sent out by campaign planners.

As opposed to the information gathering and information dissemination agendas of participatory development, culture-centered participation is rooted in the acknowledgement of the agency of local communities to define issues locally and to develop corresponding solutions and strategies that are directed toward addressing these issues (Dutta, 2006, 2007; Dutta & Basu, 2008; Dutta-Bergman, 2004a, 2004b). Culture-centered participatory processes therefore conceptualize participation within the broader framework of listening to the voices of marginalized communities that are otherwise hidden from mainstream discourses. The agenda of participation is to create avenues of expression through which the voices of local communities can be heard.

The specific objective of participatory spaces is to create opportunities for listening to unheard voices of marginalized communities and thus rupture the hegemony of the mainstream ideologies of development that exhume agency from the subaltern sectors by turning them into targets of campaigns informed by the expert knowledge of outsiders. As a starting point therefore, the goal of culture-centered processes of participatory social change is to disrupt the knowledge claims made by expert networks of knowledge production (combination of academics, practitioners, funding agencies, campaign planners, program evaluators, and so on) by co-constructing alternative rationalities and knowledge claims. These knowledge claims therefore offer the foundations for projects of social change that attend to the inequalities perpetuated by the global structures of development and modernization.

The Empowerment-based Framework

Local participation is not meaningful without taking into consideration the relationships of power that are negotiated in locally situated participatory sites and in relational spaces that constitute local communities (Conquergood, 1986; Friedman, 1992). Therefore, empowerment is the process of situating power in the local context, within the local community, in relationships, and in individuals. Individuals and their relationships are connected to the participatory spaces in the community. The empowerment of individuals is intrinsic to their engagement in processes of community participation and in articulating their voices in community platforms. For example, the empowerment of women in local contexts gives women the time to come together in collective local spaces and air their opinions. Individuals are more effectively able to participate in their communities when they are empowered, and when they feel that they have a say in the ways in which decisions are made. Noting the relevance of individuals and households to the mobilizing capacity of local communities, the concept of empowerment emphasizes the participation of individuals within families and households to participate in decisions that affect their future. Similarly, a greater level of efficacy at the household level creates a sense of confidence in participating in processes of social change and in structural transformations. Therefore, the emphasis of the empowerment-based framework is to enable the expression of agency among highly marginalized individuals, relationships, households, and communities.

Culture-Centered Approach to Participation

Participation is the cornerstone of the culture-centered approach, where the emphasis is placed on local agency as an entry point for transforming global knowledge bases and knowledge structures, along with bringing about changes in the local and global structures of organizing (Basu & Dutta, 2009; Dutta, 2007, 2008a, 2008b, 2008c, 2009; Dutta-Bergman, 2004a, 2004b). Noting the agency of cultural participants, the approach takes as its task the creation of spaces of solidarity where this agency can be enacted, and can be constituted in its politics of structural transformations. Worth noting here is the importance placed in the approach on the intersections of culture, structure, and agency as an entry point for social change. For example, in the communicative processes of social change mobilized by sex workers in the Durbar Mahila Swamanyaya Committee in Sonagachi, Kolkata, local agency was enacted in challenging structures and seeking to bring about transformations in these structures. Similarly, in the Cochabamba movement, the focus was on challenging the structures that determined the political economy of local access to water. Participation in the realm of the local shifts the structures that enable or constrain access to material resources; simultaneously, such forms of participation bring about changes in global epistemic structures and disrupt global policies. The local organizing of EZLN created openings for global transformation through the articulation of Zapatismo as an alternative interpretive and organizing framework to neoliberalism. Therefore, at the center of the localism in the culture-centered approach is its engagement with the global, its articulation of global structures of neoliberalism, and the participation of the local in global platforms with the agenda of transforming the global.

Seeking to participate in the transformative politics of social change, the culture-centered approach fundamentally attempts to interrogate the dominant structures of development and neoliberalism. It does so by creating and opening up participatory spaces for listening to the voices of local communities through journeys of co-construction. In these processes of co-construction, participatory spaces and processes are continually created that allow for the subaltern voices to emerge into the discursive spaces of knowledge and praxis, in dialogue with the researcher, scholar, or activist located at the centers of knowledge production. Discursive ruptures and disruptions of existing knowledge structures are quintessential to the culture-centered approach; these ruptures are achieved through the participation of local communities in processes of social change, articulating the narratives of subaltern sectors that have hitherto been erased from dominant discursive spaces. In creating subaltern entry points for transformative politics, culture-centered theorizing is attentive to the multiple counter-hegemonies and interplays of power as the local engages with the global. It is in these negotiations of power at various local and global intersections that possibilities of social change are constituted.

Social Capital and Community Networks

The concept of social capital has taken center stage in studies of the role of the community in processes of social change (Edwards & Foley, 2001; Kolankiewicz, 1996; Putnam, 1993, 1995). Social capital is historically defined as the degree of community participation, cohesiveness, and trust that exists within a community, and taps into the formal and informal participatory structures and networks that exist within a community. Therefore, social capital is a community-based resource, tapping into the cohesiveness and relational ties that exist within the community. Referring to the resources that exist in the relationships of trust and cooperation among people, it taps into the local structures, affiliations, and internal community processes of organizing within communities (Putnam, 1993, 1995; Saegert, Thompson, & Warren, 2001). In the context of poverty, social capital researchers observe that poorer communities lacking access to structural resources rely on networks of support and cooperation within their communities to secure access to resources (Warren et al., 2001).

As noted earlier in the book, weak social capital in the poorer sectors is situated amidst the limited structural inaccess in these sectors (Wilkinson, 1996). The flight of jobs from low-income neighborhoods also weakens the social organizations, social institutions, and youth socialization processes in these neighborhoods. Saegert et al. (2001) note that the social assets in poorer communities have greater numbers of obstacles to address, a larger number of structural issues to work with, and a larger number of threats that continually enact violence on local community ties and organizations.

Scholars studying social capital against the backdrop of processes of social change suggest that community participatory processes are crucial to the initiation, implementation, and maintenance of social change processes in communities (Basu & Dutta, 2009; Dreier, 1996; Saegert et al., 2001). The community is seen as the locus of the change initiative, and is treated as the unit of collective organizing on the basis of which communicative processes of social change are set in motion. Social capital can offer the political power for organizing among the poor, and for securing access to resources deprived from poorer communities. Furthermore, social capital in resource-deprived communities offers an entry point to making investment strategies work by placing an emphasis on a range of policies such as public health, education, housing, economic development, and education. Community-based collective organizing and networking with other outside resources and communities foster powerful alliances that may then be mobilized in processes of social change and in securing greater resources in addressing the needs of the poor (Foley, McCarthy, & Chaves, 2001). For example, the congregation-based organizing networks (CBOs) in the United States work with poor communities in building intercommunity networks, explicitly linking several congregations together, and creating entry points for social change by fostering a broader collective base for the articulation of issues and change processes (Foley et al., 2001; Warren, 1998, 2001). Similarly, Wagner and Cohen (1991) and Bradshaw and Linneker (2001) report strong networks of social ties and political organizing among the homeless and previously homeless, embodied in the tent cities, sit-ins, and years of confrontation in Washington DC led by the Coalition for Creative Non-Violence.

Community social networks and social ties are situated amidst the broader structures of political and economic organizing (Cohen, and Dawson, 1993). Poorer communities face the structural constraints imposed by the elite political sectors, and have to struggle with the impediments established by the structural configurations of the status quo (Duncan, 2001; Lopez & Stack, 2001). The struggles of organizing in marginalized communities are tied to securing political power and access to the institutional structures that determine the availability of resources. Therefore, the political power of poorer communities is facilitated through the development of institutional structures for the participation of poorer communities in processes of social change. Increasingly, critical scholars engaging with the empowerment-based processes incorporated under social capital by dominant structures such as the World Bank point toward the incorporation of community networks, community ties, and empowerment under the structures of neoliberal governance, placing the responsibility on the local communities and simultaneously co-opting the participatory capacity of local communities within the structures of neoliberalism (Sharma, 2008). The role of the state is shifted from the provision of basic services for the underserved sectors to mechanisms of empowerment that are directed toward self-reliance and self-sufficiency, where local community needs are met through participation in the market (Kahn, 2000; Menon-Sen, 2001). Culture-centered theorizing of social capital, community organizing, and participation draws attention to the tensions, complexities, and paradoxes that are constituted in the theorizing and application of participatory processes in the realm of social change communication. Furthermore, building on these tensions, spaces are explored for organizing resistance to neoliberal politics.

Culture-Centered Approach and Participatory Tensions

In the face of criticism of early development communication work, scholars across various regions of the globe raised questions about the effectiveness as well as meaningfulness of top-down development communication programs that did not take local communities into account. How are local communities constituted in development communication programs? What is the role of local communities in these programs? What are the opportunities for local communities to participate in such programs? These questions raised by development scholars and practitioners were guided by the acknowledgement that local communities need to be fundamentally involved in the communication programs and processes that are directed toward them. Furthermore, these questions were articulated against the backdrop of interrogations of the goals and agendas served by these top-down programs, and the measures of development in local communities that were actually brought about by these programs. Questions were raised about top-down articulations of development that were out of sync with the understandings of development constituted in local communities. Questions were also raised about the value-laden assumptions written into the modernization framework underlying development communication projects, and the sustainability of such projects.

Responding to the criticisms of their top-down framework configuration, development communication scholars in the dominant paradigm quickly adopted their scholarship and praxis to include participatory concepts as tools for achieving the development agendas. As noted in the previous section, the language of participation came to be included in development communication programs to serve the goals of these programs. For instance, local community participation as information resource in the form of formative research came to be widely adopted in the social marketing framework of campaigns. Gathering data about the target community became a critical part of the campaign development process. Similarly, the community came to be increasingly considered as a message dissemination channel and therefore avenues of participation came to be adopted into the intervention framework. Also, in response to this criticism, an alternative body of work emerged in development communication programs that emphasized participatory approaches to development, rooted in grassroots involvement in social change processes. These approaches to participation and social change in development communication scholarship and praxis are situated alongside grassroots-driven activist politics of social change that work through participatory spaces and local community platforms to seek out transformations in local, national, and global political spaces.

The culture-centered approach builds on subaltern studies scholarship to interrogate the discursive erasures that are achieved in mainstream discursive spaces, specifically attending to the communicative processes of erasure through which subaltern voices are placed at the peripheries of dominant discursive spaces. Therefore, the articulations of dominant structures are continually interrogated for their discursive closures, and for the ways in which they perpetuate material inequities across the globe. How are dominant structures closed to possibilities of participation? What are the communicative processes through which these closures are propagated in mainstream societies? These deconstructions of erasures in and from dominant structures offer the backdrop for theorizing and engaging with the participatory politics of social change in subaltern contexts that seek to engage the dominant structures with the goals of addressing the erasures, absences, and inequities. The role of the scholar-practitioner emerges from that of an expert developer of development knowledge to a listener-activist who tries to create discursive entry points for subaltern voices through journeys of solidarity with the subaltern sectors. Methods such as photo-essay and photovoice emerge as culture-centered tools that seek to present the voices of subaltern communities in dominant discourses.

Participatory Tensions

Participation ultimately seeks to disrupt the hegemonic control of dominant discursive spaces by creating entry points for subaltern worldviews. Therefore, it is conceptualized as a creative space for bringing about social change through the involvement of the locally situated marginalized communities in processes of change. In its transformative capacity, it attempts to invert the status quo by listening to those very voices that have been systematically erased from the status quo, and by foregrounding those voices as agents of decision-making in global policy structures. However, it is in this very relationship of the status quo with the margins that continual tensions of identities, relationships, and power are con-stituted, demonstrating the contested nature of participatory spaces as social actors strive for legitimizing their diverse worldviews in and through these spaces. In order to understand the threads of tensions in participatory processes of social change, we examine the PRSP process in Nicaragua as a case study.

In their study of the participatory PRSP process in Nicaragua, Bradshaw and Linneker (2003) note the tensions that emerge in the terrains of decision-making control as the Nicaraguan government initially engages with the Nicaraguan civil society, represented in the form of the Civil Coordinator for Emergency and Reconstruction (CCER), a meta-organization comprising 21 networks that represent the involvement of over 350 national NGOs, social movements, sectoral networks producer associations, unions, collectives, and federations to develop participatory processes for creating a Nicaraguan PRSP, which was a prerequisite for entry into the HIPC initiative that began in 1999. The government undertook an initial diagnostic as a first step and presented its initial report to the National Economic and Social Planning Council, of which CCER is a participant member; CCER questioned the poverty metrics used in the report as well as the figures presented in the report. Additionally, it argued that the data presented in the report obfuscated the changes in the distribution of poverty in Nicaragua as well as deterioration in the depth of poverty in Nicaragua. The critique offered by CCER did not influence the diagnostic tool used by the government in its report, and did not receive any response from the government, with the government noting that civil society efforts in Nicaragua ought to be focused on developing the poverty reduction strategies.

In January 2000, the government began the formal process of preparing the PRSP and presented its first draft document to CONPES; the draft included the three pillars of economic growth, human capital, and social safety nets for vulnerable populations, and was further modified to include good governance on the basis of national lobbying and international pressures. In June 2000, CCER and a number of its participant organizations were invited by the government to participate in designing the methodology to be used in the government's PRSP consultation, and the government submitted its interim PRSP for World Bank approval in July, 2000, unknown to the national civil society organizations. At the same time in July 2000, the government conducted limited consultations with member organizations of the CONPES who had suggested recommendations about consultation. Parallel to the PRSP process established by the government, CCER started its own PRSP consultation and poverty research process, seeking to create a broader participatory space around the articulations of poverty reduction strategies. In January 2001, the government was forced by the World Bank to start local consultation processes as a number of organizations sent letters to the World Bank noting that the PRSP did not have approval of social organizations and local governments. Based on its invitation–only consultations with social organizations, the government noted that these consultations had nothing new to add, and Nicaragua finally got accepted into the HIPS initiative process in June 2001. When invited to the limited participatory spaces offered by the government, CCER decided to participate in these government discussions to explore opportunities for influencing policy and simultaneously creating parallel processes of participating that rejected the government's narrow view of policy and simultaneously sought to create a broader public space for discussions of the PRSP.

The parallel PRSP process held meetings across Nicaragua which created spaces for participants to articulate their visions of the problems within their communities, the priorities, and the possible strategies and solutions needed to address them, and concrete policy recommendations. These meetings were complemented by themed meetings that discussed specific issues such as economic policy or governability. At each meeting, delegates were elected to participate in a final meeting to analyze the initial results. Two additional meetings were held to articulate the conceptualization of poverty. The CCER document that resulted from these discussions comprised two sections. The first section questioned the government's definition of poverty reduction in terms of economic growth as opposed to CCER's definition of poverty reduction as human development. It discussed the limits to the government's PRSP and why it could not succeed. The second section of the document presented specific policy recommendations arising from the consultation process, and clustered around the main pillars of the government's PRSP.

There are multiple tensions in participatory processes of decision-making that emerge in this particular case study. Negotiating the tensions between conversing with the government and responding to the needs of local civil society organizations, CCER engaged with the fundamental questions of legitimacy in terms of its participatory capacity to frame the national PRSP. On one hand, engaging with the government offered a continued opportunity for shaping the PRSP process; on the other hand, operating on the basis of consensus in general assembly meetings that were open to all civil actors created spaces for local participation and parallel definitions of poverty and poverty reduction strategies. Participating in the opportunities for discussions with the government was also situated against the backdrop of fear that participating in government processes would legitimize the government process that operated to exclude local organizations and civil society from participatory spaces and was unresponsive to civil society. Tensions also emerged among the multiple organizations represented under the umbrella of CCER, in the form of the calls for cooperation juxtaposed against the backdrop of the competing interests of these organizations that came together under the broader umbrella of CCER. Participation here is constituted in terms of the paradoxes of articulating competing interests and simultaneously seeking spaces of mutual cooperation among competing interests. These tensions within culture-centered processes of participation are noted by Basu and Dutta (2009) in their discussions of sex workers organizing in Sonagachi, a red light district in Kolkata, India, where the narratives of participation articulate multiple counter-hegemonies within participatory spaces, negotiating the tensions that emerge at the crossroads of these hegemonies. What are the entry points for articulating common visions of the collective in culture-centered processes of participation as competing agendas and interests are negotiated? It is also in this discursive realm of negotiating multiple competing interests within local collectives that questions arise about representation, voice, and access. Who gets to participate in the local participatory spaces, and who is discursively and materially situated at the margins of these spaces? How is power distributed within local communities and how do the inequities in distributions of power locally play out in the access to participatory spaces? Therefore, even as the emphasis of the culture-centered approach turns toward creating entry points for local participation, opportunities for participation are not often equally extended to all community members, often demonstrating the structural inequities in the distribution of opportunities at the local level.

Tensions also emerge in the final CCER document. The two sections of the final CCER document present the tensions that arise between CCER's vision as a radical organizing space on one hand and CCER's role in offering donor agencies an alternative policy framework to work within on the other hand. The definition used by the government's PRSP to characterize poverty and poverty reduction is fundamentally challenged. Simultaneously, solutions are offered within the definitional framework of the government and the key pillars laid out by the government's PRSP to create alternative frameworks for praxis (Bradshaw & Linneker, 2003). Even as radical grassroots movements seek to create participatory spaces for structural transformation, they engage with the dominant structures that they critique to find alternative policy formulations and alternative avenues for engaging in praxis under the existing policy guidelines. Participatory processes of social change simultaneously engage with the dominant structures and articulate reformative possibilities in those structures even as they simultaneously challenge the discursive and material hegemonies of those structures.

Co-optation versus Social Change. As the CCER case reviewed in the previous section demonstrates, participatory spaces continuously negotiate the tensions between co-optive possibilities and the possibilities of transformation. On one hand, when created within dominant structures, participatory spaces are often co-opted within the agendas of these structures; on the other hand, participatory spaces offer openings for social change through the transformative politics built into them, both in terms of the changes in policies as well as in terms of articulating a resistive politics of social transformation (Francis, 2001). It is this continual negotiation between co-optation and transformative politics that is one of the fundamental principles in participation for social change. Participatory processes feed into the agendas of transnational hegemony; simultaneously, they create openings for transforming these hegemonic configurations by opening up dominant discursive spaces in the mainstream to alternative rationalities and to alternative ways of organizing.

In situations such as UN efforts for dialoguing with indigenous communities, openings are created for listening to indigenous voices. However, these voices are filtered and edited through gatekeepers before they reach the dominant spaces of participation in the mainstream. To the extent that these voices are heard, they are often constituted within the politics and economic agendas of the mainstream, co-opted as indigenous representations in serving the interests of transnational hegemony. The entry of local voices in global spaces often turns these voices into homogeneous representations, situating the narratives at the cultural level in the broader rhetoric of multicultural tolerance, and turning problem configurations into cultural relics instead of addressing structures and deep-seated inequalities constituted in neoliberal policies. However, in other instances, participation enters into the global spaces of articulation to challenge the taken-for-granted assumptions that circulate in these spaces. The presence of subaltern voices in the mainstream and the participation of the marginalized sectors in mainstream spaces disrupt the hegemonic narratives of progress, development, and democratic participation that circulate in institutions promoting neoliberal governance.

Even as participation seeks to create spaces of involvement for local communities in social change processes, such participation often ends up serving the agendas of the status quo. Participation ends up being enlisted to serve the objectives of the dominant power structures locally, nationally, and globally, and to carry out the diffusion of specific solution configurations that are circulated in response to specific top-down strategies for identifying problems in the target communities. The rhetoric of participation and democracy serve as public relations devices that create the appearances of dialogue, equality, and participation. When the rhetoric is measured against the backdrop of the praxis of participatory processes and the outcomes associated with these participatory projects, it becomes evident that those participatory processes are promoted in the local communities that are supportive of the status quo and the broader structures reflected in this status quo. The participatory spaces that are offered to local communities are offered within the agendas of the status quo.

These negotiations between structural transformation and co-optation are evident in the widespread inclusion of participation as a strategic tool in various phases of entertainment education (E-E) programs that are then rhetorically branded as innovative and more democratic alternatives to the more traditional top-down forms of development communication campaigns of the early decades. For instance, in their culture-centered analysis of the Radio Communication Project (RCP) funded by the United States Agency for International Development and carried out by the Johns Hopkins University Center for Communication Programs (JHU/CCP), Dutta and Basnyat (2008a, 2008b) demonstrate that participatory channels for communication used by the RCP operated as strategic tools in order to serve the top-down agendas of the program as dictated by USAID and as configured by JHU/CCP. The participatory tools are simply co-opted as data-gathering tools for the purposes of formative research and as diffusion channels for carrying out the messages of family planning, as configured by the dictates of USAID, reinforcing the panopticon of the development project as well as serving to enhance the reach of the project in the local communities of the global South. Participatory spaces such as radio listener groups are constituted within the broader agendas of family planning and population control (Dutta & Basnyat, 2010). Empowerment is constituted in the realm of Eurocentric structures, and the RCP emphasizes the teaching of communication skills for the goals of empowering women. Worth noting here are the West-centric conceptualizations of these communication skills, and the modernist assumptions about the universalist characteristics of what constitutes effective communication, thus demonstrating one of the key paradoxes in the empowerment vocabulary. The widespread large-scale mass marketing of empowerment in neoliberal programs often hides the co-optive and modernist assumptions of Western superiority that continue to be reified in such programs.

Status Quo versus Structural Transformations. Whereas the roots of participatory social change communication are situated in critical interrogations of the top-down model of communication for social change and the postcolonial politics that opened up spaces for listening to the voices of local communities, participatory processes and discourses have become increasingly incorporated into the structures of neoliberal governance as mechanisms for promoting market penetration, co-opting subaltern agency, and enhancing the effectiveness and efficiency of development programs constituted under the neoliberal project (Cooke & Kothari, 2001). Increasingly, local-level participatory processes, community workshops, group discussions, and community dialogues have emerged as tools for consolidating the agendas of dominant structures in local communities in the global South.

The World Bank for instance has developed mechanisms for the incorporation of participatory processes targeting the poor in mainstream World Bank programs (Francis, 2001). In the mid-1990s, the vocabulary, rhetoric, and techniques of participatory development began to enter the mainstream operations of the World Bank. These participatory processes are constituted as management tools directed at enhancing the economic effectiveness and efficiency of the World Bank. Absent from these participatory spaces is the articulation of social contexts and structural factors. Instead, participation is framed within the World Bank objectives of optimizing economic effectiveness and efficiency in rural communities of the South by placing responsibility in the hands of the poor.

The locus of addressing poverty is situated in the individual capacities of community members, and to this extent participation is seen as a tool for enhancing economic efficiency of highly impoverished local actors. Through programs of entrepreneurship and micro-lending, for instance, rural women from the global South enter into the World Bank project of neoliberal expansion, constituted as efficient sources of labor who would not default on loans. The empowerment of rural women from the global South here is achieved within the broader agendas of SAPs and privatization of resources, ultimately circulating and reifying policies that further marginalize the poor and minimize their access to economic resources, as well as social services that were traditionally offered by the public sector. The responsibility of structural support is exhumed from the hands of the state, and the poor are further placed at the margins of the margins as these services such as education, health, and water are privatized under the free market logic.

Culture-centered communicative processes situate the relationships among culture and agency in the realm of structures of marginalization and oppression that circulate across the global South as these spaces in the South are turned into profitable entities and markets for products and services marketed by TNCs. The narratives that emerge from participatory spaces of culture-centered approaches are stories that challenge the modernist narratives of development, drawing attention to the hegemonic manipulation of participatory spaces to serve the agendas of transnational hegemony. The essentialist positions of subaltern subjects portrayed in the dominant structures are forever problematized, and subaltern narratives impurify the theoretical categories of the universalist vocabulary of development. Theories thus generated through culture-centered processes seek to transform local structures through the continual attention paid to the oppressive elements in local structures, and through the exploration of ruptures and disjunctures in the mainstream platforms that offer openings for transformation. Locally situated movements and collective organizing processes draw attention to the everyday participation of local communities in overt processes of social change directed at bringing about transformations in social structures. Simultaneously, these culture-centered theories connect with the global processes of social change by introducing alternative rationalities and forms of organizing at the global centers of neoliberal hegemony. The emergence of Zapatismo as an inspiration for populist struggles against neoliberal market economics and policies is one such example of a local theory emerging into global sites through participatory mechanisms and through networks of solidarity.

Collective Consensus versus Disagreements. Whereas much of the theoretical, methodological, and application-based focus on participatory processes of social change begins with the concept of the local community as a homogeneous collective, other projects studying local participatory processes point toward the tensions and competing interests that exist within local communities (Basu & Dutta, 2008a, 2009; Sharma, 2008). For instance, Sharma's (2008) ethnographic study of the Mahila Samakhya program, a hybrid "government-organized non-governmental organization" (GONGO) directed at collectively empowering low-caste, rural Indian women reveals the counter-hegemonies and counter-narratives that exist within discursive spaces of collective organizing. Women's gendered basis of organizing for a collective identity in Mahila Samakhya is situated amidst competing interests and tensions connected to their multiple subjectivities as mothers, wives, daughters-in-law, and landless laborers.

Amidst competing interests and agendas, communities emerge as fragmented sites where power is continually negotiated (Sharma, 2008). The negotiation of power is a dynamic and fragmented process, and often operates on the basis of traditional hierarchical markers such as class, caste, kinship, and access to vital material resources. Collective sites are materially situated and the agendas articulated at these sites therefore are intertwined amidst material tensions and competing interests located within the broader socioeconomic structures. Those with access to vital resources within these collectives also have greater opportunities of articulating the issues and agendas that are important to them. Leadership within these participatory collective spaces is often directed toward serving the interests of the dominant power structures within the local sites, and therefore those voices often emerge in discursive spaces that are articulated by the most powerful actors within local communities who already have access to resources. One of the criticisms of local forms of participation is the absence of discussions of issues of power and hegemony situated amidst the spaces of local organizing.

The culture-centered approach addresses this line of criticism by engaging with the relationships among culture, structure, and agency as fragmented and continually emerging. Agency is dynamic and is expressed in relationship to the local contexts, which in turn are continually constituted in the interactions among structure and culture. Cultural values, rules, and interpretive frameworks work hand in hand with structural configurations to constitute agency. On one hand, agency is constrained through the organizing of structures that play out through cultural mores and rituals; on the other hand, agency offers the foundation for challenging structures through the reinterpretation of cultural narratives. The culture-centered approach creates avenues for addressing structures at multiple levels, always open to the shifting structural contingencies and the ways in which these structural contingencies are negotiated by local community members.

Participatory Spaces

At the core of the culture-centered approach is the impetus to create participatory spaces for listening to the voices of local communities. These participatory spaces are fundamentally communicative as these are the sites where the local communities come together for the discussion of issues, sharing of ideas, the development of identities, and the identification and mobilization of resources. Participatory spaces within communities become sites of collective organizing and forums for the discussion, deliberation, and decisions on key issues facing local communities. The strategies and tactics for mobilizing to secure access to resources and bring about shifts in dominant structures are discussed, argued about, and decided upon in these forums of local participation. The culture-centered approach emphasizes the transitive nature of these spaces because they are situated amidst competing tensions, are often perceived as threatening to the status quo, and are constituted amidst the politics of legitimacy building and articulating change initiatives.

Participatory spaces are also vital to the linkages among the local community and other community structures situated across these dispersed sites of global organizing against globalized structures that constitute oppressive neoliberal policies. Networks connecting various sites of local struggles create cross-community spaces for the mobilization of resources, sharing of issues and ideas, and articulations of resistive politics. For example, the various linkages among local community organizations dispersed across the globe were crucial to the successful organizing of the protests against the WTO meetings in Seattle in 1999. Similarly, the successful resistance to the Multilateral Agreement on Investment (MAI) was brought about through the coordination and networking of multiple local activist groups across the globe. These global participatory spaces are locally connected, thus circulating local theories and articulations at global sites, and simultaneously informing and learning from other local sites. This criss-crossing of information across participatory spaces in resistive organizing creates a networked web of local participation that organizes against the global power of neoliberalism. The global nature of such participatory spaces also creates the impetus for drawing upon these global networks of solidarity at local sites of struggles against neoliberal policies. One group of participatory spaces are the independent media centers such as Indymedia where community members organize their own participation in mediated spheres (Carpentier, 2007). In other instances, existing organizations facilitate the participation of community members.

Also vital to the politics of social change communication is the co-creation of participatory spaces that challenge the articulations of neoliberal principles and draw attention to the inequities and injustices perpetrated by the SAPs formulated by IFIs. These spaces exist amidst the relationships among the local and the global. Local stories re-presenting alternatives to neoliberal organizing, plant seeds of processes of social change. Furthermore, resistive practices in subaltern public spheres engage with the mainstream to challenge the erasures in mainstream policy platforms, and to expose the taken-for-granted assumptions that underlie the exploitative and oppressive policies of neoliberalism. For example, the participatory spaces created by Survival International create global spaces for listening to subaltern voices and to retell stories of resistance that document the continued erasure of subaltern communities via the displacement policies of neoliberalism. Global structural transformations are created through political participation, participation at the global centers of neoliberal exploitation, and participation in policy circles that have hitherto been closed off to the subaltern sectors (Rajagopal, 2003).

Structural Transformations

Ultimately, as noted throughout this chapter, culture-centered participatory processes of social change connect local voices through participatory platforms to agendas of structural transformation. The ability to challenge structures and to bring about material changes in these structures is quintessential to the culture-centered approach. The participatory processes in the symbolic realms of the culture-centered approach are made meaningful in their relationships with the structures that constrain and enable access to economic and material resources. Therefore, the material foundations of social change processes are situated in the actual transformations in material structures and in the (in)access to economic and material resources faced by subaltern communities.

The transformative possibilities of the culture-centered approach lie in the changes in the material structures of oppression and exploitation of the subaltern sectors of the globe. In this sense, the operationalization of what constitutes social change is vitally dependent upon the articulation of tangible material changes in oppressive and exploitative structures globally, nationally, as well as locally. The argument is further extended by explicating those participatory processes that manipulate local agency with the goal of serving the goals of power and control exercised by dominant structures as opposed to the locally situated participatory processes that fundamentally position themselves in opposition to these structures, with the goal of changing these structures of oppression and exploitation.

With the increasing inequalities between the resource rich and resource poor sectors of the globe, the viability of the politics of social change ought to be measured on the basis of the structural transformations brought about by communicative processes, and the potential of these communicative processes in addressing these inequalities and in mitigating the marginalization of the poorer sectors of the globe. In this sense, the culture-centered approach is specifically concerned with interrogating the politics of change and the ways in which this change is accomplished through participatory processes that are directed toward addressing structurally situated inequalities.

Conclusion

Participation is the cornerstone of social change communication as it is through participatory processes, spaces, and techniques that local communities mobilize against oppressive social, economic, and political structures. Participation brings about social change through the presence of subaltern populations whose marginalization has been symbolically and materially achieved throughout history through their erasure from the mainstream spaces of society. The presence of these subaltern voices in the global mainstream articulates alternative rationalities that challenge the free market logics of neoliberalism, and offer alternative visions for economic, social, and political organizing. Quintessential to these culture-centered processes of participation is the interpenetration of structure and agency, connecting the spaces of local political participation with global networks, and creating local-global infrastructures for challenging and shaping local, national, and global policies through local participation.

10

MEDIATED SOCIAL CHANGE

This chapter examines the ways in which social change initiatives creatively use the media in order to draw attention to issues and reframe debates around key issues in public spaces. The chapter delves into the communication processes and strategies that are constituted in the realm of transformative politics in mediated public spheres, exploring further the intersections between dominant public spheres and subaltern public spheres in the realm of social change politics. It asks the questions: What are the roles and functions played by media in the politics of social change? How do social change processes and organizations participate in the contested terrains of the media in order to create entry points of change? What are the points of intersection between subaltern public spheres and mediated public spheres within hegemonic configurations such that agendas of change articulated through subaltern participation are voiced in mainstream public spheres? What ultimately is the role of the media in narrating the politics of social change initiated in subaltern contexts, particularly against the backdrop of the neoliberal control of global media?

We begin the chapter with an examination of the theoretical approaches to the study of media in the realm of social change. This theoretical discussion offers a framework for understanding the role and location of contemporary social change media within the broader politics of neoliberalism and globalization (Bailey, Cammaerts, & Carpentier, 2008). The intersections of mediated social change initiatives and neoliberal politics are evident in the large-scale growth of global corporate media power and global communication resources that promote neoliberalism, accompanied by the equally salient growth of media activism projects that use the very resources of neoliberal hegemony to disrupt the dominant discourses (Bennett, 2003a, 2003b). It is this contestation of power between the politics of resistance and the sites of control that is the focal point of this chapter.

Based on the discussion of the theoretical conceptualizations of the role of the media in the realm of social change, we explore the intersections of culture, structure, and agency in mediated practices of social change (Dutta, 2006, 2007, 2008a, 2008b, 2008c; Dutta & Pal, 2010). The tripod of culture, structure, and agency are continually situated in contested relationships with each other, constituting and shaping each other, and defining the terrains of a praxis of social change. The culture-centered approach, with its emphasis on disrupting the dominant discursive spaces that erase subaltern voices, creates openings for understanding the ways in which agency is played out in creating entry points for listening to the classed, raced, gendered subject whose voice has been erased from the spaces of knowledge production. Here, the role of the media is further examined in terms of the capacity of activist publics to create mediated participatory spaces that listen to subaltern voices, and disrupt the dominant narratives with subaltern rationalities that stand in resistance. The politics of change embodied in the mediated movements of social change is situated in the contestation of the status quo through the representation and circulation of images of change. Alternative rationalities and representations emerge into the discursive spaces through the contestation of dominant representations.

The intersections of structure and agency suggest the relevance of exploring cultural processes in contemporary globalization frameworks that rewrite the scripts of neoliberalism written into the dominant structures. The enactment of agency through the contestation of fluid political identities within and across national borders is made possible through the increasing permeability of mediated structures to counter-messages that flow at the very same speed as the dominant discourses of neoliberal hegemony (Bennett, 2003a, 2003b). The culture-centered approach ultimately emphasizes the communicative processes and practices through which agency is organized in order to foster social change in mediated spaces. Also, through the use of examples and case studies of mediated social change movements across the globe, this chapter discusses the communication processes through which mediated art forms protest against the oppressive politics of dominant structures, thus seeking to disrupt the hegemonic rationality that constitutes the mainstream. This chapter, on one hand, engages with the theoretical tensions that emerge at the crossroads of mainstream and subaltern public spheres, and on the other hand, draws out the key points of praxis for activist movements that participate in mediated social change politics.

Theoretical Approaches

The theoretical approaches to the study of mediated practices of social change emphasize the contested domains of power within which such practices are constituted. Furthermore, they draw our attention to the conceptualization of alternative media as sites of articulating alternative narratives and rationalities in the discursive space. In the discussions of contested terrains of power and the alternative media spheres, this section of the chapter highlights the communicative practices of organizing and solidarity building that attempt to bring about social change by questioning the hegemonic configurations in mainstream public spheres, creating multiple counter-hegemonies that offer openings for social change. Our discussion of the theoretical conceptualizations of media power and alternative media will be connected to the discussion of globalization as an overarching framework for understanding mediated processes of social change and structural transformation.

Media Power

Theories of mediated social change that examine the role of media within the broader realms of social change processes put forth the concept of media power (Couldry & Curran, 2003b). Noting the paradox in the articulations of power in the realm of mediated systems, the concept of media power not only attends to the processes through which powerful actors within social systems use the media in order to serve their agendas, but also foregrounds the powerful role of media as the catalyst of social action in contemporary complex societies, where public support for social action is contingent upon the circulation of information and images. Power therefore becomes an organizing concept, offering a framework for understanding the ways in which mediated spaces become entry points for social transformation through the articulations of alternative discourses that challenge the status quo.

Media power constitutes a dynamic and contested terrain where multiple social actors compete to have control over the representational space. Particularly in the realm of processes of social change that seek to bring about transformations in global structures, securing access to the means of media production becomes important, as it is through these mediated sites that alternative discourses are introduced into the mainstream, creating points of contestations with the hegemonic articulations within the social system (Bennett, 2003a, 2003b; Couldry, 2003; Couldry & Curran, 2003a; Downing, 2003; C. Rodríguez, 2001, 2003). The struggles that emerge in social change processes therefore are partially played out in the form of struggles over the sites and channels of representations in societies (Gitlin, 1980).

In contemporary capitalism, with media power situated in the hands of transnational corporations, the media play out their roles as tools for disseminating the mantras of capitalism and for carrying out the agendas of transnational corporations (Herman & Chomsky, 1988; Kumar, 2001; McChesney, 1997). The media, as sites of power, play a pivotal role within the United States, constituting a depoliticized citizenry that operates within the realms of selfishness and consumption as frameworks for rational choice, thus leaving tremendous openings for corporate powers to exert their influence on the mass media, determining both media agendas as well as media frames (McChesney, 1997). Media scholars document the role of the media in serving the interests of the elite, depicting a classless society and erasing the narratives of class antagonisms and labor struggles from the dominant discursive spaces (Goldman & Rajagopal, 1991). As sites of power, media represent the interests of transnational hegemony, narrating the image of a consumption-driven society, constituting individual subjectivity in consumption, and simultaneously drawing attention away from the possibilities of class struggles on the basis of the inequities perpetuated in the contemporary neoliberal configuration. However, it is within these very terrains of power that the stories of class struggles and proletarian counter-hegemonies emerge (Kumar, 2001).

In her analysis of the coverage of the United Parcel Service (UPS) workers' strike in mainstream media, Kumar (2001) noted the organizing capacity of labor to influence the coverage in traditionally pro-corporate media through the utilization of networks, interpersonal communication with publics across the country, and messages being placed in other media such as leaflets being distributed to the media, television, and the Internet. Although the initial mainstream newspaper coverage of the strike presented an anti-union pro-corporate frame where the strike was seen as disruptive, subsequent coverage shifted in tone toward covering the issues raised by the workers because of the national attention drawn by the strike, public support for the strike and general disappointment with the US economy in the 1990s that generated large profits for corporations at the cost of exploiting the workers, and the unwillingness of the US government to intervene in the strike because of the public support. Media scholars articulate that the UPS strike demonstrates the power of workers to organize and in doing so, to introduce the proletariat public sphere into a bourgeoisie public sphere, disrupting the classlessness of the dominant public spheres with narratives of class antagonisms and struggles (Kumar, 2001; Negt & Kluge, 1993).

The emphasis of social change movements then is on contesting the sites of media power both implicitly and explicitly. These movements not only question the legitimacy of the images and information circulated in the mainstream media, but also seek to create alternative interpretations and narratives mapped onto global events. This is done through processes of organizing that seek to produce and distribute alternative readings. The global Independent Media Center movement represents one such contestation of media power in its role in anti-globalization struggles (Curran & Park, 2000; Downing, 2003). In considering the goals of resistive processes to contest the increasing neoliberal control over contemporary mediated spaces, Couldry and Curran (2003b) discuss the various sources of power including the state, the market, and civil society, whose influence might be catalyzed in order to challenge the existing elite configurations that run the media system. A power-centered approach to mediated social change foregrounds the networks and relationships that are constituted in the realm of transforming social structures.

From the standpoint of the praxis of social change, activist groups working on getting coverage on issues of change participate in the contestations of power in the realms of representation, utilizing multiple points of leverage and network capacities to exert pressure on media to gain coverage of certain issues, and to influence the media frames that circulate around these issues (Kumar, 2001). The theoretical conceptualization of power in mediated sites of social change elucidates the paradoxical relationship between structure and agency (more on this later), as organizations participating in social change processes engage with those very structures that perpetuate the instrumentalities of control. For instance, the global communication networks that seek to promote neoliberal discourses across the globe also become the very sites of resistive organizing and communication for disrupting the very same neoliberal discourse, as evident in the protests organized in Seattle against the World Trade Organization (Bennett, 2003a, 2003b; Couldry & Curran, 2003b). Globalization processes directed at increasing the power and control of TNCs across the globe (Sassen, 1988) have also created spaces for global activist networks that question the mass media power exerted globally (Bennett, 2003a, 2003b).

Alternative Media

Drawing upon the notion of media power that conceptualizes the competing interests and struggles that play out over the question of representation, alternative media represent the many sites of media production that exist outside the realms of traditionally controlled mainstream media, often challenging the very discourses that are circulated in the mainstream (Atton, 2002; Castells, 2001; McKay, 1996). In this case, the mainstream captures the mass media products that are widely available and widely consumed across the globe, often concentrated in the hands of a few transnational media houses; alternative media then are situated in opposition to these mainstream forms of media, offering an alternative to the mainstream forms of media consumption in a given society (Atton, 2002; Castells, 2001; Waltz, 2005). In defining what constitutes this opposition, media theorists establish the following criteria: first, delivering content presenting points of view that are not usually presented in the mainstream media; second, serving communities that are not usually served by the mainstream mass media; third, being created and disseminated in ways that are radically different from the mainstream business practices of corporate media houses; fourth, being organized and operated in alternative frameworks that depart from the traditional formats of media organizing; and fifth, advocating some form of social change that seeks to bring about transformations in the contemporary mainstream structures (Waltz, 2005).

An example of an alternative medium that not only presents alternative viewpoints to its somewhat non-mainstream audiences, but also embodies an alternative form of organizing built on an alternative model for media production is the publication *Z Magazine*, founded by the alternative media theorist Michael Albert (2003). Albert's vision of alternative media is built upon the concept of an alternative economic production and organizing framework, termed participatory economics, where media products are created and distributed by the people who make them, organized in the form of democratic workers' councils. The organizing of Z Magazine is based on participatory principles of decision-making where everyone in the organization is involved in decision-making, having access to all the necessary information before participating in decision-making, as well as being encouraged and supported to share their views openly and effectively. The emphasis is on democratic decision-making rather than on hierarchical decision-making; similarly, everyone working in an alternative media organization should earn the same amount of income for the same amount of work, irrespective of job titles. These participatory principles of internal organizing are also extended to the interactions of the organization with its audiences on the basis of the same principles of democratic organizing (Waltz, 2005). Furthermore, Albert (2003) notes the importance of alternative media to reach out to a large audience based on the foundations of a broad appeal and build networks of solidarity that support and nurture other forms of alternative media, as opposed to the market-based model of competition that drives the mainstream media environment.

At a global level, the seeds of alternative media are evident in the UNESCO project on the New World Information and Communication Order (NWICO) with its objectives of balancing the inequities in media ownership by placing electronic media and necessary resources in the hands of citizens who have been previously denied access to the capabilities for producing and distributing mediated messages (I. Rodríguez, 2001). The inequities in communicative opportunities in the 1970s were noted in the global North-South divides, with much of the information about the Third World being created and circulated by a few transnational communications corporations that were mostly located in the United States and in Western Europe. This placing of the capabilities of producing media messages in the hands of the local communities that have traditionally been subalternized creates a discursive space that disrupts the status quo. Clemencia Rodríguez (2001) notes:

> I could see how producing alternative media messages implies much more than simply challenging the mainstream media with *campesino* correspondents as new communication and information sources. It implies having the opportunity to create one's own images of self and environment; it implies being able to recodify one's own identity with the signs and codes that one chooses, thereby disrupting the traditional acceptance of those imposed by outside sources; it implies becoming one's own storyteller, regaining one's own voice; it implies reconstructing the self portrait of one's own community and one's own culture; it implies exploring the infinite possibilities of one's own body, one's own face, to create facial expressions (a new codification of the face) and non-verbal languages (a new codification of the body) never seen before; it implies taking one's own languages out of their usual hiding places and throwing them out there, into the public sphere.
>
> (C. Rodríguez, 2001, p. 3)

What becomes evident in Rodríguez's concept of citizens' media is the location of agency within the subaltern community not only in terms of defining its identities and narratives, but also in terms of having a voice in the hegemonic spaces.

Borrowing from Mouffe and McClure's theory of radical democracy (Mouffe, 1993), Clemencia Rodríguez (2001) proposes the concept of community media, noting the organic, dynamic, and fragmented processes through which individuals as well as collectives enact their agency as they gain access to and reclaim their own media. Individual participants become active citizens as they engage in the processes of articulating their views and enacting their agency. In this sense, the concept of the citizens' media takes into account the processes of empowerment, conscientization, and fragmentation of power that take place as citizens come to take charge of their lives, the mediated representations that narrate their stories, and disrupt the traditional structures of decision-making that take their agency for granted. Through the processes of conscientization and empowerment, citizens' media participants enact their agency in making decisions about their lives, communities, and cultures. For Rodríguez (2001), inherent in the idea of citizens' media is progressive thinking that challenges the status quo and offers spaces for enactment of agency among marginalized communities across the globe. Similarly, O'Sullivan's (1994) conceptualization of alternative media is based on its capacity to articulate spaces of radical social change and to create entry points for political action directed at these goals of social change on the basis of democratic and collectivistic processes of production that pursue alternative content, design, and delivery styles.

Along similar lines, Waltz (2005) defines activist media as those media sites that encourage their readers to take action. In other words, inherent in the conceptualization of activist media is the capacity of such media to emerge as spaces for political action, pushing readers to participate in processes of social change. There exists a wide range of debate regarding what constitutes activist media, based on the categorization of the nature of calls for political action issued by the media. Scholars suggest that media calls for mainstream political action such as voting and volunteering do not constitute activism as they do not fall outside the realm of the mainstream. In other words, the nature of the action proposed by the media is important in considering the categorization of the media as activist media.

Increasingly, the globalization of new media technologies and the availability of platforms for the expression of alternative political opinions have also created emerging sites for the development, production, and dissemination of political content that resists the mainstream. As noted in Chapter 7 on performing social change, the widespread accessibility of the Internet has also opened up alternative sites that serve as spaces for the articulation of contentious politics. Major resistance campaigns operate through websites, posting information about issues facing the marginalized populations, creating frames around these issues, mobilizing spaces and strategies of support for these issues, and connecting the online participation to offline forms of participation in activist projects. Listservs, blogs, and social media such as Facebook also serve as platforms for posting information and mobilizing resources for participatory processes of social change.

Platforms such as YouTube have emerged as sites for distribution of videos that document the structural and material violence in the subaltern sectors, bringing local stories to global audiences, often narrated by local participants at sites of contention, and thus also documenting the narratives of violence and control enacted by the military industrial complex and its collaborators in the neoliberal project. For example, the organization Survival: The Movement for Tribal Peoples works on changing public opinion about tribal issues; seeking to create global platforms for listening to local tribal voices; engaging these voices with dominant actors such as corporations, governments, extremist missionaries, banks, and experts who violate the rights of tribal peoples (www.survivalinternational.org/info). Survival strategically utilizes YouTube to disseminate its messages of change, directly bringing to public platforms in mainstream society the voices of tribal people in marginalized spaces, and creating spaces for listening to the tribal voices as entry points for disrupting the neoliberal hegemony that operates on the basis of constructing the tribal culture as a passive relic of the past on its way to extinction. The campaigns run by Survival use a variety of techniques such as letter writing campaigns, reports, bulletins, community radio, and new media platforms to disseminate the messages of tribal populations in dominant discursive spaces, particularly targeting the public in the West and the global North, with the goal of educating the West about the relevance of the tribal cosmology to the contemporary world. Web projects developed by Survival use video clips, films, and pictures to create communicative spaces for listening to tribal voices that disrupt the hegemony of the mainstream, and simultaneously for enlisting public support against the implementation of neoliberal policies that threaten tribal life and displace tribal populations from the spaces they call home. Furthermore, Survival utilizes social media to connect the web projects with specific campaigns and specific calls for action.

Simultaneously, projects of social change have started focusing on the development of alternative media sites and distribution channels for the delivery of alternative content to the public, with the goals of raising public opinion about social-economic-political issues and creating spaces of social change. For example, Link TV operates as a television cable channel, drawing its revenues from donations, grants, and viewer support, and delivering alternative conceptualizations of politics, economics, and society that challenge neoliberal policies, and seeking to activate viewers to participate in processes of social change (www.linktv.org/whoweare/mission). The non-profit organization Link Media sees its role as creating spaces for alternative views that are typically inaccessible in mainstream media, create a platform for listening to the voices of those communities that are traditionally unheard in dominant public spheres, connecting the local to the global, promoting dialogues, promoting action through offering access to tools and connections for action, and networking with global organizations at the grassroots to create collaborative spaces of change. Link TV programming is available on cable and satellite; Link Media also has a presence on the web, as well as a blog. Similarly, Pacifica Radio is the oldest public national radio network in the United States, with over a hundred affiliated radio stations and five non-commercial listener supported radio stations that seek to create alternative spaces of political action, resistance, and social change (www.pacificafoundation.org/). The A-Infos Radio Project provides compressed audio files that can be downloaded by listeners to their computers, and serves as a site for grassroots activists, free radio journalists, grassroots broadcasters, and cyberactivists to share their programs over the Internet, with the goal of promoting democratic and participatory communicative spaces that challenge the dominant structures of contemporary hegemony (www.radio4 all.net/index.php/about/).

Alternative media are also constituted in the presence of alternative distribution channels, platforms, and resources for reaching out to the public with content on issues that challenge the hegemony of the neoliberal framework that continues to occupy most of mainstream media. For example, the Magic Lantern Foundation is a nonprofit organization that serves as a resource for film production, film training, and film education, and as an archive for dissemination of resistance films, working with a revenue panel to sustain itself. The production and distribution of alternative films creates spaces for the articulation of alternative voices that exist in the peripheries of neoliberal hegemony and are simultaneously the subjects of neoliberal exploitation. In essence then, distribution channels such as Magic Lantern create spaces for the articulation of subaltern voices in the mainstream that challenge and resist the dominant free market logic of neoliberalism. In the context of subaltern displacements and movements of resistance, such distribution channels open up avenues for engaging public opinion with alternative viewpoints that interrogate the hegemonic narratives of TNCs and the narratives sponsored by the state.

Yet another way for creating alternative spaces is by democratizing the access to the creation of media content in underserved communities that have historically been rendered voiceless in mediated public spheres. The Rural Media Company (RMC) based in Hereford (www.ruralmedia.co.uk) works on co-creating mediated spaces with marginalized youth from rural contexts, equipping them with skill sets and technologies to become media creators rather than passive media audiences or subjects of occasional reports. The narratives that are articulated through the project voice the issues and concerns facing rural youth and the ways in which they engage with these issues and concerns. Locating the participatory capacity within the ambits of the local community creates spaces of change by engaging parents, education authorities, teachers, policy-makers, and others through the public sphere.

New Media

As noted in the previous section, one of the key markers of globalization has been the compression of time and space through the presence of new communication technologies that bring about new communication infrastructures and opportunities for publics to communicate across the globe through networks of organizing (Castells, 1996, 1997, 1998). These information and communication technologies (ICTs) have been critical in the consolidation of power in the hands of global power structures, bringing local sites across the globe under the purview of TNCs and their control. The "new subalterns" have been constituted within the exploitative structures of neoliberalism precisely because of these new infrastructures of communication and modalities for bringing global spaces under the control of centrally operated communicative processes and practices. However, even as these communication technologies of control have enhanced the reach and penetration of TNCs, they have also created spaces for connecting subaltern organizing with global sites of change, co-creating subaltern narratives in global spaces that challenge neoliberal hegemony (Donk, Loader, Nixon, & Rucht, 2004).

ICTs play a vital role in social movements, as social movements use email, newsgroups, mailing lists, forums, websites, streaming, blogs, social media, and hacktivism to communicate with each other, to communicate with key stakeholders, to present an identity to outside stakeholders, and to challenge dominant structures and the rationalities perpetuated in these structures (Donk et al., 2004; Grignou & Patou, 2004). The Internet has emerged as a strategic platform for social movements to mobilize and organize protest, to communicate with members of the public, and to put forth resistive strategies that question the legitimacy of the narratives circulated in the dominant structures (Warkentin, 2001). In tackling global problems, movements such as the Climate Action Network develop networks of transnational cooperation and strategically harness the capacity of the Internet for disseminating information quickly to mobilize groups all across the globe (Donk et al., 2004).

The reach and immediacy of the Internet are essential to global mobilization for groups such as Earth Action that utilize the medium for alerting its worldwide constituency to action targeting political leaders on important political issues. The Internet also serves as a tool for providing alternative information that is typically suppressed by mainstream media, thus creating spaces for alternative narratives, ideologies, and voices that challenge the dominant structures (Grignou & Patou, 2004). For example, Indymedia (www.indymedia.org) is a loose network of leftist-oriented media that are located in different countries and offer alternative stories of events that challenge the stories circulated in mainstream media.

One of the earliest examples of subaltern resistance organized, networked, and articulated through the Internet is the Zapatista movement (H. Cleaver, 1998). The movement utilized the Internet not only to distribute information about local oppressions and struggles in the Zapatista communities, but also to create networks of solidarity across the globe with other indigenous actors as well as actors in the environmental and feminist sectors (H. Cleaver, 1998; Garrido & Halavais, 2003; Schulz, 1998). In doing so, it developed a model of solidarity among indigenous communities for resisting the dominant global-national-local structures that perpetrated their exploitation and erasure, and connected these indigenous struggles with issues of environmental activism and women's rights. The success of the movement was attributed to its capacity to utilize the Internet to globally situate a grassroots struggle of resistance in a marginalized community, to build linkages with struggles that bypassed and often resisted national policies of structural adjustment, to create a global base of support and public opinion for the local Zapatista struggle, and to place into the mainstream public spheres of globalization local models of alternative rationality, participatory processes, and organizing that stood in opposition to the values and organizing principles of neoliberalism. Noting the revolutionizing role of the EZLN in creating a global network of grassroots solidarity utilizing the web, a network analysis conducted by Garrido and Halavais (2003) demonstrated that Zapatista-related sites are central to the global NGO networks and play a pivotal role in binding them together.

Along similar lines, the Internet emerged as a key site of mobilization, information dissemination, public opinion formation, and expression in resistance to the Multilateral Agreement on Investment (MAI) in 1998. Mobilization by NGOs across the globe connected through the Internet and protesting the MAI ultimately led to its failure (Ayres, 1999, 2001). Similarly, the Association for the Taxation of Financial Transactions for the Aid of Citizens (ATTAC) was created in 1998, mobilizing activist communities throughout the globe using the Internet to create a people's education movement seeking to generate awareness and transparency of the economic policies of neoliberalism and the economic procedures of decision-making in neoliberal governance (della Porta, Kreisi, & Rucht, 1999; Grignou & Patou, 2004). Having started in France with approximately 250 local communities that were represented, ATTAC gained international support, with over 35 separate movements that were created all across the world including in Brazil, Japan, and Senegal (Grignou & Patou, 2004). At the top of ATTAC's organizational chart is a scientific community of approximately 20 academics and researchers who publish key concepts in ATTAC books and provide intellectual and conceptual fodder for ATTAC campaigns. These ideas offer counter-expertise to dominant narratives of neoliberalism and provide entry points for targeted action for local activist movements.

The local sites of activism are connected to the global platforms of activist politics through new media platforms such as web pages, bulletin boards, and discussion groups, through social media such as Facebook, and through audio-visual tools such as YouTube. For example, the Save Niyamgiri project seeks to organize public opinion and support against the development of a mining project in the Niyamgiri hills of Orissa, India, that threatens to displace large populations of the Kondh tribals who live in the area. The project has a Facebook presence through which it shares important news directly from the site, compiles a variety of media stories, as well as connects with videos that narrate through the voices of the tribals the experiences they face against the backdrop of the mining project, the threats to their life posed by the London-based Vedanta Corporation, the violence enacted by the corporation, and the state-sponsored police violence on tribal protests.

Globalization, Media, and Social Change

Globalization is defined by Tomlinson (1999) as a *complex connectivity*, as a rapidly developing and increasingly deepening network of interconnections and dependencies across time and space. Appadurai (1996) notes that contemporary globalization processes and global spaces are marked by the two concepts of flow and disjuncture, both playing central roles in the theorizing of communicative processes of social change. Central to the many definitions of globalization is the increasing speed and volume of flow of people, capital, ideas, goods, images, and services that connect actors across national borders (Appadurai, 1996, 2001; Keohane, 2002; McMichael, 2005, 2008). Simultaneously, these relationships of flows across global borders are played out in the form of disjunctures in the pathways and vectors taken by the goods, labor, ideas, images, and services that flow across the borders, creating multiple points of interruptions, frictions, and possibilities of resistance within global systems (Appadurai, 2001). These disjunctures are constituted by the "different speeds, points of origin and termination, and varied relationships to institutional structures in different regions, nations or societies" (Appadurai, 2001, p. 6), creating new opportunities for the articulation of resistance in the contemporary global landscape. For Appadurai (2001), the fundamental problems of equity, suffering, social justice, and governance are products of the disjunctures between the various vectors of the current global configuration. Therefore, inherent in the politics of power and control in globalization are the possibilities of resistance that disrupt these spaces of power and control (Pal & Dutta, 2008a, 2008b).

The same networks and mediated spaces that serve the functions of consolidating power and control in the hands of TNCs also bring together fluid networks of solidarity constituted around issues and ideologies, collectively organized as sites of resistance to the hegemony of TNCs. Within the framework of globalization, the rise in activist movements demonstrates the global opportunities for organizing movements across borders and for international mobilization (della Porta & Diani, 2006; della Porta & Tarrow, 2005). These activist movements draw our attention to the necessity to theorize about the ways in which resistance is enacted in complexly connected sites that weave the global with the local, played out through the collective organizing sites of new media (Bennett, 2003a, 2003b). Resistance becomes a communicative space connected with individual and collective practice through which the interplay of the global and local becomes situated in the realm of transformative politics played out through new media networks. For example, the Argentine protests were triggered by the pressures of international financial institutions but were directed at local institutions (Auyero, 2003). Simultaneously, movement organizations often become involved supranationally in order to create international alliances for nationally weak social movements (Keck & Sikkink, 1998). With their Eurostrike in 1997, Spanish, French, and Belgian Renault workers protested the closing of the Renault factory of Vilvorde in Belgium at the EU level (Lefebure & Lagneau, 2002).

The practice of global activism brings to the forefront the global connectivity of issues, demonstrating that issues are no longer situated within locally isolated spaces, but rather are interconnected globally with global processes and practices. The WTO protests, for instance, brought to our attention the ways in which global policies impact local actors, and the processes through which the opportunities of participation by geographically dispersed local actors bring about globally situated resistance to powerful social actors (in this instance, the WTO). The local is impacted by events that happen in the realm of the global, and simultaneously influences the processes that continue to take place globally. Local issues and the possibilities for how these issues are implemented are impacted by the global policies in the realm of which they are situated. For instance, the framing of policies related to the pharmaceutical industry in the local realm is impacted by the articulation and implementation of health policies in the global arena that govern the innovation, dissemination, and use of health products.

Drawing upon this emphasis on transnational resistance, critical public relations scholars explore the ways in which the public relations strategies of powerful global actors influence global and local policies, and the lives of locally situated publics, and the opportunities of resistance they create (Dutta, 2009). Furthermore, critical scholarship interrogates the ways in which the framing of global issues is influenced by the flow of power and control in the realm of globalization. Specifically, in the area of public policies and the construction of global risks, it would be worthwhile to examine the global processes through which these risks are constituted and policies developed to control, manage, and evaluate them. For communication practitioners, this has brought about the relevance of communicating with globally dispersed publics that are situated locally and yet connected globally through sets of issues that offer the substratum for their cohesiveness. For example, global HIV/AIDS activist groups have emerged that mobilize locally as well as globally to shape global HIV/AIDS policies. This suggests the relevance for engaging in globally situated issues management that is sensitized to the continuous interpenetration of the local and the global. From a critical standpoint, this suggests the importance of interrogating the global power structures within which issues are framed and policies are managed. This local-global interflow in globalization processes is accompanied by time-space compression in global organizations, and the complex interplay among the various scapes of social life within which the human experience is organized, and human activism becomes possible.

Reflecting upon this complexity of global processes and the possibilities of resistance that are written into the very structures of control that seek to fold global spaces under the market logics of TNCs, Appadurai (1990) writes "the new global cultural economy has to be understood as a complex, overlapping, disjunctive order." In understanding the fluidity in globalization processes played out at the sites of the media, he proposes the concept of the mediascape. Mediascape refers to the conglomeration of media entities that carry mediated information across borders, providing images that depend on several interests of global actors and playing out the functions of representing the interests of transnational global actors. The concentration of media ownership in a few hands suggests the need to explore how global media ownership patterns interplay with the public relations messages of transnational corporations, and the connections between powerful global actors and the access to media agenda setting and issue framing secured by public relations practitioners. Simultaneously, it is in these very mediascapes spread across time and space that pathways are created for transnational activism that seeks to disrupt the dominance of the global hegemony.

In summary, the global shift, associated with the creation of world markets and with international communication and media flows, has profound implications for the way people make sense of their lives and of the changing world, and the ways in which they resist the dominant global configurations (Robins, 2000). Robins (2000, p. 198) notes that globalization "is provoking new senses of disorientation and of orientation, giving rise to new experiences of both placeless and placed identity." In essence, most of the globalization theories explain globalization in terms of diversity and difference rather than in terms of homogenization. It is within this simultaneity of diversity and difference that is at once situated and displaced that activist theorists and practitioners must locate a set of resistive practices that are meaningful to the global publics dispersed across various local sites around the globe, and serve as means of global organizing.

National identities are no longer marked by simplistic concepts such as collectivism and individualism that offer polar opposites to locate national cultures based on the notion of static cultures that can be delimited within the geographical definitions of nation states. Cultures exist in continuous flux, continuously interpreted and reinterpreted through human interactions, and embedded within the context of the lives of the members of the cultures. Culture is both a carrier of traditions and a site of transformation. It is within this dialectical tension between tradition and transformation that identities and relationships become meaningful, suggesting the necessity of conceptualizing social change communication within an organic framework of evolving relationships rather than within a simplistic modernist frame that seeks to develop the best strategy for a national culture based on predefined markers such as individualism/collectivism, power distance, uncertainty avoidance, and masculinity/femininity. The complex interplay of the global–local tension accompanied by the dynamic interactions among the five scapes offers theoretical and pragmatic entry points for exploring the ways in which resistance is enacted in the realm of global activism. In other words, globalization cannot be understood as a singular condition or in terms of linear development logic. It is multifaceted, weaving intricate networks between communities, states, international institutions, NGOs, and TNCs. Amidst these complex networks, globalization provides a new context for thinking of issues of power and domination, and resistance to such dominance (Ganesh et al., 2005) particularly in the context of the growing strength of collective movements to resist neoliberal policies both at local as well as global sites.

Culture-Centered Approach to Mediated Social Change

The culture-centered approach offers a meta-theoretical framework for understanding the role of communication in bringing about structural transformations, particularly in the context of listening to the voices of local communities that create spaces of global structural transformations (Basu & Dutta, 2009). Of interest to culture-centered scholars is the act of listening to subaltern voices that have been rendered subaltern precisely because of the politics of erasure embedded in the mainstream public spheres and the systems of knowledge production within these public spheres. Challenging the expertise-based knowledge articulations in mainstream media spheres that legitimize the oppression and exploitation of the subaltern sectors, subaltern articulations in mediated spheres offer alternative rationalities, document the narratives of structural oppressions, and co-create spaces for enacting subaltern agency at global sites where public opinion as well as knowledge about policies and interventions are circulated.

The culture-centered approach ruptures the hegemonic narrative of neoliberal expansion by emphasizing the creation of mediated public spheres that narrate stories of social change and social transformation. These public spheres become sites of information sharing as well as spaces of collective mobilization, identity building, and organizing. Ultimately, the culture-centered approach brings about theoretical and practical changes in the ways in which we think of media in the politics of social change. It does so by first noting the communicative processes of marginalization in the dominant corporatized media spheres that delegitimize cultural voices of local communities living under poverty across the globe, and subsequently articulating the possibilities of resistance that are written into the marginalizing practices of the dominant media spheres (Couldry & Curran, 2003b; Dutta, 2009; Dutta & Pal, 2010). On one hand, as Bennett (2003a) notes, the increasing consolidation of media power in the hands of a few global media networks have placed the uses of these networks toward the public relations strategies and strategic communications agendas of TNCs; on the other hand, new media configurations such as mobile phones, the Internet, streaming technologies, wireless networks, as well as the publishing and dissemination capacities of the World Wide Web have opened up new possibilities for resistive organizing across geographic and media boundaries.

These competing processes are articulated within the domain of social, political, and economic structures, amidst the constraining and enabling functions of social structures, and their dialectical relationship with agency. Structures are at once determinative in their influences on everyday living experiences and are simultaneously fluid in their ability to metamorphose through the enactment of agency. Inherent in the power configurations of dominant structures are the possibilities for the enactment of agency (Bennett, 2003a, 2003b). Those very structures that carry out the agendas of the status quo also create new avenues for participation, for activism, and for projects of transformative politics (Aelst & Walgrave, 2004; Bennett, 2004).

Negotiating Structure and Agency

What the intersections of the alternative, activist, and new media presented above point toward is the continuous negotiation between structure and agency in the terrains of globalization (Aelst & Walgrave, 2004; Bennett, 2004). The seamless flow of transnational power through the formulation and adoption of neoliberal policies is disrupted by the voices of resistance articulated by subaltern communities at the global sites, thus creating fissures and fragments within the structures of neoliberal hegemony, and offering openings for listening to the voices of the poorest sectors of the globe that are being continually erased by the increasing global inequities and the neoliberal policies promoting these inequities (Couldry & Curran, 2003b; Dutta, 2009).

For example, the Zapatista movement operated through the structures of new media technologies and turned these structures into spaces of organizing support for the local movement against the Mexican nation state and its neoliberal policies, thus bypassing the power of the state in enacting its power and control over local indigenous people. The movement not only engaged the dominant structures with local agency, but also introduced a locally situated rationality of Zapatismo into the dominant discursive spaces of globalization politics. What becomes evident is the central role of the Zapatista network in serving as a fulcrum for the Internet-based mobilization of transnational projects of social change, offering an alternative epistemological and ontological basis for collective organizing (Grignou & Patou, 2004).

Along similar lines, the Internet served a key function in the mobilization of the worldwide protests against the WTO meeting in Seattle in 1999 (Aelst & Walgrave, 2004). At one level, the Internet emerged as a key resource through which both local as well as globally distributed activist groups coordinated and planned their actions from long before the actual date of the meetings. The presence of the anti-WTO campaign on the Internet raised awareness about the issues and recruited participants into the campaign that was conducted throughout 1999. One of the key media resources utilized for mobilization was the StopWTO Round distribution list. Furthermore, various websites operated on the Internet to coordinate action, with the anti-WTO coalition occupying much of the mediated space. The Internet-based communication network facilitated the distribution of labor globally, with the local groups focusing on direct action and the international partners playing pivotal roles in providing frames and information to sustain the collective action of resistance (George, 2001).

The articulations of agency in the domain of new media structures also create avenues for questioning the structures of neoliberal governance. For example, videos posted on YouTube documenting United Nations meetings draw attention to the ways in which these meetings silence the voices of indigenous communities through their procedures and rules, in spite of the rhetoric of indigenous rights that resonates throughout the UN. In one specific instance, a video documenting a meeting of the United Nations Framework Convention on Climate Change (UNFCCC) on December 10, 2008, documents the ways in which indigenous community participants were not allowed to articulate their resistive position to global environmental policies on the basis of references to procedural issues (www.youtube.com/watch?v=brsqUgbBHu0&playnext_from=TL&videos=o9E MMWZ9TFM). The expression of agency of a community participant who pointed out the hypocrisy of a meeting that silenced indigenous voices in spite of its rhetoric of indigenous rights challenges the structures of neoliberal governance that have widely adopted the symbolic languages of democracy, participation, and listening in the broader approach to indigenous peoples while at the same time promoting the erasure of indigenous voices through their participation in neoliberal economic policies. In this instance, the specific video documented within the mediated global structures notes the resistive capacity of agency to challenge and disrupt the narratives of the dominant structure.

Cultural Negotiations of Structures

Structures are negotiated via cultural practices and artifacts, through the co-optation and juxtaposition of corporate images against the backdrop of the narratives of oppression and violence carried out by TNCs (Bennett, 2003a, 2003b). Images that circulate culturally are constituted within activist projects to challenge the structures of neoliberalism. Neoliberal logics are disrupted through the adoption of the symbols of neoliberalism within alternative cultural logics that narrate resistive stories seeking to transform global structures. New media forms create opportunity structures across time and space to circulate alternative cultural stories that co-opt and interrogate the symbolic images that are otherwise used by the dominant structures. Furthermore, such forms of new media discourse find their way into 24/7 traditional media through the news and commercial values embedded in them (Bennett, 2003a, 2003b).

Memes are images that are imitated and transmitted across social networks, thus drawing upon the corporate image and identity of a well-established brand, and reconstituting the brand image in an alternative cultural story that questions and seeks to change unfair corporate practices. For example, culture jammer Jonah Peretti visited Nike's corporate shopping website and used its personalized shopping tool that promises customized shoes to request shoes branded with the term "sweatshop." The effectiveness of the resistive Nike meme operated on the basis of the positioning of Nike's promise of personal freedom amidst the exploitative labor practices of the organization. Peretti's exchanges with Nike executives about the transaction were forwarded to a dozen friends via email, who then forwarded the message to their networks, and through such viral communication, it reached many thousands of people. Such forms of culture jamming achieve their effectiveness through the deployment of cultural symbols that traditionally serve the dominant structure to articulate alternative values and rationalities, finding coverage in mainstream media.

Similar movement of messages of social change from micro media such as email, lists, and personal blogs into mass media such as newspapers, TV talk shows, and cable broadcasts is achieved through the strategic use of cultural symbols that communicate the resistive message to a large audience (Bennett, 2003a, 2003b). The group Global Exchange utilized the Internet to mobilize a campaign against Nike's sweatshops by coordinating demonstrations featuring a speech by an Indonesian factory worker in front of Nike stores across the United States. This Internet-based campaign was accompanied by the use of publicity materials directed toward the media, and attempting to shape media agendas and frames around the issue. The success of the campaign drew upon the uses of cultural symbols in traditional as well as new media, effectively turning the Nike image as synonymous with "sweatshop" (Bennett, 2003a, 2003b).

Using platforms such as Facebook, YouTube, and wesbites, the "Save Niyamgiri" online campaign is founded on the articulation of local cultural voices of the indigenous people residing in the Niyamgiri hills of Orissa, India, who are threatened to be displaced by the neoliberal project of bauxite mining to be set up by the London-based Vedanta Corporation. The links to articles and videos, as well as organizing information posted by activists situated both locally and across the globe on the site, create a space for the articulation of local indigenous voices in the discursive space that resist the neoliberal rhetoric of development that is utilized to build the bauxite mining project. These local voices of indigenous people of Niyamgiri, who have and continue to be erased from the mainstream public spheres of neoliberal media, narrate the stories of the Niyamgiri God who protects the Dongria Kondh tribals living in the region, the harmonious relationship between the mountain and the indigenous people, the tremendous health and economic threats to the local communities posed by the Vedanta mining project, and the epistemic violence carried out by the project in writing over the local indigenous knowledge in the Niyamgiri communities about the sacredness of the mountain.

Here, the epistemology and ontology of a cultural narrative is articulated in a mediated public sphere through locally situated voices authoring these narratives, directly challenging the grand narrative of development perpetrated by the state, the corporate social responsibility programs of Vedanta, and the public relations practices of Vedanta. Culture enters into the global structures to disrupt the universal logics of development and modernization, thus forever rendering "impure" the hegemonic narrative of development put forth by neoliberalism. Social change is achieved through the disruption of hegemonic structures through the articulation of locally situated cultural stories. The epistemic violence embodied in the universalizing rhetoric of development is deconstructed, and it is on the basis of this deconstruction that the viewer, reader, listener, or public is invited to participate in the co-creation of an alternative narrative.

Culture in Agency

Agency is expressed on mediated platforms through the adoption of cultural symbols and cultural artifacts (Downing, 2001). Culturally situated aesthetic performances such as poems, songs, dances, and plays documented in alternative and new media platforms narrate the stories of oppression and exploitation carried out by dominant structures, and also narrate resistive articulations, strategies, and tactics through the adoption of cultural symbols (Coyer, Dowmount, & Fountain, 2007). Culturally narrated stories reproduced and co-constructed through mediated spaces deconstruct the oppressive politics of neoliberalism, disrupt the stories of development that are narrated by the dominant structures, and offer as hope culturally situated stories based on cultural knowledge bases. Culture here emerges through media platforms not as a relic of the past, but instead as an active, meaning-making agent that dynamically constructs the stories of contemporary politics and change. The re-storying of issues and agendas from local cultural viewpoints offers entry points into the politics of structural transformation. Social change is co-constructed in the discursive spaces through the foregrounding of the local cultural context as the backbone for emerging meanings.

In other words, agency plays out in mediated public spheres through the circulation of several cultural symbols; cultural symbols are exchanged and shared in mediated spheres to create entry points for meaning making. These shared meanings, drawing upon the cultural frameworks of interpretation, offer the foundations on which agency is enacted. For example, the resistance to the exploitations of labor in sweatshops is expressed through the adoption of mimetic cultural symbols.

Furthermore, it is through agency that local knowledge bases are expressed, simultaneously bringing forth the cultural foundations of West-centered universal notions of modernity and development. When individuals and their communities become the producers of media content that is then globally distributed through new media platforms, they create opportunities for social change. The presence of the subaltern voices from Niyamgiri in the "Save Niyamgiri" campaign present a cultural logic that privileges living in harmony with the environment as a desired lifestyle as opposed to the lifestyle based on the exploitation and pollution of natural resources, reiterated in the rhetoric of development.

Conclusion

In summary, the media exist at the intersections of neoliberal hegemony and the grassroots-driven politics of change that seeks to dislocate this hegemony. In their consolidated power as public relations devices of neoliberalism, they carry out the exploitative agendas of TNCs and embody the neoliberal principles of bringing the entire planet under the capitalist logics of profiteering and exploitation in the hands of TNCs. The languages of capitalism, privatization, minimal state involvement, and attaining democracy through free market continue to inundate the corporate media houses. Simultaneously, they open up avenues for exposing the hypocrisies of neoliberalism, attending to the exploitations of the subaltern sectors, and serving as spaces for enabling the resistive capacities of locally situated practices of social change to emerge on the global arena and disrupt the monolithic narratives of development, economic efficiency, and progress embedded in capitalism. The widespread activist networks of social change seek to bring about changes in political, economic, and social structures by interrogating the stories told by the neoliberal configuration. Locally narrated stories offer insights into alternative rationalities, alternative forms of economic organizing, and alternative renderings of events, thus creating spaces for listening to subaltern voices, witnessing the stories of oppression, and creating entry points for global connections against the marginalization and oppression of the subaltern sectors of the globe.

11

EPILOGUE

The Praxis of Social Change Communication

This book has reviewed the margins of the globe that are created via the programs of development, modernization, privatization, commoditization, and free market economics embodied in neoliberalism. This examination of the margins was set up as the foundation for studying the processes of communication embodied in the politics of social change. What roles then can academics in communication play in global processes of social change? What is the future of communication for social change, especially against the backdrop of the increasing inequalities across the globe in response to the large-scale adoption of neoliberal policies? This concluding chapter offers some theoretical, methodological, and applied entry points for the students and scholars of social change to think about as they embark on journeys of working toward social justice, equality, and access. The emphasis therefore is specifically on exploring the work that can be done at academic sites and through academic engagement toward participating in the broader politics of transformative politics that's taking place across the globe.

Of specific concern in this chapter is the role that scholars and teachers can play in processes of social change, in standing beside the poor, and in creating entry points for social action (Frey & Carragee, 2007; Papa et al., 2006). The impetus here is to ask: What is the relevance of theory to the study and practice of social change? As theorists and practitioners who continually participate in the production and reproduction of knowledge that constitutes the terrains of communication for social change, what are the possibilities for academic participation in social change processes? As universities are continually being brought under the purviews of the neoliberal project to serve the agendas of transnational hegemony, what roles can communication scholars play in creating avenues for structural transformation, in effectively interrogating neoliberal policies, in challenging these policies, in creating spaces of resistive politics that seek to rupture the universalist discourse of neoliberalism, and in addressing the material inequities that are produced by neoliberal development? And most importantly, what is the role played by theory in the context of the praxis of change. In summarizing the several elements of communicative processes of social change, it is my hope to conclude this book by highlighting the centrality of theory to the praxis of social change and to the dangers of a-theoretical engagement in a world where the industry-state-academic partnership has emerged as the cornerstone for carrying out the interests of transnational elites. Critical theorizing lies at the heart of the project of transformative politics that challenges neoliberalism by interrogating the very assumptions of altruism and human development that are utilized to serve the agendas of the status quo, and by continually drawing attention to the contradictions in the development paradigm that uses the language of development to create oppressive structural conditions for the poor. Of vital importance is the translation of such critical theorizing both inside and outside the classroom through participation in a variety of forums and spaces.

Methodologically, the culture-centered approach foregrounds the importance of deep reflexivity in the study and practice of social change communication, especially as it engages with questions of truth, and participates collaboratively with the subaltern sectors in the politics of making truth claims to co-create spaces of structural transformations. Reflexivity refers to the turning of the lens on the self and on the methods of knowing that have created the academic expert, to question the capacity of methods to dialogically engage with subaltern communities. It engages with the politics of co-creating possibilities of transformation, being fully aware of the impossibilities of dialogue as the spaces of dialogue are continually erased and violently disrupted through the very acts of knowledge production. Being aware of the violence embodied in the reductionist systems of knowledge production, reflexivity engages with the material politics of marginalization to resist the profound forms of material inequities and marginalization that are being carried out by the neoliberal project. It is through their method that activist scholars carve out a journey of solidarity, imbued with the deep awareness of "privilege as loss," and equipped with the sense of turning this privilege into a rallying point for articulating a politics of social change that foregrounds a subaltern rationality. Co-constructions of subaltern rationalities turn the lens inward as opposed to outward; the radical politics of methodology lies in its overturning of the subject of knowledge, interrogating those very spaces of knowledge production that have historically remained hidden in their universal presence as producers of truth about the subaltern and as manufacturers of development interventions. The truth claims as well as the politics of these truth claims become the subject of knowledge production, connecting participatory spaces in the subaltern sectors to these centers of truth claims, and representing subaltern politics at the centers of knowledge production. Culture-centered dialogues engage with the articulations of knowledge in dominant structures with values such as cooperation and collective harmony that are resistive to the politics of neoliberalism, contradicting the values of human greed, competition, and control built into the neoliberal project. Epistemologically, the participation of the scholar or activist in the processes of social change is colored with the continual tensions between contradictory impulses of deconstruction and co-constructions, charting out a pathway for action that consistently works through these impulses.

As demonstrated throughout the book, the theorizing and study of processes of social change are deeply intertwined with the practice of social change. Historically, academic sites of knowledge production have been crucial to carrying out the agendas of the status quo. From the early days of development communication work reflected in the works of communication scholars such as Daniel Lerner, Wilbur Schramm, and Everett Rogers, knowledge about development has been at the center of producing the science of development, policies related to development, the design of development interventions, and evaluative criteria for measuring development. Therefore, the theoretical interrogation of the development paradigm and the roots of neoliberal ideology embodied in it is vital to the structural transformation of the field of development. Academic work, on one hand, needs to engage with the praxis of policy-making and intervention development, and on the other hand, continually engage in the field in solidarity with the subaltern sectors. The praxis of communication for social change is situated amidst the continual negotiation of this relationship between the margins and the spaces of policy-making and intervention development at the center.

The Academic Politics of Social Change Communication

As noted throughout the book, the paradoxes and tensions constituted around the politics of social change are intertwined with the ways in which we define social change. Therefore, in this section, we examine the broader linkages among academic sites of knowledge production and the underlying political processes that are actively at play in portraying these sites as apolitical and value free, while at the same time constituting these academic linkages to serve the agendas of transnational hegemony.

Academics, Privatized Knowledge Production, and Neoliberalism

Increasingly, universities are emerging as spaces for producing capitalist knowledge, having been incorporated within neoliberal structures of profiteering, privatization, and corporate management. As corporate structures and partnerships emerge onto the sites of knowledge production, an increasing number of academic projects are driven toward serving the needs of TNCs. The line between knowledge production and knowledge management blurs as academics increasingly participate in creation of knowledge commodities that would sell in the free market. For example, federally funded projects of geography map out indigenous spaces across the globe so that these spaces can be used to serve the geostrategic and market-based interests of the status quo. Similarly, anthropological projects of gathering indigenous knowledge about local agricultural and healing systems are utilized for the purposes of stealing indigenous knowledge bases so that they can be patented by TNCs, and gradually be turned into commodities sold in the global market by these TNCs. Projects of community dialogue and participatory communication are funded by global structures so that the participation of the poor can be co-opted toward serving the interests of TNCs in mining resources, building dams, and building manufacturing units of TNCs. Academic-industry partnerships under frames such as corporate social responsibility, sustainable management, and critical management studies have evolved to use the data gathering and strategic communication expertise of the academic sector to carry out the agendas of transnational hegemony.

The neoliberal structures of contemporary academe have created incredible opportunities for communication scholars working on projects such as nation branding, public diplomacy, civil society building, nation building, and democracy promotion, where knowledge of strategic communication, publicity, public affairs, and community organizing are put together to serve the agendas of transnational hegemony (Dutta, 2009; Dutta & Pal, 2010). The academic participation in processes of communicating transnational agendas not only lends the creed of scientific credibility to these neocolonial interventions, but also creates new opportunities for building academic-industry partnerships toward the goal of serving so-called global problems. The altruism of solving global crises becomes the driving point for the partnerships, simultaneously erasing the economic and political agendas served by these partnerships. The term "social change" has become a buzzword for justifying market interventions and for building the reach of global TNCs. Programs such as the President's Emergency Plan for AIDS Relief (PEPFAR) have emerged on the global landscape as models of academic-government-industry partnerships that serve the dual purposes of combating HIV/AIDS and increasing the global penetration of global brand products. Against the backdrop of neocolonial interventions, such as the US invasion and occupation of Iraq, requests for proposals have been issued and grants have been awarded to democracy promotion, civil society building, and democracy promotion initiatives that would refashion Iraq into a neoliberal space. Grants on building educational institutions, civil society, and media institutions in Iraq have been given out under the broader agendas of turning Iraq into a pro US, pro free market state.

In the domains of health and development communication, academia has enjoyed a partnership with funding agencies as well as the private sector. Programs such as public diplomacy and business diplomacy have embodied this collaborative relationship between academia, industry, and the nation state (Dutta-Bergman, 2005a, 2005b). The concept of democracy promotion for instance has been deployed through specific funded programs of nation building in co-opting subaltern participation and in opening up nation states across the globe to TNCs, based in the nation states carrying out the so-called altruistic missions of enlightening the subaltern sectors of the globe with the mantras of democracy.

Similarly, as noted by Prasad (2009), knowledge production through programs such as clinical trials have emerged as new forms of imperialism, turning Third World subjects as bodies with diverse gene pools to be tested and manipulated as guinea pigs in clinical trials carried out by TNCs. With the increasing efforts of funding agencies therefore to recruit communication scholars who would be deployed to use their knowledge of persuasion and strategic communication for the purposes of recruiting participants for clinical trials, it is critical to interrogate the ethics of clinical trials and to situate the politics of clinical trials within the broader geopolitics of the agendas of transnational hegemony. Critical interrogations of academic practices raise questions such as: Whose agendas are served by the knowledge we produce? What are the ethical implications of our participation in carrying out these agendas? Digging beneath the veil of altruistic claims that shroud the political and economic agendas of the structures of knowledge production, critical engagement with the politics of social change continually questions the circulation of power in dominant knowledge structures and the ways in which this power is played out through seemingly altruistic missions that adopt the language of change and rhetorically frame themselves as the messiahs of enlightenment and empowerment.

Reclaiming the Agenda of Social Change

Reclaiming the agenda of social change within academia is fundamentally a political project. The essence of communication for social change lies in the articulation that knowledge production is fundamentally a political exercise. Embedded in the production of knowledge is the political agenda of the dominant power structures in manufacturing subaltern subjectivity and in exploiting this subjectivity to perpetuate the power and control of neoliberal hegemony. In order to reclaim the agenda of social change, critical communication theorists and scholars draw attention to the hegemonic narratives of capitalism and neoliberalism, and continually disrupt these hegemonic narratives theoretically, methodologically and in praxis.

Essential to the academic politics of social change are the negotiations of power structures and spaces of legitimacy in order to be able to make alternative knowledge claims based on these positions of legitimacy. The scholar studying social change in this sense becomes a mediator, forever making impure the dominant spaces of knowledge production and informing the theories at the center through critical interrogations committed to the politics of change. Her engagement with subaltern contexts challenges the epistemic structures within academia, questioning the very categories of knowledge that are circulated to reify the status quo and to increase the market penetration of neoliberal hegemony.

Spaces of Change

As noted in the previous section, the role of academia at the sites of development and social change is played out in the realms of theory, methodology, and praxis. In this section, we explore the interconnections among the theory, methodology, and praxis of communication for social change.

Social Change Theory

The wide-ranging theories of social change that circulate in the academic literature and inform the practices in the field vary greatly in their conceptualizations of change. The chapters presented in this book note the various tensions and paradoxes that play out in these definitional terrains of social change communication. The culture-centered approach engages with the ways in which local agency challenges local, national, and global structures through the strategic mobilization of cultural symbols in communicative processes. Therefore, one of the central ideas presented in this book is the key role played by the agency of local participants, with the communicative processes of social change participating in creating entry points for listening to these voices that have been historically erased from the dominant platforms of knowledge production and praxis.

It is worth highlighting here that whereas historically the concept of social change has been used to label top-down interventions carried out within the logics of development and modernization, the articulation of social change as narrated in this book is focused on those processes that challenge dominant structures and seek to bring about changes in them. As opposed to the individual-level behavioral focus of development communication interventions, resistive social change practices seek to disrupt these dominant structures and bring about transformations in them. Engaging with the culture-centered approach in theorizing about social change brings attention to the location of theory within the dominant structures, and the ways in which theory can then serve the agendas of structural transformation.

As deconstruction, the culture-centered approach interrogates the dominant modes of knowledge production and the ways in which these modes of knowledge production have served the interests of the dominant structures. Under the name of social change, mainstream processes of development communication have served the status quo, diffusing Eurocentric concepts of development and modernization based on assumptions of universal progress, serving the interests of the status quo, and playing the roles of public relations for dominant development institutions, transnational powers, funding agencies, and nation states. Such deconstructions of social change processes under development approach it as a political entity, negotiated amidst the political and economic interests of transnational hegemony. Culture-centered deconstructions of social change communication ultimately point toward the ways in which the labeling of social change strategically co-opts the possibilities of transformative politics, instead focusing on policies and interventions that carry out the agendas of the status quo. Close interrogation of the vocabulary of participation, civil society building, nation building, empowerment, and democracy promotion draw attention to the paradoxes in the naming and practice of these terms, suggesting that the emancipatory rhetoric of these terms often serves as a cover for co-opting and delegitimizing subaltern participation, and for carrying out the agendas of transnational power structures.

For communication scholars engaging in social change projects, reflexive deconstructions at the theoretical level interrogate not only the relevance of a specific communicative theory applied toward attaining certain pre-established objectives, but also, and more fundamentally, the ways in which problems and solutions are defined for the purposes of the change initiative. Such interrogations would engage with the questions of ethics and values in understanding problem configurations and solution developments. Rather than taking for granted the inherent value of the interventions being proposed, a deconstructive lens questions the value of the intervention and critically situates it amidst broader understandings of the ways in which it will bring about change. Questions such as "Who defines development?," "For whose purposes?," and "Who benefits from development?" need to be continually asked. Asking such questions creates entry points for engaging with the oppressive elements of the institutions of development, and the ways in which development has emerged as a tool in the hands of power structures. For instance, critical interrogations attend to the ways in which development consolidates the interests of power structures globally, in usurping indigenous knowledge bases and indigenous resources across the globe, and in turning global spaces into markets for TNCs under the vocabulary of development.

Methodological Issues

Challenging the criteria of effectiveness and efficiency that are circulated as measures of success in the mainstream, students and scholars of social change ought to engage with the possibilities of listening to subaltern communities that have been historically erased by the very knowledge structures that they inhabit. Fundamental to the politics of social change is the creation of spaces for local participation, the connection of these spaces to resources, infrastructures, and political processes, and the articulation of local rationalities at dominant sites of knowledge production. Countering the wholesale commoditization of academia for the purposes of TNCs through think tanks, grants, and consultancies serving the status quo, the academic politics of social change achieves its resistive potential by creating alternative spaces of critical interrogations both within these very powerful structures of knowledge production as well as outside of them. The methodological tools presented here summarize the key points about methodological engagement with the politics of social change raised throughout the book.

Authenticity. As noted throughout several chapters of the book, one of the questions that perennially comes up for the culture-centered scholar working on processes of social change is the question of authenticity (Basu & Dutta, 2008a, 2008b, 2009; Dutta, 2008a, 2008b, 2008c; Tihuwai Smith, 2006; Tomaselli et al., 2008). Authenticity reflects the degree of truth that is narrated in the projects of change, in the relationship of scholars to their project, to the local community that they participate with, to the academic community that they are members of, and to their relationships and values as human beings. The personal intersects with the politics of knowledge production (Conquergood, 1986; Dutta, 2008c; Harter et al., 2009; Singhal, 2001, 2004). The resistive politics of social change lies in the participation in research with subaltern communities that create entry points for making truth claims that challenge the truth claims made by the dominant platforms through the deployment of research that justifies the oppression of subaltern communities in the name of development and progress (Tihuwai Smith, 2006). Tihuwai Smith (2006, p. 122) notes:

> For some indigenous groups the formal claims process demanded by tribunals, courts and governments has required the conducting of intensive research projects resulting in the writing of nation, tribe, and family histories. These "histories" have a focus and purpose, that is, to establish the legitimacy of the claims being asserted for the rest of time. Because they have been written to support claims to territories and resources or about past injustices, they have been constructed around selected stories.

Methodologies such as the *testimonio* insert themselves into the dominant structure to interrogate the politics of the dominant structure not only in terms of the stories of violence over the indigenous sectors that have been omitted from these structures, but also in terms of interrogating the viability of the dominant methods that have been utilized to document subaltern voices. Witnessing violence and narrating these stories of violence through co-constructions become vital tools in creating spaces of social change.

In the face of the continuing violence in subaltern contexts across the globe, the authenticity of culture-centered communication scholarship of social change ought to be measured in terms of its ability to foreground the stories of violence, atrocities, and displacement that are being performed across the globe in order to carry out the agendas of TNCs in collusion with the state and the IFIs. The field of truth claims emerges as a political field with specific agendas, and it is amidst this field that discursive claims need to be documented to narrate the stories of indigenous marginalization and violence enacted on the poor. It is also amidst this field of truth claims in the neoliberal regime that entry points need to be created for listening to subaltern actors for constituting subaltern knowledge bases that challenge the agendas of neoliberalism. Authenticity in co-creating alternative truths of structural violence and exploitation embodied in transnational hegemony is expressed through forums such as the Independent People's Tribunal organized in India in April 2010 by activists, scholars, and civil society groups on land acquisition, resource grab, and Operation Green Hunt in India that has displaced and continues to threaten the displacement of tribal populations in Central and Eastern India so that tribal land can be exploited by neoliberal projects carried out by corporations and supported by the government through the deployment of police and paramilitary forces (www.navdanya.org/events/92-independent-peoples-tribunal).

As a critical project, the culture-centered approach is fundamentally interested in questions of truth, arguing that the material truths of exploitation and oppression of the subaltern sectors remain hidden amidst the culturally produced truths of categories and causal linkages that are produced through the instruments of the social sciences (Tihuwai Smith, 2006). The continual search for the material truth underlies the emphasis on the deconstructions of the material realities of inequality and marginalization that are written into the apparently value-free structures of knowledge that produce truths about development. These truths are contested through the presence of subaltern voices, based on the argument that authentic relationships with the marginalized sectors create openings for the telling of narratives that bring forth the structural violence written into the dominant structures of development and modernization. These relationships of authenticity narrate the various forms of marginalizing practices that are embedded into the hypocrisy of dominant knowledge circles and their truth claims about social change.

Commitment. Commitment reflects the continued and sustained relationship with the subaltern contexts in which communication students and scholars participate in order to bring about structural transformations. As opposed to research tourism in mainstream communication research when it engages with marginalized populations, the criterion of commitment calls for projects that build sustainable and long-term relationships with local communities. It questions the value and meaningfulness of scholarship that issues empirical claims on the basis of minimal interactions with local communities, instead suggesting that these relationships with local communities are partnerships that are optimally influential over the long-term processes of social change.

The practice of social change requires continual conversations and dialogues with communities, explorations of structural resources in order to create avenues for engagement, and the undertaking of professional and personal risks in order to make arguments that are considered unfashionable among the neoliberal structures of academia. These sustainable relationships offer the foundations for participating in collaborative processes that take time to build, building relationships on the foundations of trust and mutual respect, and working tirelessly to bring about transformations in local, national, and global structures.

Commitment also means that we question the viability of the platforms and the methods of knowledge productions in which we engage to produce knowledge

(A. Singhal, personal communication, 2010). As suggested by Harter et al. (2009), alternative rationalities offer entry points for reconsidering and reconstituting the ways in which knowledge claims are made and the kinds of stimuli that are included as knowledge. In doing so, multiple avenues of embodied performance emerge as sites and processes of doing scholarship. Through forms such as dance, art, songs, and poetry, scholars co-create stories of change.

Reflexivity. As noted earlier in the book, as a methodological device and as a criterion, reflexivity is indicative of the extent to which a methodology critically turns the lens toward the author/scholar and toward the academic practices of knowledge production (Basu & Dutta, 2008a, 2009; Dutta, 2007, 2008a, 2008b, 2008c; Dutta-Bergman, 2004a, 2004b; Holman Jones, 2005). Situated amidst critical interrogations of the intersections of the positions of class, race, gender, and nationality, reflexivity offers a lens into the privileged position of the scholar researchers, questioning the ways in which this privilege and the practices attached to it produce the conditions at the margins.

As a political act, reflexivity shifts the gaze of research from the "other" to the "self," asking "What is it that we can learn about ourselves through our interactions with the other?" The interaction of the other as a performance then opens up the discursive space to challenging the broader fabric of knowledge production and the ways in which this fabric serves the interests of the status quo. Continually questioning this relationship with the status quo then, the scholar researcher seeks out entry points for participating in processes and politics of social change in solidarity with subaltern communities. Reflexivity embodies in it humility and openness to learning from other ways of knowing that have been silenced through the colonizing methods of knowledge production. In writing about "going outside the colonizer's cage," McCaslin and Breton (2009) note:

> As indigenous peoples, we can call on the deep, abiding currents of our traditions, cultures, and communities. Some indigenous peoples feel these currents more strongly than others, depending on the access we have to elders, traditional family structures, and culturally rooted communities. These currents align us to who we are as indigenous peoples and help us respond in good, sustainable ways to the colonial onslaughts. Our culture, traditions, and communities give us energy, hope, and direction as we do our best to negotiate rough waters.
>
> *(McCaslin & Breton, 2009, p. 515)*

Indigenous or native researchers can learn about and from their past only through the continual interrogation of the colonizing knowledge structures and through openness to learning from the pasts and from sources of wisdom and knowledge that have been undermined and devalued by dominant, scientific, modernist, and colonizing knowledge structures as primitive, unscientific, pre-modern, and backward.

Epistemological reflexivity calls for continual interrogations of these categories and labels and the deconstructions of the ways in which these dichotomies have been utilized to perpetrate violence on subaltern sectors across the globe. It is through reflexivity that openings for dialogue are created, articulating philosophies such as *sarvodaya* (welfare for all) and earth democracy as alternative political, economic, and social rationalities. Reflexivity also embodies the urgency to interrogate the silences amidst dominant structures, coming face to face with the impossibilities and vulnerabilities of dialogue as scholars weave through narrative co-constructions to make sense of subaltern narratives of loss, dispossession, agency, and dignity. One such example is put forth by Krog, Mpolweni-Zantsi, and Ralete (2008) who describe the disjunctures in the incoherences and understandings of subaltern testimonies based on their dialogic engagement with Mrs. Zabonka Konile, the mother of a young man who had joined the military wing of the African National Congress and was killed in an ambush by the security forces:

> within a postcolonial context, a woman may appear either incoherent because of severe suffering or unintelligible because of oppression—while in fact she is neither. Within her indigenous framework, she is logical and resilient in her knowledge of her loss and its devastating consequences in her life. She is not too devastated to make sense; she is devastated because she intimately understands the devastation that has happened to her. However, the forum she finds herself in and the way narratives are being read make it very hard for her to bring the depth of this devastation across.
>
> *(Krog et al., 2008, p. 544)*

Reflexively engaging in the politics of social change implies the continual negotiations of the limits to knowing and narrative coherence that are imposed by the contingency of dialogues in subaltern contexts. The fragmented, incoherent, and difficult to comprehend sites of interactions with subaltern knowledge point toward the vitality of commitment as scholars continue to reflexively engage with the violent erasures that have happened through the very knowledge structures that they inhabit.

Solidarity. Solidarity as a methodological tool or criterion invites researchers and scholars to participate in journeys of co-construction with subaltern communities. These journeys are intrinsically tied to reflexivity and the realization of the power and privileges attached to the positions occupied by scholars. Solidarity embodies the building of relationships as sojourners and co-participants in order to leverage the privileges one inhabits as a researcher in order to create spaces of change. In constituting research as solidarity, the scholar does not speak to or proclaim to speak for the margins, but rather creates openings for building relationships on the basis of trust, mutual respect, humility, and a commitment to bring about changes in the structures of oppression.

In this sense, solidarity simply does not end at listening to the subaltern narratives, but instead attends to the necessity of working through these stories of oppression and exploitation to shift structures and transform them. Solidarity maps out a pathway for participating in the politics of change as an actively involved subject, drawing upon the privileges of the position of enunciation of the researcher, and simultaneously unlearning this privilege in order to listen to subaltern voices as a co-participant, to open up spaces that might otherwise be closed off because of the expertise-driven narrowness of the tools and methods that one has been trained in.

Issues of Praxis

The praxis of communication for social change is achieved through the active participation of scholars in theoretical and methodological deconstructions at the very sites of neoliberal knowledge production that they inhabit. Theory is quintessential to the practice of social change as it is through theory that the dominant epistemic structures and their knowledge claims are challenged. This connection between theory and activist praxis is eloquently exemplified by Zoller (2005) in the call for resistance to the dominant power relationships that influence health negatively. Similarly, the work of critical policy and legal theorists with the subaltern sectors focuses on deconstructing theoretically the erasures written into the dominant legislative and juridical structures, and finds entry points for co-constructing alternative policy narratives based on the voices of subaltern participants (Santos & Rodríguez-Garavito, 2005).

One of the dismissive moves made by the dominant structure in ensuring its status quo is embodied in the delegitimizing of critical theory, pointing toward the pessimism and lack of application in critical theory. As the various chapters throughout this book demonstrate, theory lies at the heart of the oppressions and exploitations carried out by the neoliberal project. Neoliberal theory operates on the basis of certain assumptions of the free market, and these assumptions have percolated throughout the dominant global policy institutions as well as university structures, shaping the meta-theories as well as the specific localized theories and methodologies that shape the practical terrains of policies and interventions carried out globally.

It is ultimately on the foundations of theory that the oppressions and inequalities across the globe are created, tied to the free market logic, and consistently backgrounded within this logic to emphasize the participation of the individual in the free market in order to secure resources through participation in the market. Global and national funding agencies and policy structures such as the World Bank, IMF, WHO, UNICEF, UNAIDS, UNDP, UNESCO, NIH, NSF, CDC, and USAID are situated within the broader meta-theoretical frame of neoliberalism, and it is this meta-theoretical frame that shapes the science and technology of knowledge production and intervention development that happen within the purviews and discursive fields of these major institutions. It is because of this primacy of theory to the perpetuation of the neoliberal project that the project also needs to be fundamentally opposed at a theoretical level, creating entry points for alternative theories and alternative rationalities for organizing the education, health, agricultural, and industrial sectors. The culture of neoliberalism as embodied in the "Science" of communication interventions needs to be fundamentally deconstructed through sophisticated theoretical engagement that interrogates the ways in which specific legitimized knowledge configurations and relationships of power are embodied in these interventions. Navarro (1999) notes:

> We can see that neoliberalism and globalization, for example, are the political and ideological instruments of class domination. Demystifying them, and introducing an analysis of the power relations in our society, is of the utmost urgency. It is not just sufficient but wrong to analyze the determinants of our populations' health without analyzing the reproduction of power relations (exploitation and domination), of which class, gender, and race relations are of overwhelming importance . . . I invite you to study, for example, how different power relations configure societies and the level of well-being of their populations, and how labor movements and other allied forces in both developed and developing countries are the most important forces in improving the health and wellbeing of much of the human race . . . I am aware that neither the international agencies nor the research-funding agencies will be willing to fund this type of research, and it is quite likely that those daring to engage in such research will be silenced and ignored.
>
> *(Navarro, 1999, pp. 224–225)*

Attention is drawn not only to the politics of knowledge production and the participation of funding agencies in such forms of knowledge production, but also to the risks faced by critical interrogations and alternative articulations. It is this politics of legitimacy and risks to legitimacy that the praxis of social change communication has to negotiate.

The praxis of social change also involves the creation and exploration of participatory spaces within dominant structures so that voices of the subaltern sectors may be heard. Such forms of participatory interventions, however, can remain constrained as cultural projects narrating the exotic other under the multicultural and diversity-based agendas of neoliberalism, unless they are mobilized structurally to create spaces of change through subaltern involvement. The intersections of culture, structure, and agency in the praxis of communication for social change create avenues for transformative politics through subaltern participation in interrogating the hegemonic practices of power and control in the dominant structures.

For example, the practice of mobilizing for social change in the Navdanya movement worked with global opportunity structures to resist the biopirating of

Neem by the United States and a US-based multinational (Shiva, 2007). In this case, structural change was achieved through the agency of subaltern participants at the structures of knowledge production and regulation. Similarly, in the face of the large-scale theft of indigenous knowledge in the form of biopiracy promoted by TRIPS, co-constructive journeys of social change can create alternative knowledge structures that resist the claims of TNCs to indigenous knowledge by documenting oral indigenous knowledge, wisdom, and art as prior knowledge, and by resisting the efforts to turn such knowledge into commodities owned by TNCs without the involvement of indigenous actors. Transnational networks of these alternative knowledge structures can emerge as global organizing points for monitoring biopiracy and bioprospecting, for monitoring the involvement of academic sectors and funding agencies in carrying out the agendas of TNCs, and for mobilizing local-global support to organize against such forms of exploitation.

The publishing of white papers, creation of research sites, training in methodologies, recording of voices and narratives at sites of oppression and resistance, documentations in fact finding missions are academic tools through which the dominant structures of oppression can be engaged and challenged. The practice of scholarship is connected with the production of knowledge that can then be utilized in making empirical claims amidst dominant structures, and in drawing attention to the oppressions in these structures. Global political structures and institutional resources such as human rights networks and institutions can be critically engaged in order to create internal and external pressures through institutional structures, engage public opinions, and discursively shape the agendas and frames in mainstream public spheres. Organizations and institutions within states and globally can be critically engaged through the politics of scholarship in order to create and sustain spaces of social change and transformative social justice.

Conclusion

In conclusion, this chapter wraps up the book with the questions of what it means to engage in the politics of social change as a communication student, scholar, or researcher. The theoretical, methodological, and practical issues raised in this chapter draw attention to the complexities of engaging in research in a complex field of knowledge production about structural oppressions, exploitations, and erasures. For the communication scholar working with the subaltern sectors, the scholarship of social change is tied to the practice of social change. Theory, research, and practice are intrinsically intertwined. Whereas on one hand, theoretical journeys in subaltern contexts create vital entry points for the praxis of social change, on the other hand, it is through praxis that theoretical entry points are created, foregrounded, and placed within dominant structures in order to challenge these structures. This dynamic relationship between theory and practice is vital to creating global spaces of social change politics through communication scholarship (Frey & Carragee, 2007).

NOTES

Introduction

1   Neoliberalism is a form of political economic organizing that operates under the assumption that human development is best achieved when individual entrepreneurial freedoms are liberated within the institutional frameworks of property rights, free markets, and free trade (Harvey, 2005).

2   The term subaltern refers to the condition of being under, played out in the context of race, class, gender, caste, nationality, occupation, and position within the social structure.

3   The term "Third World" is used through the book to refer to the geopolitics of contemporary neocolonial and neoliberal politics that continue to play out the geographic terrains of material inequalities in the context of the circulation of the symbolic markers of the Enlightenment project. Therefore, the choice of the term Third World is a political choice precisely to imbue the global South with the politics of social change against the backdrop of West-centric processes of domination and control that continue to operate through the mechanisms of international financial institutions, nation states, and TNCs.

2 Poverty at the Margins

1   Santalis are an indigenous tribe in the eastern part of India, located at the margins of contemporary Indian society, with minimum access to the resources of development and simultaneously being displaced from their natural spaces of livelihood through state-sponsored projects of industrialization and development.

3 Agriculture and Food: Global Inequalities

1   Any restriction imposed on the free flow of trade is a trade barrier. Trade barriers can either be tariff barriers (i.e., a levy of ordinary customs duties) or non-tariff barriers (i.e., any trade barriers other than the tariff barriers, such as import policy barriers; standards,

testing, labeling and certification requirements; and anti-dumping and countervailing measures, services barriers, etc.).

2 "Most-favored-nation treatment" (MFN) requires parties to accord the most favorable tariff and regulatory treatment given to the product of any one contracting party for import or export to all "like products" of other contracting parties. For example, if contracting party A agrees with contracting party B to reduce the tariff on the product X to 5 percent, this same "tariff rate" must apply to all other contracting parties for products that are the same as X (i.e., like products). In other words, if a country gives most-favored-nation treatment to one country regarding a particular issue, it must handle all other countries equally regarding the same issue.

3 One of the most important aspects of the Agreement on Agriculture is tariffication. This requires countries with non-tariff measures, such as quantitative restrictions and import licensing, to abolish them by transferring the non-tariff measures to the tariff equivalents and adding these into fixed tariffs. The tariff equivalent was calculated based on average world market price of the product to which non-tariff measures were applied traditionally.

4 The Common Agricultural Policy is a system of European Union agricultural subsidies that guarantees a minimum price to producers and provides direct payment of a subsidy for crops planted. The Common Agricultural Policy has been providing some economic certainty for EU farmers and production of a certain quantity of agricultural goods.

5 The ACP is comprised of seventy-eight nations, of which the twelve traditional banana producing ACP countries are Cameroon, Cape Verde, Ivory Coast, Madagascar, Somalia, Jamaica, Belize, St. Lucia, St. Vincent, Grenada, Dominica, and Suriname.

9 Participation, Social Capital, Community Networks, and Social Change

1 Social capital refers to the community ties, trust, interpersonal relationships, community networks, and participatory forums that exist within communities, thus tapping into the existing community capacities for bringing about transformations in structures and seeking out access to resources. Social capital catalyzes participation by creating the spaces for participation.

REFERENCES

Abramovitz, M. (1956). Resource and output trends in the United States since 1870. *American Economic Review, 46,* 5–23.

Acharya, L., & Dutta, M. (2010). *Constructions of HIV/AIDS in Koraput tribal: A critical interrogation.* Paper presented at the Annual Convention of the National Communication Association, San Francisco, CA.

Aelst, P., & Walgrave, S. (2004). New media, new movements? The role of the internet in shaping the "anti-globalization" movement. In W. V. Donk, B. Loader, P. Nixon, & D. Rucht (Eds.), *Cyberprotest: New media, citizens, and social movements* (pp. 97–122). London: Routledge.

Afshar, H. (1944). *Islam and feminisms: An Iranian case study.* New York: St. Martin's Press.

Agacino, R., & Escobar, P. (1997). Empleo y pobreza: Uncomentario sobre la experiencia chilena. *Revista Aportes, 2,* 5.

Agency for Healthcare Research and Quality. (2008). *National Health Disparities Report 2008.* Rockville, MD: Agency for Healthcare Research and Quality.

Airhihenbuwa, C. (1995). *Health and culture: Beyond the Western paradigm.* Thousand Oaks, CA: Sage.

Albert, M. (2003). What makes alternative media alternative? Toward a federation of alternative media activists and supporters—FAMAS. *Z Magazine.* Retrieved May 29, 2005 from www.zmag.org/zmag/articles

Algranati, C., Seoane, J., & Taddei, E. (2004). Neoliberalism and social conflict: The popular movements in Latin America. In F. Polet (Ed.), *Globalizing resistance: The stage of struggle* (pp. 112–135). London: Pluto.

Amis, P. (2001). Attacking poverty: But what happened to urban poverty and development. *Journal of International Development, 13,* 353–360.

Amkpa, A. (2003). *Theatre and postcolonial desires.* New York: Routledge.

Anderson, R., & Cissna, K. N. (1996). Criticism and conversational texts: Rhetorical bases of role, audience, and style in the Buber-Rogers dialogue. *Human Studies, 19,* 85–118.

Anderson, R., & Cissna, K. N. (1997). *The Martin Buber-Carl Rogers dialogue: A new transcript with commentary.* Albany, NY: State University of New York Press.

Anderson, R., & Cissna, K. N. (2008). Fresh perspectives in dialogue theory. *Communication Theory, 18,* 1–4.

Anderson, R., & Morrison, B. (Eds.) (1982). *Science, politics and the agricultural revolution in Asia.* Boulder, CO: Westview, for the American Association for the Advancement of Science.

Anderson, R., Baxter, L. A., & Cissna, K. N. (Eds.) (2004). *Dialogue: Theorizing difference in communication studies.* Thousand Oaks, CA: Sage.

Anuradha, R. V., Taneja, B., & Kothari, A. (2001). *Experiences with biodiversity policy making and community registers in India.* London: International Institute for Environment and Development.

Appadurai, A. (1990). Disjuncture and difference in the global cultural economy. *Public Culture, 2,* 1–24.

Appadurai, A. (1995). Disjuncture and difference. In B. Ashcroft, G. Griffiths, & H. Tiffin (Eds.), *The post-colonial studies reader* (2nd ed., pp. 468–472). New York: Routledge.

Appadurai, A. (1996). *Modernity at large.* Minneapolis, MN: University of Minnesota Press.

Appadurai, A. (2001). *Globalization.* Durham, NC: Duke University Press.

Arnett, R. C. (1982). Toward a phenomenological dialogue. *Western Journal of Speech Communication, 46,* 358–372.

Arnett, R. C. (1993). *Dialogic education: Conversation about ideas and between persons.* Carbondale, IL: Southern Illinois University Press.

Arnett, R. C. (2001). Civility as pragmatic ethical praxis: an interpersonal metaphor for the public domain. *Communication Theory, 11,* 315–338.

Artz, L. (2006). On the material and the dialectic: Toward a class analysis of communication. In L. Artz, S. Macek, & D. Cloud (Eds.), *Marxism and communication studies: The point is to change it* (pp. 5–51). New York: Peter Lang.

Atton, C. (2002). *Alternative media.* Thousand Oaks, CA: Sage.

Auyero, J. (2003). *Contentious lives: Two Argentine women, two protests, and the quest for recognition.* Durham, NC: Duke University Press.

Ayres, J. M. (1999). From the streets to the Internet: The cyber-diffusion of contention. *Annals of the American Academy of Political and Social Science, 566,* 132–143.

Ayres, J. M. (2001).Transnational political processes and contention against the global economy. *Mobilization, 6,* 55–68.

Bailey, O., Cammaerts, B., & Carpentier, N. (2008). *Understanding alternative media.* New York: Open University Press.

Bakhtin, M. (1981). *The dialogic imagination: Four essays* (J. M. Holquist, Trans.). Austin: University of Texas Press.

Banana Link (2004). *Banana Link Website.* Retrieved May 5, 2004 from www.banana link.org.uk/

Baquet, C. (2002). What is "health disparity"? *Public Health Report, 17,* 426–429.

Bartley, M., Power, C., Blane, D., Davey Smith, G., & Shipley, M. (1994). Birthweight and later socioeconomic disadvantage: Evidence from the 1958 British cohort study. *British Medical Journal, 309,* 1475–1478.

Basu, A. (Ed.) (1995). *The challenge of local feminisms: Women's movements in global perspectives.* Boulder, CO: Westview.

Basu, A. (2004). Women's movements and the challenge of transnationalism. *Curricular Crossings: Women's Studies and Area Studies.* Retrieved October 12, 2010 from www3.amherst.edu/~mrhunt/womencrossing/basu.html

Basu, A. (2005). *Women, political parties, and social movements in South Asia.* United Nations Research Institute for Social Development (UNRISD) Occasional Paper. Geneva: UNRISD.

Basu, A. (2009). Women, political parties, and social movements in South Asia. In A. M. Goetz (Ed.), *Women's political effectiveness in contexts of democratization and governance reform* (pp. 87–111). New York: Routledge.

Basu, A., & Dutta, M. (2008a). Participatory change in a campaign led by sex workers: Connecting resistance to action-oriented agency. *Qualitative Health Research, 18,* 106–119.

Basu, A., & Dutta, M. (2008b). The relationship between health information seeking and community participation: The roles of motivation and ability. *Health Communication, 23,* 70–79.

Basu, A., & Dutta, M. (2009). Sex workers and HIV/AIDS: Analyzing participatory culture-centered health communication strategies. *Human Communication Research, 35,* 86–114.

Baxter, L. A., & Montgomery, B. M. (1996). *Relating: Dialogues and dialectics.* New York: Guilford.

Beltran, L. R. (1979). *A farewell to Aristotle: "Horizontal" communication.* Paris: Unesco International Commission for the Study of Communication Problems.

Benford, R. D., & Snow, D. A. (2000). Framing processes and social movements: An overview and assessment. *Annual Review of Sociology, 26,* 611–639.

Bennett, W. L. (2003a). New media power: The Internet and global activism. In N. Couldry & J. Curran (Eds.), *Contesting media power* (pp. 17–37). Lanham, MD: Rowman & Littlefield.

Bennett, W. L. (2003b). Branded political communication: Lifestyle politics, logo campaigns, and the rise of global citizenship. In M. Micheletti, A. Follesdal, & D. Stolle (Eds.), *The politics behind products.* New Brunswick, NJ: Transaction.

Bennett, W. L. (2004). Communicating global activism: Strengths and vulnerabilities of networked politics. In W. V. Donk, B. Loader, P. Nixon, & D. Rucht (Eds.), *Cyberprotest: New media, citizens, and social movements* (pp. 123–146). London: Routledge.

Benston, G. J. (1980). *Conglomerate mergers: Causes, consequences, and remedies.* Washington, DC: American Enterprise Institute for Public Policy.

Berkman, L. F. (1995). The role of social relations in health promotion. *Psychosomatic Medicine, 57,* 245–254.

Beverley, J. (1999). *Subalternity and representation: Arguments in critical theory.* Durham, NC: Duke University Press.

Beverley, J. (2001). The impossibility of politics: Subalternity, modernity, hegemony. In I. Rodríguez (Ed.), *The Latin American subaltern studies reader* (pp. 47–63). Durham, NC: Duke University Press.

Beverley, J. (2004a). *Subalternity and representation: Arguments in cultural theory.* Durham, NC: Duke University Press.

Beverley, J. (2004b). *Testimonio: On the politics of truth.* Minneapolis, MN: University of Minnesota Press.

Bhabha, H. (1994). *The location of culture.* New York: Routledge.

Bhattacharya, A. (2009). *Singur to Lalgarh via Nandigram: Rising flames of people's anger against displacement, destitution and state terror.* Retrieved March 8, 2010 from www.no2 displacement.com/attachments/121_Lalgarh%20Book.pdf Visthapan Virodhi Jan Vikas Andolan.

Blane, D. (1995). Social determinants of health: Socioeconomic status, social class, and ethnicity. *American Journal of Public Health, 85,* 903–905.

Blaser, M., Feit, H., & McRae, G. (2004). *In the way of development: Indigenous peoples, life projects, and globalization.* London: Zed.

Boal, A. (1979). *Theatre of the oppressed*. New York: Urizen.

Boal, A. (1992). *Games for actors and non-actors*. New York: Routledge.

Boal, A. (1995). *The rainbow of desire: The Boal method of theatre and therapy*. New York: Routledge.

Boal, A. (1998). *Legislative theatre: Using performance to make politics*. London: Routledge.

Bodekar, G. (2003). Traditional medical knowledge, intellectual property rights, and benefit sharing. Symposium: traditional knowledge, intellectual property, and indigenous culture. *Cardozo Journal of International and Comparative Law, 11*, 785–814.

Bogad, L. M. (2003). Facial insufficiency: Political street performance in New York City and the selective enforcement of the 1845 Mask Law. *Drama Review, 47*, 75–84.

Bradshaw, S., & Linneker, B. (2001). Challenging poverty, vulnerability and social exclusion in Nicaragua: Some considerations for poverty reduction strategies. *Nicaraguan Academic Journal, 2*, 2, 186–224. Managua, Nicaragua, Ave Maria College of the Americas, San Marcos, Carazo, Nicaragua, www.avemaria.edu.ni

Bradshaw, S., & Linneker, B. (2003). Civil society responds to poverty reduction strategies in Nicaragua. *Progress in Development Studies, 3*, 147–158.

Braidotti, R., Charkiewicz, E., Häusler, S., & Wieringa, S. (1994). *Women, the environment and sustainable development: Towards a theoretical synthesis*. London: Zed.

Braveman, P. (2006). Health disparities and health equity: Concepts and measurement. *Annual Review of Public Health, 27*, 167–194.

Brecher, J., Costello, T., & Smith, B. (2000). *Globalization from below: The power of solidarity*. Cambridge, MA: South End Press.

Brenner, J., Ross, J., Simmons, J., & Zaidi, S. (2000). Neoliberal trade and investment and the health of Maquiladora workers on the US–Mexico border. In J. Y. Kim, J. V. Millen, A. Irwin, & J. Gershman (Eds.), *Dying for growth: Global inequality and the health of the poor* (pp. 261–290). Monroe, ME: Common Courage Press.

Broadfoot, K. J., & Munshi, D. (2007). Diverse voices and alternative rationalities: Imagining forms of postcolonial organizational communication. *Management Communication Quarterly, 21*, 249–267.

Brock-Utne, B. (2000). *Whose education for all? The recolonization of the African mind*. New York: Falmer.

Browne, S., & Morris, C. (Eds.) (2006). *Readings on the rhetoric of social protest*. State College, PA: Strata.

Buber, M. (1958). *I and Thou* (2nd ed.; R. G. Smith, Trans.). New York: Scribner.

Buber, M. (1965). *Between man to man* (M. Friedman, Ed.; R. G. Smith, Trans.). New York: Macmillan.

Burbach, R. (1994). Roots of the postmodern rebellion in Chiapas. *New Left Review, 205*, 113–124.

Burkey, S. (1993). *People first: A guide to self-reliant, participatory rural development*. London: Zed.

Burt, J. M., & Mauceri, P. (2004). Introduction. In J. M. Burt & P. Mauceri (Eds.), *Politics in the Andes: Identity, conflict, reform* (pp. 1–14). Pittsburgh, PA: University of Pittsburgh Press.

Carawan, G., & Carawan, C. (1963). *We shall overcome: Songs of the Southern Freedom Movement*. New York: Oak.

Cardoso, F. H., & Faletto, E. (1979). *Dependency and development in Latin America*. Los Angeles, CA: University of California Press.

Carpentier, N. (2007). Theoretical frameworks for participatory media. In N. Carpentier, P. Pruulmann-Vengerfeldt, K. Nordenstreng, M. Hartmann, P. Vihalemm, B.

Cammaerts, & H. Nieminen (Eds.), *Media technologies and democracy in an enlarged Europe* (pp. 105–122). Tartu, Estonia: Tartu University Press.

Castells, M. (1996). *The rise of network society*. Oxford: Blackwell.

Castells, M. (1997). *The power of identity*. Oxford: Blackwell.

Castells, M. (1998). *End of millennium*. Oxford: Blackwell.

Castells, M. (2001). *The internet galaxy: Reflections on the Internet, business and society*. Oxford: Oxford University Press.

CBS. (April 26, 2008). *Agricultural giant battles small farmers: Monsanto goes to great lengths to protect its patents on genetically modified crops*. Retrieved March 1, 2010 from www.cbsnews. com/stories/2008/04/26/eveningnews/main4048288.shtml

Chalmers, D., Vilas, C., Hite, K., Martin, S., Piester, K., & Segarra, M. (1997). *The new politics of inequality in Latin America: Rethinking participation and representation*. Oxford: Oxford University Press.

Chambers, R. (1983). *Rural development: Putting the last first*. Lagos: Longman.

Chambers, R. (1994a). The origins and practice of participatory rural appraisal. *World Development, 22,* 953–969.

Chambers, R. (1994b). Participatory rural appraisal (PRA): Analysis and experience. *World Development, 22,* 1253–1268.

Chambers, R. (1994c). Participatory rural appraisal: Challenges, potentials, and paradigms. *World Development, 22,* 1437–1454.

Chambers, R. (1997). *Whose reality counts? Putting the last first*. London: ITDG.

Chatterjee, P. (1982). Agrarian relations and communalism in Bengal. In R. Guha (Ed.), *Subaltern studies I: Writings on South Asian history and society* (pp. 9–38). Delhi: Oxford University Press.

Chatterjee, P. (1983). More on modes of power and the peasantry. In R. Guha (Ed.), *Subaltern studies II: Writings on South Asian history and society* (pp. 311–349). Delhi: Oxford University Press.

Chaturvedi, V. (2000). *Mapping subaltern studies and the postcolonial*. New York: Verso.

Cheney, G., & Cloud, D. (2006). Doing democracy, engaging the material: Employee participation and labor activity in an age of market globalization. *Management Communication Quarterly, 19,* 501–540.

Choi, C. (1995). Transnational capitalism, national imaginary, and the protest theater in South Korea. *Boundary, 2, 22,* 235–261.

Cissna, K. N., & Anderson, R. (1996). Dialogue in public: Looking critically at the Buber-Rogers dialogue. In M. Friedman (Ed.), *Martin Buber and the human sciences* (pp. 191–206). Albany, NY: State University of New York Press.

Cissna, K. N., & Anderson, R. (1998). Theorizing about dialogic moments: The Buber-Rogers position and postmodern themes. *Communication Theory, 8,* 63–104.

Clark, H. R. (2002). WTO banana dispute settlement: Implications for trade relations between the United States and the European Union. *Cornell International Law Journal, 35,* 291–305.

Clarkson, M. B. E. (1995). A stakeholder framework for analyzing and evaluating corporate social performance. *Academy of Management Review, 20,* 1, 92–117.

Cleaver, F. (1999). Paradoxes of participation: questioning participatory approaches to development. *Journal of International Development, 11,* 4, 597–612.

Cleaver, H. (1982). Technology as political weaponry. In R. Anderson & B. Morrison (Eds.), *Science, politics and the agricultural evolution in Asia*. Boulder, CO: Westview, for the American Association for the Advancement of Science.

Cleaver, H. (1998). The Zapatista effect: The Internet and the rise of an alternative political fabric. *Journal of International Affairs, 5*, 621–640.

Cloud, D. (2001). Laboring under the sign of the new. *Management Communication Quarterly, 15*, 2, 268–278.

Cloud, D. (2005). Fighting words: Labor and the limits of communication at Staley, 1993 to 1996. *Management Communication Quarterly, 18*, 509–542.

Cloud, D. (2006). Change happens: Materialist dialectics and communication studies. In L. Artz, S. Macek, & D. Cloud (Eds.), *Marxism and communication studies: The point is to change it* (pp. 53–70). New York: Peter Lang.

Cloud, D. (2007). Corporate social responsibility as oxymoron: Universalization and exploitation at Boeing. In S. May, G. Cheney, & J. Roper (Eds.), *The debate over corporate social responsibility* (pp. 219–231). New York: Oxford University Press.

Coburn, A. F. (2002). Rural long-term care: What do we need to know to improve policy and programs? *Journal of Rural Health, 18*, 256–269.

Coburn, D. (2000). Income inequality, social cohesion and the health status of populations: The role of neoliberalism. *Social Science and Medicine, 51*, 135–146.

Coburn, D. (2004). Beyond the income inequality hypothesis: Class, neo-liberalism, and health inequalities. *Social Science and Medicine, 58*, 41–46.

Cockburn, A., St. Clair, J., & Sekula, A. (2000). *Five days that shook the world: Seattle and beyond.* London: Verso.

Cohen, C. J., & Dawson, M. (1993). Neighborhood poverty and African American politics. *American Political Science Review, 87*, 286–302.

Cohen-Cruz, J., & Schutzman, M. (2006). *A Boal companion: Dialogues on theatre and cultural politics.* London: Routledge.

Conquergood, D. (1986). Between experience and meaning: Performance as paradigm for meaningful action. In T. Colson (Ed.), *Renewal and revision: The future of interpretation* (pp. 26–59). Denton, TX: Omega.

Cooke, B., & Kothari, U. (Eds.) (2001). *Participation: The new tyranny?* (pp. 16–35). London: Zed.

Cornia, G. A., & Kiiski, S. (2001). *Trends in income distribution in the post-World War II period.* United Nations University: World Institute for Development Economics Research. Retrieved September 20, 2010 from http://website1.wider.unu.edu/publications/dps/dp2001-89.pdf

Couldry, N. (2003). *Media rituals: A critical approach.* New York: Routledge.

Couldry, N., & Curran, J. (2003a). *Media power: Alternative media in a networked world.* Oxford: Rowman & Littlefield.

Couldry, N., & Curran, J. (2003b). The paradox of media power. In N. Couldry & J. Curran (Eds.), *Contesting media power* (pp. 3–15). Lanham, MD: Rowman & Littlefield.

Cousineau, P. (2009). *Earth wisdom for a world in crisis* [interviews transcript]. Link TV. Retrieved October 12, 2010 from www.linktv.org/video/3824/earth-wisdom-for-a-world-in-crisis

Coyer, K., Dowmunt, T., & Fountain, A. (2007). *The alternative media handbook.* London: Routledge.

Curran, J., & Park, M. J. (2000). Beyond globalization theory. In J. Curran & M-J. Park (Eds.), *De-westernizing media studies* (pp. 3–18). New York: Routledge.

Dagdeviren, H., & Fine, B. (2004). *Privatization in the Asia-Pacific.* Draft thematic summary on privatization for the Asia-Pacific Regional Programme on the Macroeconomics of Poverty Reduction, May.

Daniels, N. (2008). *Just health: Meeting health needs fairly*. Cambridge: Cambridge University Press.

De, K. (2009). Lalgarh: An icon of adivasi defiance. *Racism and National Consciousness News/Commentary*, January 3. Retrieved March 1, 2010 from http://racismandnational consciousnessnews.wordpress.com/2009/01/03/lalgarh-an-icon-of-adivasi-defiance-koustav-de/

Deetz, S. (1992). *Democracy in an age of corporate colonization*. Albany, NY: State University of New York Press.

Deetz, S. (1995). *Transforming communication, transforming business: Building responsive and responsible workplaces*. Cresskill, NJ: Hampton.

Deetz, S., & Simpson, J. (2004). Critical organizational dialogue. Open formation and the demand of "otherness". In R. Anderson, L. A. Baxter, & K. N. Cissna (Eds.), *Dialogue: Theorizing difference in communication studies* (pp. 141–158). Thousand Oaks, CA: Sage.

della Porta, D. (2009). Global justice movement organizations: The organizational population. In D. della Porta (Ed.), *Democracy in social movements* (pp. 16–43). Basingstoke: Palgrave Macmillan.

della Porta, D., & Diani, M. (2006). *Social movements: An introduction*. Malden, MA: Blackwell.

della Porta, D., & Tarrow, S. (2005). *Transnational protest and global activism*. Oxford: Rowman & Littlefield.

della Porta, D., Kreisi, H., & Rucht, D. (Eds.) (1999). *Social movements in a globalizing world*. London: Macmillan.

Dellacioppa, K. Z. (2009). *This bridge called Zapatismo: Building alternative political cultures in Mexico City, Los Angeles, and beyond*. Lanham, MD: Rowman & Littlefield.

Denzin, N. (2003). *Performance ethnography: Critical pedagogy and the politics of culture*. New Delhi: Sage.

Desai, M. (2005). Transnationalism: The face of feminist politics post-Beijing. *International Social Science Journal*, *184*, 319–330.

Deshpande, S. (2007). *Theatre of the streets: The Jana Natya Manch experience*. New Delhi: Jana Natya Manch.

Desmarais, A. (2007). *La Via Campesina: Globalization and the power of peasants*. Halifax, NS: Fernwood.

DeSouza, R., Basu, A., Kim, I., Basnyat, I., & Dutta, M. (2008). The paradox of "fair trade": The influence of neoliberal trade agreements on food security and health. In H. M. Zoller & M. Dutta (Eds.), *Emerging perspectives in health communication: Interpretive, critical and cultural approaches* (pp. 411–430). Mahwah, NJ: Lawrence Erlbaum Associates.

Diani, M. (1996). Linking mobilization frames and political opportunities: Insights from regional populism in Italy. *American Sociological Review*, *61*, 1053–1069.

Diani, M. (2005). *Movements, networks, and social movement theory: What relevance for Middle-East societies?* Paper for the workshop Cooperation across Ideological Divides in the Middle East, Rockefeller Foundation, Bellagio, Italy, August 8–13.

Dietz, H. (1980). *Land invasion and consolidation: A study of working poor/governmental relations in Lima, Peru*. Austin, TX: University of Texas Press.

Dietz, H. (1998). *Urban poverty, political participation, and the state: Lima 1970–1990*. Pittsburgh, PA: University of Pittsburgh Press.

Dirlik, A. (1994). The postcolonial aura: Third World criticism in the age of global capitalism. *Critical Inquiry*, *20*, 328–356.

Dirlik, A. (1997). *The postcolonial aura: Third World criticism in the age of global capitalism*. Boulder, CO: Westview.

Dirlik, A. (2000). Globalization as the end and the beginning of history: The contradictory implications of a new paradigm. *Rethinking Marxism, 12*, 4–22.

Donk, W. V., Loader, B., Nixon, P., & Rucht, D. (Eds.) (2004). *Cyberprotest: New media, citizens, and social movements*. London: Routledge.

Downing, J. (2001). *Radical media: Rebellious communication and social movements*. Thousand Oaks, CA: Sage.

Downing, J. (2003). Audiences and readers of alternative media: The absent lure of the virtually unknown. *Media, Culture, and Society, 25*, 625–645.

Dreier, P. (1996). Community empowerment strategies: The limits and potential of community organizing in urban neighbourhoods. *Cityscape, 2*, 121–159.

Duncan, C. M. (2001). Social capital in America's poor rural communities. In S. Saegert, J. P. Thompson, & M. R. Warren (Eds.), *Social capital and poor communities* (pp. 60–88). New York: Russell Sage Foundation.

Dutta, M. (2006). Theoretical approaches to entertainment education: A subaltern critique. *Health Communication, 20*, 221–231.

Dutta, M. (2007). Communicating about culture and health: Theorizing culture-centered and cultural-sensitivity approaches. *Communication Theory, 17*, 304–328.

Dutta, M. (2008a). Participatory communication in entertainment education: A critical analysis. *Communication for Development and Social Change: A Global Journal, 2*, 53–72.

Dutta, M. (2008b). A critical response to Storey and Jacobson: The co-optive possibilities of participatory discourse. *Communication for Development and Social Change: A Global Journal, 2*, 81–90.

Dutta, M. (2008c). *Communicating health: A culture-centered approach*. Cambridge: Polity.

Dutta, M. (2009). Theorizing resistance: Applying Gayatri Chakravorty Spivak in public relations. In Ø. Ihlen, B. van Ruler, & M. Fredriksson (Eds.), *Social theory on public relations* (pp. 278–300). London: Routledge.

Dutta, M. (2010). Culture-centered interrogation of public relations in the global landscape. In K. Sriramesh (Ed.) *Culture approaches to public relations*. New York: Taylor & Francis.

Dutta, M. (in press). Public relations in a global context: Postcolonial thoughts. In N. Bardhan & K. Weaver (Eds.), *Public relations in global cultural contexts*. London: Routledge.

Dutta, M., & Basnyat, I. (2008a). Interrogating the Radio Communication Project in Nepal: The participatory framing of colonization. In H. Zoller & M. Dutta (Eds.), *Emerging perspectives in health communication: Interpretive, critical and cultural approaches* (pp. 247–265). Mahwah, NJ: Lawrence Erlbaum Associates.

Dutta, M., & Basnyat, I. (2008b). The Radio Communication Project in Nepal: A culture-centered approach to participation. *Journal of Health Education and Behavior, 35*, 4, 442–454.

Dutta, M., & Basnyat, I. (2008c). Rebuttal. The Radio Communication Project in Nepal: A culture-centered approach to participation. *Journal of Health Education and Behavior, 35*, 4, 445–460.

Dutta, M., & Basnyat, I. (2010). The Radio Communication Project in Nepal: Culture, power and meaning in constructions of health. In L. K. Khiun (Ed.), *Liberalizing, feminizing and popularizing health communications in Asia* (pp. 151–176). Burlington, VT: Ashgate.

Dutta, M., & Basu, A. (2007a). Health among men in rural Bengal: Approaching meanings through a culture-centered approach. *Qualitative Health Research, 17*, 38–48.

Dutta, M., & Basu, A. (2007b). Centralizing context and culture in the co-construction of health: Localizing and vocalizing health meanings in rural India. *Health Communication, 21*, 187–196.

Dutta, M., & Basu, A. (2008). Meanings of health: Interrogating structure and culture. *Health Communication, 23*, 560–572.

Dutta, M., & Pal, M. (2007). The Internet as a site of resistance: The case of the Narmada Bachao Andolan. In S. Duhe (Ed.), *New media and public relations* (pp. 203–215). New York: Peter Lang.

Dutta, M., & Pal, M. (2010). Public relations in a global context: Postcolonial thoughts. In N. Bardhan & K. Weaver (Eds.), *Public relations in global cultural contexts.* London: Routledge.

Dutta, M., Bodie, G. D., & Basu, A. (2008). Health disparity and the racial divide among the nation's youth: Internet as an equalizer? In A. Everett (Ed.), *MacArthur Foundation series on digital media and learning: Race and ethnicity* (pp. 175–197). Cambridge, MA: MIT Press.

Dutta-Bergman, M. (2004a). Poverty, structural barriers and health: A Santali narrative of health communication. *Qualitative Health Research, 14*, 1–16.

Dutta-Bergman, M. (2004b). The unheard voices of Santalis: Communicating about health from the margins of India. *Communication Theory, 14*, 237–263.

Dutta-Bergman, M. (2004c). An alternative approach to entertainment education. *Journal of International Communication, 10*, 93–107.

Dutta-Bergman, M. (2005a). Civil society and communication: Not so civil after all. *Journal of Public Relations Research, 17*, 3, 267–289.

Dutta-Bergman, M. (2005b). Theory and practice in health communication campaigns: A critical interrogation. *Health Communication, 18*, 2, 103–112.

Dutta-Bergman, M. (2006). U.S. public diplomacy in the Middle East: A critical approach. *Journal of Communication Inquiry, 30*, 102–124.

Edwards, B., & Foley, M. W. (2001). Civil society and social capital: A primer. In B. Edwards, M. W. Foley, & M. Diani (Eds.), *Beyond Tocqueville: Civil society and the social capital debate in comparative perspective* (pp. 1–14). Hanover, NH: University Press of New England.

Edwards, M., & Hulme, D. (1995). Introduction. In M. Edwards & D. Hulme (Eds.), *NGO performance and accountability: Beyond the magic bullet* (pp. 3–16). London: Earthscan.

Ehrlich, P. (1968). *The population bomb.* New York: Ballantine.

Eisenberg, E. M. (1990). Jamming: Transcendence through organizing. *Communication Research, 17*, 139–164.

Eisenberg, E. M. (1994). Dialogue as democratic discourse: Affirming Harrison. In S. A. Deetz (Ed.), *Communication Yearbook, 17* (pp. 275–284). Thousand Oaks, CA: Sage.

Eisenberg, E. M., & Goodall, H. L. (1997). *Organizational communication: Balancing creativity and constraint* (2nd ed.). New York: St. Martin's Press.

Ellinor, L., & Gerard, G. (1998). *Dialogue: Rediscover the transforming power of conversation.* New York: J. Wiley & Sons.

Ellis, C., & Bochner, A. (2000). Autoethnography, personal narrative, reflexivity. In N. K. Denzin & Y. Lincoln (Eds.), *The Sage handbook of qualitative research* (pp. 733–768). Thousand Oaks, CA: Sage.

England, K., & Ward, K. (2007). *Neoliberalization: States, networks, peoples.* Malden, MA: Wiley-Blackwell.

Escobar, A. (1995). *Encountering development: The making and unmaking of the Third World.* Princeton, NJ: Princeton University Press.

Escobar, P. (2003). The new labor market: The effects of the neoliberal experiment in Chile. *Latin American Perspectives, 30*, 70–78.

Esteva, G., & Suri, M. (1992). Grassroots resistance to sustainable development: Lessons from the banks of the Narmada. *Ecologist, 22*, 45–45.

Fair, J. E. (1989). 29 years of theory and research on media and development: The dominant paradigm impact. *Gazette, 44*, 129–150.

Fair, J. E., & Shah, H. (1997). Continuities and discontinuities in communication and development research since 1958. *Journal of International Communication, 4*, 2, 3–22.

Fanon, F. (1963). *The wretched of the Earth.* New York: Grove.

Fanon, F. (1968). *Black skin, white masks.* New York: Grove.

Farmer, P. (1988a). Bad blood, spoiled milk: Bodily fluids as moral barometers in rural Haiti. *American Ethnologist, 15*, 131–151.

Farmer, P. (1988b). Blood, sweat, and baseballs: Haiti in the West Atlantic system. *Dialectical Anthropology, 13*, 83–99.

Farmer, P. (1992). *AIDS and accusation: Haiti and the geography of blame.* Berkeley, CA: University of California Press.

Farmer, P. (1999). *Infections and inequalities: The modern plagues.* Berkeley, CA: University of California Press.

Farmer, P. (2003). *Pathologies of power: Health, human rights and the new war on the poor.* Berkeley, CA: University of California Press.

Farmer, P., & Bertrand, D. (2000). Hypocrisies of development and the health of the Haitian poor. In J. Kim, J. Millen, A. Irwin, & J. Gershman (Eds.), *Dying for growth: Global inequality and the health of the poor* (pp. 65–89). Monroe, ME: Common Courage Press.

Fernandez, L. A. (2008). *Policing dissent: Social control and the anti-globalization movement.* Rutgers, NJ: Rutgers University Press.

Ferree, M. M. (2006). Globalization and feminism: Opportunities and obstacles for activism in the global arena. In M. M. Ferree & A. M. Tripp (Eds.), *Global feminism: Transnational women's activism, organizing, and human rights* (pp. 3–23). New York: New York University Press.

Ferree, M. M., & Tripp, A. M. (Eds.) (2006). *Global feminism: Transnational women's activism, organizing, and human rights.* New York: New York University Press.

Ferrel, J. (2001). Reclaim the streets. In J. Ferrel, *Tearing down the streets: Adventures in urban anarchy* (pp. 131–141). New York: Palgrave.

Finley, M. (2003). The bitter with the sweet: The impact of the World Trade Organization's settlement of the banana trade dispute on the human rights of Ecuadorian banana workers. *New York Law School Review, 48*, 4, 815–846.

Fiszbein, A., & Lowden, P. (1999). *Working together for a change: Government, civic, and business partnerships for poverty reduction in Latin America and the Caribbean.* Washington, DC: Economic Development Institute of the World Bank.

Foley, M. W., McCarthy, J. D., & Chaves, M. (2001). Social capital, religious institutions, and poor communities. In S. Saegert, J. P. Thompson, & M. Warren (Eds.), *Social capital and poor communities* (pp. 215–245). New York: Russell Sage Foundation.

Food and Agriculture Organization (FAO). (1999). *FAOSTAT 98 (Food and Agriculture Organization, United Nations, Rome).* Rome: FAO.

Foster, S. (Ed.) (1996). *Corporealities: Dancing knowledge, culture and power.* New York: Routledge.

Fowler, A. (2000). Beyond partnership: Getting real about NGO relationships in the aid system. *IDS Bulletin of Development Studies, 31*, 3, 1–13.

Francis, P. (2001). Participatory development at the World Bank: The primacy of process. In B. Cooke & U. Kothari (Eds.), *Participation: The new tyranny?* (pp. 72–87). London: Zed.

Freire, P. (1970). *Pedagogy of the oppressed.* New York: Seabury.

Freire, P. (1973). *Education for critical consciousness*. New York: Continuum.

Frey, L., & Carragee, K. (2007). *Communication activism: Communication for social change*. Cresskill, NJ: Hampton.

Friedman D. (1992). *Empowerment: The politics of alternative development*. Oxford: Blackwell.

Gadamer, H. G. (1982). *Truth and method*. New York: Crossroad.

Gagliardi, P. (2006). A role for humanities in the formation of managers. In P. Gagliardi & B. Czarniawska (Eds.), *Management education and humanities* (pp. 3–9). Northampton: Edward Elgar.

Gamson, W. (1992). *Talking politics*. New York: Cambridge University Press.

Ganesh, S., Zoller, H., & Cheney, G. (2005). Transforming resistance, broadening our boundaries: Critical organizational communication meets globalization from below. *Communication Monographs, 72*, 169–191.

Garrido, M., & Halavais, A. (2003). Mapping networks of support for the Zapatista movement. In M. McCaughey & M. D. Ayers (Eds.), *Cyberactivism: Online activism in theory and practice* (pp. 165–184). New York: Routledge.

Gates Foundation (2008). *Off the beaten track: Avahan's experience in the business of prevention among India's long-distance truckers*. New Delhi: Bill & Melinda Gates Foundation.

Geertz, C. (1994). *Readings in the philosophy of social science*. Cambridge, MA: MIT Press.

George, S. (2001). *The global citizen's movement: A new actor for a new politics*. Paper presented at the Conference on Reshaping Globalization, Central European University, Budapest, October.

Gershman, J., & Irwin, A. (2000). Getting a grip on the global economy. In J. Y. Kim, J. V. Millen, A. Irwin, & J. Gershman (Eds.), *Dying for growth: Global inequality and the health of the poor* (pp. 11–43). Monroe, ME: Common Courage Press.

Gitlin, T. (1980). *The whole world is watching: Mass media in the making and unmaking of the New Left*. Los Angeles, CA: University of California Press.

Giugni, M. (2002). Examining cross-national similarities among social movements. In J. Smith & H. Johnston (Eds.), *Globalization and resistance: Transnational dimensions of social movements* (pp. 13–29). New York: Rowman & Littlefield.

Giugni, M. (2004). *Social protest and policy change: Ecology, antinuclear, and peace movements in comparative politics*. Lanham, MD: Rowman & Littlefield.

Giugni, M., McAdam, D., & Tilly, C. (Eds.) (1998). *From contention to democracy*. Lanham, MD: Rowman & Littlefield.

Giugni, M., McAdam, D., & Tilly, C. (Eds.) (1999). *How social movements matter*. Minneapolis, MN: University of Minnesota Press.

Godalof, I. (1999). *Against purity: Rethinking identity with Indian and Western feminisms*. New York: Routledge.

Goldman, R., & Rajagopal, A. (1991). *Mapping hegemony: Television news coverage of industrial conflict*. Norwood, NJ: Ablex.

Gollnick, B. (2008). *Reinventing the Lacandón: Subaltern representations in the rainforest of Chiapas*. Tucson, AZ: University of Arizona Press.

Gómez-Peña, G. (1993). *Warrior for Gringostroika*. St Paul, MN: Graywolf.

Gómez-Peña, G. (1996). *The new world border*. San Francisco, CA: City Lights.

Gómez-Peña, G. (2000). *Dangerous border crossers*. London: Routledge.

Gonzalez, C. G. (2002). Institutionalizing inequality: The WTO agreement on agriculture, food security, and developing countries. *Columbia Journal of Environmental Law, 27*, 447–449.

Griffin, K. (2003). Economic globalization and institutions of global governance. *Development and Change, 34*, 789–808.

Griffin, P. (2009). *Gendering the World Bank: Neoliberalism and the gendered foundations of global governance*. New York: Palgrave Macmillan.

Grignou, B., & Patou, C. (2004). Attac(k)ing expertise: Does the Internet really democratize knowledge? In W. V. Donk, B. Loader, P. Nixon, & D. Rucht (Eds.), *Cyberprotest: New media, citizens, and social movements* (pp. 164–179). London: Routledge.

Grunig, J., & Hunt, T. (1984). *Managing public relations*. New York: Holt, Rinehart & Winston.

Guha, R. (Ed.) (1981). *Subaltern studies I: Writings on South Asian history and society*. Delhi: Oxford University Press.

Guha, R. (Ed.) (1983). *Subaltern studies II: Writings on South Asian history and society*. Delhi: Oxford University Press.

Guha, R. (2001). Subaltern studies: Projects for our time and their convergence. In I. Rodríguez (Ed.), *The Latin American subaltern studies reader* (pp. 35–46). Durham, NC: Duke University Press.

Guha, R., & Spivak, G. (Eds.) (1988). *Selected subaltern studies*. New Delhi: Oxford University Press.

Guidry, J., Kennedy, M., & Zald, M. (2000). *Globalizations and social movements*. Ann Arbor, MI: University of Michigan Press.

Gumucio-Dagron, A., & Tufte, T. (Eds.) (2006). *Communication for social change anthology: Historical and contemporary readings*. South Orange, NJ: Communication for Social Change Consortium.

Habermas, J. (1989). *The theory of communicative action*. Boston, MA: Beacon.

Habermas, J. (1996a). *The philosophical discourse of modernity*. Cambridge, MA: MIT Press.

Habermas, J. (1996b). *Between facts and norms: Contributions to a discourse theory of law and democracy*. Cambridge, MA: MIT Press.

Hammond, C., Anderson, R., & Cissna, K. (2003). The problematics of dialogue and power. *Communication Yearbook*, *27*, 125–157.

Harman, E. S., & Chomsky, N. (1988). *Manufacturing consent: The political economy of the mass media*. New York: Pantheon.

Harris, R. L., & Seid, M. J. (2004). Globalization and health in the new millennium. *Perspectives on global development and technology*, *3*, 1–46.

Harter, L., Sharma, D., Pant, S., Singhal, A., & Sharma, Y. (2007). Catalyzing social reform through participatory folk performances in rural India. In L. Frey & K. Carragee (Eds.), *Communication and social activism* (pp. 285–314). Cresskill, NJ: Hampton.

Harter, L., Dutta, M. J., Ellingson, L., & Norander, S. (2009). The poetic is political . . . and other notes on engaged communication scholarship. In L.M. Harter & M. J. Dutta (Eds.), *Communicating for social impact: Engaging communication theory, research, and practice* (pp. 33–46). Cresskill, NJ: Hampton.

Harvey, D. (1995). Globalization in question. *Rethinking Marxism*, *8*, 1–17.

Harvey, D. (2001). City and justice: Social movements in the city. In D. Harvey, *Spaces of capital: Towards a critical geography* (pp. 188–207). London: Routledge.

Harvey, D. (2005). *A brief history of neoliberalism*. Oxford: Oxford University Press.

Hashmi, S. (2007). The first ten years of street theatre: October 1978–October 1988. In S. Deshpande (Ed.), *Theatre of the streets: The Jana Natya Manch experience* (pp. 11–16). Delhi: Jana Natya Manch.

Herman, E., & Chomsky, N. (1988). *Manufacturing consent: The political economy of the mass media*. New York: Pantheon.

Herrick, C. (2008). The Southern African famine and genetically modified food aid: The ramifications for the United States and European Union's trade war. *Review of Radical Political Economics*, *40*, 50–66.

Hindustan Times. (February 24, 2010). Moratorium on Bt Brinjal. *Hindustan Times.* Retrieved March 10, 2010 from www.hindustantimes.com/PM-upholds-moratorium-on-Bt-Brinjal/H1-Article1-512522.aspx

Holman Jones, S. (2005). Autoethnography: Making the personal political. In N. K. Denzin & Y. Lincoln (Eds.), *The Sage handbook of qualitative research* (pp. 763–791). Thousand Oaks, CA: Sage.

Hossfeld, K. J. (1990). "Their logic against them": Contradictions in sex, race, and class in silicon valley. In K. Ward (Ed.), *Women workers and global restructuring* (pp. 149–178). Ithaca, NY: ILR Press, School of Industrial and Labor Relations, Cornell University.

House, J. S., Landis, K. R., & Umberson, D. (1988). Social relationships and health. *Science, 241*, 540–545.

Hubbard, M. (2001). Attacking poverty: A strategic dilemma for the World Bank. *Journal of International Development, 13*, 293–298.

Hudec, R. E. (1988). Legal issues in US–EC trade policy: GATT litigation 1960–1985. NBER Chapters. In *Issues in US–EC Trade Relations* (pp. 15–64). National Bureau of Economic Research. Retrieved October 9, 2010 from www.nber.org/chapters/c5955.pdf.

India Together. (March 31, 2009). Suicides in Chattisgarh. Chattisgarh, *India Together.* Retrieved March 1, 2010 from www.indiatogether.org/2009/mar/agr-chsui.htm

Inkeles, A. (1966). The modernization of man. In M. Weiner (Ed.), *Modernization: The dynamics of growth* (pp. 138–150). New York: Basic Books.

Inkeles, A. (1969). Making men modern: On the causes and consequences of individual change in six countries. *American Journal of Sociology, 75*, 208–225.

Inter-American Development Board (IDB). (1997). *Economic and social progress in Latin America: Latin America after a decade of reforms.* Washington, DC: IDB.

Inter-American Development Board (IDB). (1998a). *Economic and social progress in Latin America.* Washington, DC: IDB.

Inter-American Development Board (IDB). (1998b). *Facing up to inequality in Latin America: Economic and social progress in Latin America 1998–1999 report.* Washington, DC: IDB.

Johnston, H. (2009). Protest cultures: Performance, artifacts, and ideations. In H. Johnston (Ed.), *Culture, social movements, and protest* (pp. 3–29). Burlington, VT: Ashgate.

Johnston, H., & Noakes, J. (2005). *Frames of protest: Social movements and the framing perspective.* Lanham, MD: Rowman & Littlefield.

Jones, M. (2003). Globalisation and the organisation(s) of exclusion. In S. Clegg & R. Westwood (Eds.), *Debating organisation theory* (pp. 265–271). London: Macmillan.

Josling, T. E., Tangermann, S., & Warley, T. K. (1996). *Agriculture in the GATT.* London: Macmillan.

Kabeer, N. (1994). *Reversed realities: Gender hierarchies in development thought.* London: Verso.

Kanbur, R. (1987). Measurement and alleviation of poverty: With an application to the effects of macroeconomic adjustment. *I.M.F. Staff Papers, 30*, 60–85.

Kanbur, R. (1990a). *Poverty and the social dimensions of structural adjustment in Cote d'Ivoire.* SDA Working Paper Series. Washington, DC: World Bank.

Kanbur, R. (1990b). Poverty and development: The Human Development Report and the World Development Report, 1990. In R. van der Hoeven and R. Anker (Eds.), *Poverty monitoring: An international concern* (pp. 1–27). New York: St. Martin's Press.

Kanbur, R., & Mukherjee, D. (2007). Premature mortality and poverty measurement. *Bulletin of Economic Research, 59*, 4, 339–359.

Kar, S. B., Alcalay, R., & Alex, S. (2001). *Health communication: A multi-cultural perspective.* Delhi: Sage.

Katz, N. & Kemnitzer, D. (1983). Fast forward: The internationalization of Silicon Valley. In J. Nash & M. Fernandez-Kelly (Eds.) *Women, men and the international division of labor* (pp. 332–345). Albany, NY: State University of New York Press.

Kawachi, I., & Kennedy, B. (1997). Health and social cohesion: Why care about income inequality? *British Medical Journal, 314*, 1037–1040.

Kawachi, I., & Wamala, S. (2007). Globalization and health: Challenges and prospects. In I. Kawachi & S. Wamala (Eds.), *Globalization and health*. New York: Oxford University Press.

Kawachi, I., Kennedy, B., Lochner, K., & Prothrow-Stith, D. (1997). Social capital, income inequality, and mortality. *American Journal of Public Health, 87*, 1491–1498.

Kawachi, I., Kennedy, B., & Wilkinson, R. (1999). *Income inequality and health: A reader.* New York: New Press.

Kawachi, I., Wilkinson, R., & Kennedy, B. (1999). *The society and population health reader: Income inequality and health*. New York: New Press.

Keck, M. E., & Sikkink, K. (1998). *Activists beyond borders: Advocacy networks in international politics*. Ithaca, NY: Cornell University Press.

Kelsey, J. (2005). *A people's guide to the Pacific's Economic Partnership Agreement*. Suva, Fiji: Women's Crisis Centre (WCC), March.

Kennedy, B., Kawachi, I., & Prothrow-Stith, D. (1996). Income distribution and mortality: Cross-sectional ecological study of the Robin Hood Index in the United States. *British Medical Journal, 312*, 1004–1007.

Keohane, R. O. (2002). *After hegemony: Cooperation and discord in the world political economy*. Princeton, NJ: Princeton University Press.

Kershaw, B. (1992). *The politics of performance: Radical theatre as cultural intervention*. London: Routledge.

Kessler, R. (2003). *The bureau: The secret history of the FBI*. New York: St. Martin's Press.

Kessler, R. (2004). *The CIA at war: Inside the secret campaign against terror*. New York: St. Martin's Press.

Kim, I. (2008). *Voices from the margin: A culture-centered look at public relations of resistance*. Unpublished doctoral dissertation, Purdue University, West Lafayette, IN.

Kim, I., & Dutta, M. (2009). Studying crisis communication from the subaltern studies framework: Grassroots activism in the wake of Hurricane Katrina. *Journal of Public Relations Research, 21, 2*, 142–164.

King, K. (1994). *Theory in its feminist travels: Conversations in US women's movements*. Bloomington, IN: Indiana University Press.

Klandermans, B., & de Weerd, M. (2000). Group identification and political protest. In S. Stryker, T. Owens, & R. White (Eds.), *Self, identity and social movements* (pp. 66–90). Minneapolis, MN: University of Minnesota Press.

Kolankiewicz, G. (1996). Social capital and social change. *British Journal of Sociology, 47*, 427–441.

Korten, D. C. (1995). *When corporations rule the world*. Bloomfield, CT: Kumarian.

Korten, D. C. (1999). *The post-corporate world*. San Francisco, CA: Kumarian.

Kreps, G. (2005). Disseminating relevant information to underserved audiences: Implications from the Digital Divide Projects. *Journal of the Medical Library Association, 93*, S68–S73.

Kreuter, M. W., & Haughton, L. T. (1996). Integrating culture into health information for African American women. *American Behavioral Scientist, 49*, 794–811.

Kreuter, M. W., & McClure, S. M. (2004). The role of culture in health communication. *Annual Review of Public Health, 25*, 439–455.

Krog, A., Mpolweni-Zantsi, N., & Ralete, K. (2008). The South African Truth and Reconciliation Commission (TRC): Ways of knowing Mrs. Konile. In N. Denzin, Y. Lincoln, & L. Tuhiwai Smith (Eds.), *Handbook of critical and indigenous methodologies* (pp. 531–545). Thousand Oaks, CA: Sage.

Kuh, D. H., & Cooper, C. (1992). Physical activity at 36 years: Patterns and childhood predictors in a longitudinal study. *Journal of Epidemiology and Community Health, 46*, 114–119.

Kuh, D. H., & Wadsworth, M. E. J. (1993). Physical status at 36 years in a British national birth cohort. *Social Science and Medicine, 37*, 905–916.

Kumar, D. (2001). Mass media, class, and democracy: The struggle over newspaper representation of the UPS strike. *Critical Studies in Media Communication, 18*, 285–302.

Labonte, R. (2001). Globalization and reform of the World Trade Organization. *Canadian Journal of Public Health, 92*, 4, 248–249.

Labonte, R., & Torgerson, R. (2002). *Frameworks for analyzing the links between globalization and health.* Saskatoon, SK: University of Saskatchewan.

Lal, V. (2001). Subaltern studies and its critics: Debates over Indian history. *History and Theory, 40*, 135–148.

Lal, V. (2005). Travails of the nation. *Third Text, 19*, 177–187.

Landry, D., & MacLean, G. (Eds.) (1996). *The Spivak reader: Selected works of Gayatri Chakravorty Spivak* (pp. 15–28). New York: Routledge.

Lappé, F. M., Collins, J., & Rosset, P., with L. Esparza (1998). *World hunger. Twelve myths* (2nd ed.). New York: Grove.

Lappé, M., & Bailey, B. (1998). *Against the grain: Biotechnology and the corporate takeover of your food.* Monroe, ME: Common Courage Press.

Lefebure, P., & Lagneau, E. (2002). Le Moment volvorde: Action protestataire et espace publique européen. In R. Balme & D. Chabanet (Eds.), *L'Action collective en Europe* (pp. 495–529). Paris: Presses de Sciences.

Lepecki, A. (2006). *Exhausting dance: Performance and the politics of movement.* New York: Routledge.

Lerner, D. (1958). *The passing of traditional society.* Glencoe, IL: Free Press.

Lerner, D. (1964). The transformation of institutions. In W. B. Hamilton (Ed.), *The transfer of institutions* (pp. 1–26). Durham, NC: Duke University Press.

Lerner, D. (1967). International cooperation and communication in national development. In D. Lerner & W. Schramm (Eds.), *Communication and change in the developing countries* (pp. 103–125). Honolulu, HI: East-West Center Press.

Lerner, D. (1968). *The passing of traditional society: Modernizing the Middle East.* New York: Free Press.

Lerner, D. (1969). *Communication and change in the developing countries.* Honolulu, HI: East-West Center Press.

Lerner, D. (1976). International cooperation and communication in national development. In D. Lerner & W. Schramm (Eds.), *Communication and change in the developing countries* (pp. 103–125). Honolulu, HI: East-West Center Press.

Lewis, S. J., Kaltofen, M., & Ormsby, G. (1991). *Border trouble: Rivers in peril. A report on water pollution due to industrial development in Northern Mexico.* Boston, MA: National Toxics Campaign Fund.

Lofland, J. (1996). *Social movement organizations: Guide to research on insurgent realities.* Hawthorne, NY: Walter de Gruyter.

Lopez, M. L., & Stack, C. B. (2001). Social capital and the culture of power: Lessons from the field. In S. Saegert, J. P. Thompson, & M. R. Warren (Eds.), *Social capital and poor communities* (pp. 31–59). New York: Russell Sage Foundation.

Lora, E. (2001). *Structural reforms in Latin America: What has been reformed and how to measure it.* Inter-American Development Bank Working Paper 466. Washington, DC: Inter-American Development Bank.

Lora, E., & Panizza, U. (2002). *Structural reforms in Latin America under scrutiny.* Inter-American Development Bank Working Paper 470. Washington, DC: Inter-American Development Bank.

Lucero, J. A. (2008). *Struggles of voice: The politics of indigenous representation in the Andes.* Pittsburgh, PA: University of Pittsburgh Press.

Maciunas, G. (1965). *Manifesto on art/Fluxus art amusement.* Retrieved February 26, 2010 from www.artnotart.com/fluxus/gmaciunas-artartamusement.html

Madeley, J. (1999). *Big business, poor peoples: The impact of transnational corporations on the world's poor.* London: Zed.

Madeley, J. (2000). *Hungry for trade.* London: Zed.

Mahadevia, D. (2002). The impact of structural adjustment programme on land and water resources of Gujarat. In V. Shiva & G. Bedi (Eds.), *Sustainable agriculture and food security: The impact of globalization* (pp. 121–160). New Delhi: Sage.

Majid, A. (2000). *Unveiling traditions: Postcolonial Islam in a polycentric world.* Durham, NC: Duke University Press.

Majid, A. (2008). The postcolonial bubble. In R. Krishnaswamy & G. C. Hawley (Eds.), *The postcolonial and the global* (pp. 134–155). Durham, NC: Duke University Press.

Marmot, M. (2005). Social determinants of health inequalities. *The Lancet, 365,* 1099–1104.

Martin, R. (1998). *Critical moves: Dance studies in theory and politics.* Durham, NC: Duke University Press.

Marx, K. (1970). *Critique of the Gotha program.* New York: International.

Marx, K. (1975). *Early writings.* London: Penguin.

Marx, K. (2007). *Das Kapital.* Synergy International of the Americas.

McAdam, D., & Rucht, D. (1993). The cross-national diffusion of movement ideas. *Annals of the American Academy of Political and Social Sciences, 528,* 56–74.

McAdam, D., McCarthy, J., & Zald, M. (Eds.) (1996a). *Comparative perspectives in social movements: Political opportunities, mobilizing structures, and cultural framings.* Cambridge: Cambridge University Press.

McAdam, D., McCarthy, J., & Zald, M. (1996b). Introduction: Opportunities, mobilizing structures and framing processes. In D. McAdam, J. McCarthy, & M. Zald (Eds.), *Comparative perspectives in social movements: Political opportunities, mobilizing structures, and cultural framings* (pp. 1–20). Cambridge: Cambridge University Press.

McCaslin, W., & Breton, D. (2008). Justice as healing: Going outside the colonizers' cage. In N. Denzin, Y. Lincoln, & L. Tuhiwai Smith (Eds.), *Handbook of critical and indigenous methodologies* (pp. 511–529). Thousand Oaks, CA: Sage.

McChesney, R. W. (1997). *Corporate media and the threat to democracy.* New York: Seven Stories Press.

McKay, G. (1996). *Senseless acts of beauty: Cultures of resistance since the sixties.* London: Verso.

McKinley, T. (2004). *Economic policies for growth and poverty reduction: PRSPs, neoliberal conditionalities and "post-consensus" alternatives.* Paper presented at the International Conference on the Economics of New Imperialism, New Delhi, India.

McMichael, A. J., & Beaglehole, R. (2000). The changing global context of public health. *The Lancet, 356,* 495–499.

McMichael, P. (2005). Global development and the corporate food regime. In T. Marsden (Ed.), *Research in rural sociology and development, 11,* 265–299.

McMichael, P. (2008). *Development and social change: A global perspective.* New Delhi: Sage.

McPhail, C., & McCarthy, J. D. (2004). Who counts and how: Estimating the size of protests. *Contexts, 3,* 12–18.

McPhail, C., & McCarthy, J. D. (2005). Protest mobilization, protest repression, and their interaction. In C. Davenport, H. Johnston, & C. Mueller (Eds.), *Repression and mobilization* (pp. 3–32). Minneapolis, MN: University of Minnesota Press.

Melkote, S. (2000). Reinventing development support communication to account for power and control in development. In K. Wilkins (Ed.), *Redeveloping communication for social change: Theory, practice, and power* (pp. 39–53). Lanham, MD: Rowman & Littlefield.

Melkote, S., & Steeves, L. (2001). *Communication for development in the Third World.* New Delhi: Sage.

Melucci, A. (1996). *Challenging codes: Collective action in the information age.* Cambridge: Cambridge University Press.

Menon-Sen, K. (2001). The problem: Toward equality. A symposium on women, feminism, and women's movements. *Seminar, 505,* 12–15.

Meur, M. (2000). Are markets like mushrooms? And other neoliberal quandaries. *Review of Radical Political Economics, 32,* 461–469.

Meyer, D., & Staggenborg, S. (1996). Movements, countermovements, and the structure of political opportunity. *American Journal of Sociology, 101,* 1628–1660.

Mies, M. (1982). *The lace makers of Narsapur: Indian housewives produce for the world market.* London: Zed.

Mies, M. (1986). *Patriarchy and accumulation on a world scale.* London: Zed.

Mike, E. (July 11, 2009). *Revolution in India: Lalgarh's hopeful spark.* Retrieved March 8, 2010 from http://kasamaproject.org/2009/07/11/sam-shell-lagarhs-hopeful-spark/

Milanovic, B. (2005). *Worlds apart: Measuring international and global inequality.* Princeton, NJ: Princeton University Press.

Millen, J., & Holtz, T. (2000). Dying for growth, Part I: Transnational corporations and the health of the poor. In J. Y. Kim, J. V. Millen, A. Irwin, & J. Gershman (Eds.), *Dying for growth: Global inequality and the health of the poor* (pp. 177–223). Monroe, ME: Common Courage Press.

Millen, J., Irwin, A., & Kim, J. (2000). Introduction: What is growing? Who is dying? In J. Y. Kim, J. V. Millen, A. Irwin, & J. Gershman (Eds.), *Dying for growth: Global inequality and the health of the poor* (pp. 3–10). Monroe, ME: Common Courage Press.

Miller, M. J. (2006). Biodiversity policy making in Costa Rica: Pursuing indigenous and peasant rights. *Journal of Environment Development, 15,* 359–381.

Miraftab, F. (2004). Public-private partnerships: The Trojan Horse of neoliberal development? *Journal of Planning Education and Research, 24,* 89–101.

Miyoshi, M. (2005). The university, the universe, the world, and "globalization". *Australasian Journal of Process Thought, 6,* 29–41.

Moghadam, V. (2009). *Globalization and social movements.* Lanham, MD: Rowman & Littlefield.

Mohanty, C. (2006). *Feminism without borders: Decolonizing theory, practicing solidarity.* Durham, NC: Duke University Press.

Montefiore, J. (1995). *Feminism and poetry.* London: Pandora.

Moraga, C., & Anzaldua, G. (Eds.) (1981). *This bridge called my back: Writings of radical women of color.* Watertown, MA: Persephone.

Mosley, P. (2001). Attacking poverty and the "Post-Washington consensus." *Journal of International Development, 13,* 3, 307–314.

Mosse, D. (2001). People's knowledge, participation and patronage: Operations and representations in rural development. In B. Cooke & U. Kothari (Eds.), *Participation: The new tyranny?* (pp. 16–35). London: Zed.

Mouffe, C. (1993). *The return of the political.* London: Verso.

Moure-Eraso, R., Wilcox, M., & Punnett, L., et al. (1994). Back to the future: Sweatshop conditions on the Mexico–US border I. Community health impact of Maquiladora industrial activity. *American Journal of Industrial Medicine, 25,* 311–324.

Moure-Eraso, R., Wilcox, M., & Punnett, L., et al. (1997). Back to the future: Sweatshop conditions on the Mexico–US border II. Community health impact of Maquiladora industrial activity. *American Journal of Industrial Medicine, 31,* 587–599.

Muñoz Ramírez, G. (2008). *The fire and the word: A history of the Zapatista movement.* San Francisco, CA: City Lights.

Munshi, D., & Kurian, P. (2007). The case of the subaltern public: A postcolonial investigation of corporate social responsibility's (o)missions. In S. May, G. Cheney, & J. Roper (Eds.), *The debate over corporate social responsibility* (pp. 438–447). New York: Oxford University Press.

Mychalejko, C., & Ryan, R. (2009). US military funded mapping project in Oaxaca: Geographers used to gather intelligence? *Z Magazine, 22,* 17–22.

Naples, N., & Desai, M. (2002). Women's local and translocal responses: An introduction to the chapters. In N. Naples & M. Desai (Eds.), *Women's activism and globalization* (pp. 11–33). New York: Routledge.

Narayan, D., & Petesch, P. (2002). *Voices of the poor: From many lands.* Washington, DC: World Bank.

Narayan, D., Patel, R., Schafft, K., Rademacher, A., & Koch-Schulte, S. (1999a). *Dying for change: Poor people's experience of health and ill-health.* Washington DC: World Bank.

Narayan, D., Patel, R., Schafft, K., Rademacher, A., & Koch-Schulte, S. (1999b). *Voices of the poor: Can anyone hear us?* Washington, DC: World Bank.

National Crime Records Bureau. (1998). *Accidental deaths and suicide in India.* New Delhi: National Crime Records Bureau. Ministry of Home Affairs, Government of India.

Navarro, V. (1999). Health and equity in the world in the era of "globalization." *International Journal of Health Services, 29,* 215–226.

Navlakha, G. (2010). Days and nights in Maoist heartland. *Economic and Political Weekly, 15,* 38–47.

Negt, O., & Kluge, A. (1993). *Public sphere and experience: Towards an analysis of the bourgeois and proletarian public sphere.* Minneapolis, MN: University of Minnesota Press.

Nixson, F., & Walters, B. (2003). *Privatization, income distribution and poverty: Mongolian experience.* Sydney: Asia-Pacific Press.

Noakes, J. A., & Johnston, H. (2005). Frames of protest: A road map to a perspective. In H. Johnston & J. Noakes (Eds.), *Frames of protest: Social movements and the framing perspective* (pp. 1–29). Lanham, MD: Rowman & Littlefield.

Oakley, P., Bichmann, W., & Rifkin, S. (1999). CIH: Developing a methodology. In H. M. Kahssey & P. Oakley (Eds.), *Community involvement in health development: A review of the concept and practice* (pp. 114–144). Geneva: World Health Organization.

O'Brien, R., Goetz, A., Schotle, J., & Williams, M. (2000). *Contesting global governance: Multilateral economic institutions and global social movement.* Cambridge: Cambridge University Press.

Oguamanam, C. (2007). Tensions on the farm fields: The death of traditional agriculture? *Bulletin of Science Technology Society, 27,* 260–273.

Olivera, O., with Lewis, T. (2004). *Cochabamba! Water war in Bolivia.* Cambridge, MA: South End Press.

O'Sullivan, T. (1994). *Key concepts in communication and cultural studies.* New York: Routledge.

Padhi, R., Pradhan, P., & Manjit, D. (2010). How many more arrests will Orissa see? *Economic and Political Weekly, 45,* 10, 24–26.

Pal, M. (2008). *Fighting from and for the margin: Local activism in the realm of global politics.* Unpublished doctoral dissertation, Purdue University, West Lafayette, IN.

Pal, M., & Dutta, M. (2008a). Public relations in a global context: The relevance of critical modernism as a theoretical lens. *Journal of Public Relations Research, 20,* 159–179.

Pal, M., & Dutta, M. (2008b). Theorizing resistance in a global context: Processes, strategies and tactics in communication scholarship. *Communication Yearbook, 32,* 41–87.

Papa, M. J., Singhal, A., & Papa, W. H. (2006). *Communication for social change: A dialectic journey of theory and praxis.* New Delhi: Sage.

Payer, C. (1974). *The debt trap: The IMF and the Third World.* New York: Monthly Review Press.

Peet, R. (2003). *Unholy trinity: The IMF, the World Bank, and the WTO.* London: Zed.

Pezzullo, P. (2004). Toxic tours: Communicating the "presence" of chemical contamination. In S. Depoe, J. Delicath, & M. Aepli Elsenbeer (Eds.), *Communication and public participation in environmental decision making* (pp. 235–254). New York: State University of New York Press.

Pogge, T., & Reddy, S. (2006). Unknown: Extent, distribution and trend of global income poverty. *Economic and Political Weekly, 41,* 2241–2247. Retrieved October 1, 2010 from www.socialanalysis.orf

Pollack, A. (2001). Cross-border, cross-movement alliances in the late 1990s. In P. Hamel, J. Lustier-Thaler, N. Pieterse, & S. Roseneil (Eds.), *Globalization and social movements* (pp. 183–205). Basingstoke: Palgrave Macmillan.

Polletta, F. (2006). *It was like a fever: Storytelling in protest and politics.* Chicago, IL: University of Chicago Press.

Porter, G. (2003). NGOs and poverty reduction in a globalizing world: Perspectives from Ghana. *Progress in Development Studies, 3,* 131–145.

Portes, A. (1976). On the sociology of national development: Theories and issues. *American Journal of Sociology, 82,* 1, 55–85.

Potter, B. (2007). Constricting contestation, coalitions, and purpose: The causes of neoliberal restructuring and its failures. *Latin American Perspective, 34,* 3–24.

Prakash, G. (1992). Postcolonial criticism and Indian historiography. *Social Text, 31–32,* 8–19.

Prakash, G. (1994). *After colonialism: Imperial histories and postcolonial displacements.* Princeton, NJ: Princeton University Press.

Prasad, A. (2003). *Postcolonial theory and organizational analysis: A critical engagement.* New York: Palgrave Macmillan.

Prasad, A. (2009). Capitalizing disease: Biopolitics of drug trials in India. *Theory, Culture, and Society, 26,* 1–29.

Putnam, R. (1993). *Making democracy work: Civic transitions in modern Italy.* Princeton, NJ: Princeton University Press.

Putnam, R. (1995). Bowling alone: America's declining social capital. *Journal of Democracy, 6,* 65–78.

Rahnema, M. (1993). Poverty. In W. Sachs (Ed.), *The development dictionary: A guide to knowledge as power* (pp. 158–176). London: Zed.

Raina, V. (2004). Political diversity, common purpose: Social movements in India. In F. Polet (Ed.), *Globalizing resistance: The stage of struggle* (pp. 3–14). London: Pluto.

Rajagopal, B. (2003). *International law from below: Development, social movements, and third world resistance*. Singapore: Cambridge University Press.

Reagon, B. J. (1975). *Songs of the civil rights movement, 1955–1965: A study in culture history*. PhD dissertation, Howard University, Washington, DC.

Reclaim the Streets. (n.d.). *Privatization of public space*. Retrieved February 26, 2010 from http://rts.gn.apc.org/prop05.htm

Reclaim the Streets. (n.d.). *Won't the streets be better without cars?* Retrieved February 26, 2010 from http://rts.gn.apc.org/prop07.htm

Reddy, S., & Pogge, T. W. (2007). How *not* to count the poor. In S. Anand & J. Stiglitz (Eds.), *Measuring global poverty*. Oxford: Oxford University Press. Retrieved October 2, 2010 from www.socialanalysis.org

Reed, T. V. (2005). *The art of protest: Culture and activism from the civil rights movement to the streets of Seattle*. Minneapolis, MN: University of Minnesota Press.

Reimann, K. D. (2002). Building networks from the outside in: Japanese NGOs and the Kyoto Climate Change Conference. In J. G. Smith, J. Smith, & H. Johnston (Eds.), *Globalization and resistance: Transnational dimensions of social movements* (pp. 173–190). Lanham, MD: Rowman & Littlefield.

Robertson, R. (1992). *Globalization: Social theory and global culture*. London: Sage.

Robins, K. (2000). En-countering globalisation. In D. Held & A. Mc Grew (Eds.), *The great globalisation debate: An introduction*. Cambridge: Polity.

Robinson, W. I. (2009). Globalization and the sociology of Immanuel Wallerstein: A critical appraisal. *Sociological Analysis, 3*, 75–95.

Rodgers, G. B. (1979). Income and inequality as determinants of mortality: An international cross-section analysis. *Population Studies, 33*, 2, 343–351.

Rodríguez, C. (2001). *Fissures in the mediascape: An international study of citizens' media*. Cresskill, NJ: Hampton.

Rodríguez, C. (2003). The bishop and his star: Citizens' communication in Southern Chile. In N. Couldry & J. Curran (Eds.), *Contesting media power: Alternative media in a networked world* (pp. 177–194). Oxford: Rowman & Littlefield.

Rodríguez, I. (2001). Reading subalterns across texts, disciplines, and theories: From representation to recognition. In I. Rodríguez (Ed.), *The Latin American subaltern studies reader* (pp. 35–46). Durham, NC: Duke University Press.

Rogers, E. M. (1962). *Diffusion of innovations*. New York: Free Press.

Rogers, E. M. (1971). *Social change in rural society*. Englewood Cliffs, NJ: Prentice Hall.

Rogers, E. M. (1973). *Communication strategies for family planning*. New York: Free Press.

Rogers, E. M. (1974). Communication in development. *Annals of the American Academy of Political and Social Science, 412*, 44–54.

Rogers, E. M. (1983). *Diffusion of innovations*. New York: Free Press.

Rogers, E. M. (1995). *Diffusion of innovations*. New York: Free Press.

Rogers, E. M. (2003). *Diffusion of innovations*. Singapore: Free Press.

Rogers, E. M., & Svenning, L. (1969). *Modernization among peasants: The impact of communication*. New York: Holt, Rinehart, & Winston.

Rose, H. (2001). Epilogue: Women's work is never done. In M. Lederman & I. Bartsch (Eds.), *The gender and science reader* (pp. 483–490). London: Routledge.

Ross, J. (1995). *Rebellion from the roots: Indian uprising in Chiapas*. Monroe, ME: Common Courage Press.

Rossem, R. V. (1996). The world-system paradigm as general theory of development: A cross-national test. *American Sociological Review, 61*, 508–527.

Rothman, F., & Oliver, P. (1999). From local to global: The anti-dam movement in southern Brazil. *Mobilization: An International Quarterly, 4*, 41–57.

Rothman, F., & Oliver, P. (2002). From local to global: The anti-dam movement in Southern Brazil, 1979–1992. In J. Smith & H. Johnston (Eds.), *Globalization and resistance: Transnational dimensions of social movements* (pp. 115–149). Lanham, MD: Rowman & Littlefield.

Routledge, P. (1993). *Terrains of resistance: Nonviolent social movements and the contestation of place*. Westport, CT: Praeger.

Routledge, P. (2000). "Our resistance will be as transnational as capital": Convergence space and strategy in globalizing resistance. *Geo Journal, 52*, 25–33.

Runyan, A. S. (1999). Women in the neoliberal "frame." In M. K. Meyer & E. Prugl (Eds.), *Gender politics in global governance* (pp. 210–220). Lanham, MD: Rowman & Littlefield.

Ryan, B., & Gross, N. (1943). The diffusion of hybrid seed corn in two Iowa communities. *Rural Sociology, 8*, 15–24.

Sachs, J. (2005). *The end of poverty: Economic possibilities for our time*. New York: Penguin.

Sachs, W. (1992). *The development dictionary*. London: Zed.

Saegert, S., Thompson, J. P., & Warren, M. R. (Eds.) (2001). *Social capital and poor communities*. New York: Russell Sage Foundation.

Said, E. (1979) *Orientalism*. Vintage.

Said, E. (1988). Foreword. In R. Guha & G. C. Spivak (Eds.), *Selected subaltern studies* (pp. v–xii). New York: Oxford University Press.

Sainath, P. (February 3, 2010). Farm suicides: A 12-year saga. *India Together*. Retrieved March 2, 2010 from www.indiatogether.org/2010/feb/psa-suicides.htm

Sanger, K. (1995). *When the spirit says sing! The role of freedom songs in the civil rights movement*. New York: Garland.

Santos, B., & Rodríguez-Garavito, C. A. (2005). *Law and globalization from below: Towards a cosmopolitan legality*. Cambridge: Cambridge University Press.

Sassen, S. (1988). *The mobility of labor and capital: A study in international investment and labor flow*. Cambridge: Cambridge University Press.

Sastry, S., & Dutta, M. (in press). Postcolonial deconstructions of US media portrayals of HIV/AIDS in India. *Health Communication*.

Sawyer, S. (2006). Disabling corporate sovereignty in a transnational lawsuit. *PoLAR: Political and Legal Anthropology Review, 29*, 23–43.

Schramm, W. (1964). *Mass media and national development*. Stanford, CA: Stanford University Press.

Schramm, W. (1968). *Communication satellites for education, science, and culture*. Paris: Unesco.

Schramm, W., & Lerner, D. (1976). *Communication and change: The last ten years and the next*. Honolulu, HI: University Press of Hawaii.

Schulz, M. (1998). Collective action across borders: Opportunity structures, network capacities, and communicative praxis in the age of advanced globalization. *Sociological Perspectives, 4*, 597–610.

Seidman, G. (2000). Adjusting the lens. In J. A. Guidry, M. D. Kennedy, & M. B. Zald (Eds.), *Globalizations and social movements: Culture, power, and the transnational public sphere* (pp. 339–357). Ann Arbor, MI: University of Michichigan Press.

Sen, A. (1988). *On ethics and economics*. Malden, MA: Blackwell.

Sen, A. (1992). *Inequality re-examined*. Oxford: Clarendon Press.

Sen, A. (1999). *Development as freedom*. Oxford: Oxford University Press.

Sen, A. (2005a). Human rights and capabilities. *Journal of Human Development, 6,* 151–166.

Sen, A. (2005b). *Culture and captivity*. Address to the Fifth Annual Conference of the Human Development and Capability Association, Unesco, Paris, September 11.

Shakow, A., & Irwin, A. (2000). Terms reconsidered: Decoding development discourses. In J. Y. Kim, J. V. Millen, A. Irwin, & J. Gershman (Eds.), *Dying for growth: Global inequality and the health of the poor* (pp. 44-61). Monroe, ME: Common Courage Press.

Sharma, A. (2008). *Logics of empowerment: Development, gender, and governance in neoliberal India*. Minneapolis, MN: University of Minnesota Press.

Shepherd, A. (2001). Consolidating the lessons of 50 years of development. *Journal of International Development, 13,* 315–320.

Shiva, V. (1988). Reductionist science as epistemic violence. In A. Nandy (Ed.), *Science, hegemony, and violence*. New Delhi: Oxford University Press.

Shiva, V. (1989). *Staying alive: Women, ecology, and development*. London: Zed.

Shiva, V. (1991). *The violence of the green revolution: Third World agriculture, ecology and politics*. London: Zed.

Shiva, V. (2000). *Stolen harvest: The hijacking of the global food supply*. Cambridge, MA: South End Press.

Shiva, V. (2001). Democratizing biology: Reinventing biology from a feminist, ecological, and Third World perspective. In M. Lederman & I. Bartsch (Eds.), *The gender and science reader* (pp. 447–465). London: Routledge.

Shiva, V. (2002). Seeds of suicide: The ecological and human cost of globalization of agriculture. In V. Shiva & G. Bedi (Eds.), *Sustainable agriculture and food security: The impact of globalization* (pp. 169–183). New Delhi: Sage.

Shiva, V. (2005). *Earth democracy: Justice, sustainability and peace*. Cambridge, MA: South End Press.

Shiva, V. (2007). *Wheat biopiracy: The real issues the government is avoiding*. Retrieved May 15, 2010 from www.zcommunications.org/wheat-biopiracy-the-real-issues-the-government-is-avoiding-by-vandana2-shiva.pdf

Shiva, V. (January 12, 2010). Press statement on Bt. Brinjal and GM foods. Retrieved March 1, 2010 from www.navdanya.org/news/81-press-statement-on-bt-brinjal-a-gm-foods

Shiva, V., & Bedi, G. (2002). *Sustainable agriculture and food security: The impact of globalization*. New Delhi: Sage.

Shiva, V., & Jafri, A. H. (2003). *Failure of the GMOs in India*. Retrieved March 1, 2010 from www.mindfully.org/GE/2003/India-GMO-Failure-Shiva31may03.htm

Shiva, V., Anderson, P., Schücking, H., Gray, A., Lohmann, L., & Cooper, D. (1991). *Biodiversity: Social and ecological perspectives*. London: Zed.

Shiva, V., Jafri, A. H., Emani, A., & Pande, M. (2002). *Seeds of suicide: The ecological and human costs of globalization stone, biotechnology and suicide in India of agriculture* (Rev. ed.). New Delhi: Research Foundation for Science, Technology and Ecology.

Shome, R., & Hegde, S. R. (2002). Postcolonial approaches to communication: Charting the terrain, engaging the intersections. *Communication Theory, 12,* 249–270.

Simpson, J. L. (2008). The color-blind double bind: Whiteness and the (im)possibility of dialogue. *Communication Theory, 18,* 139–159.

Singhal, A. (2001). *Facilitating community participation through communication*. New York: Unicef.

Singhal, A. (2004). Entertainment education through participatory theater: Frierean strategies for empowering the oppressed. In A. Singhal, M. Cody, E. Rogers, &

M. Sabido (Eds.), *Entertainment education and social change: History, research, and practice.* Mahwah, NJ: Lawrence Erlbaum Associates.

Smith, C. (February, 2004). "Whose streets?" Urban social movements and the politicization of social movements. In J. Holland & L. Hunter (Eds.), *Proceedings of the Second Annual Canadian Association of Cultural Studies Conference.* Retrieved February 26, 2009 from www.culturalstudies.ca/proceedings04/proceedings.html

Smith, J. (2002). Globalizing resistance: The Battle of Seattle and the future of social movements. In J. Smith & H. Johnston (Eds.), *Globalization and resistance: Transnational dimensions of social movements* (pp. 207–228). Lanham, MD: Rowman & Littlefield.

Smith, J., & Johnston, H. (2002). Globalization and resistance: An introduction. In J. Smith & H. Johnston (Eds.), *Globalization and resistance: Transnational dimensions of social movements* (pp. 1–10). Lanham, MD: Rowman & Littlefield.

Snow, D. A., & Benford, R. D. (1988). Ideology, frame resonance, and participant mobilization. *International Social Movement Research, 1,* 197–217.

Snow, D. A., & Benford, R. D. (1992). Master frames and cycles of protest. In A. Morris & C. M. Mueller (Eds.), *Frontiers of social movement theory* (pp. 133–155). New Haven, CT: Yale University Press.

Snow, D. A., & Benford, R. D. (1998). Ideology, frame resonance, and participant mobilization. *International Social Movement Research, 1,* 197–218.

Snow, D. A., Rochford, B., Worden, S. K., & Benford, R. D. (1986). Frame alignment processes, micromobilization, and movement participation. *American Sociological Review, 51,* 464–481.

Speidel, J. J., Sinding, S., Gillespie, D., Maguire, E., & Neuse, M. (2009) *Making the case for US international family planning.* Retrieved September 30, 2010 from www.jhsph.edu/gatesinstitute/pdf/policy_practice/Papers/MakingtheCase.pdf

Spivak, G. C. (1988). Can the subaltern speak? In G. Nelson & L. Grossberg (Eds.), *Marxism and the interpretation of culture* (pp. 120–130). Urbana, IL: University of Illinois Press.

Spivak, G. C. (1996). Bonding in difference: Interview with Alfred Arteaga. In D. Landry & G. MacLean (Eds.), *The Spivak reader: Selected works of Gayatri Chakravorty Spivak* (pp. 15–28). New York: Routledge.

Spivak, G. C. (1999). *A critique of postcolonial reason: Toward a history of the vanishing present.* Cambridge, MA: Harvard University Press.

Spivak, G. C. (2003). *Death of a discipline.* New York: Columbia University Press.

St. Clair, A. (2004a). The role of ideas in the United Nations Development Programme. In M. Boas & D. McNeill (Eds.), *Global institutions and development: Framing the world?* (pp. 178–192). London: Routledge.

St. Clair, A. (2004b). *Ideas in action: Human development and capability as boundary objects.* Working Paper, Department of Sociology, University of Bergen, Norway.

St. Clair, A. (2006a). The World Bank as a transnational expertise institution. *Global Governance, 12,* 77–95.

St. Clair, A. (2006b). Global poverty: The co-production of knowledge and politics. *Global Social Policy, 6,* 57–77.

Staggenborg, S. (1986). Coalition work in the pro-choice movement: Organization and environmental opportunities and obstacles. *Social Problems, 33,* 374–390.

Staggenborg, S. (1988). Consequences of professionalization and formalization in the pro-choice movement. *American Sociological Review, 53,* 585–606.

Staggenborg, S. (1989). Stability and innovation in the women's movement. *Social Problems, 36,* 75–92.

Staggenborg, S. (1991). *The Pro-Choice Movement.* New York: Oxford University Press.

Starr, A. (2005). *Global revolt: A guide to the movements against globalization.* London: Zed.

Statham, L. (February 20, 2009). Indigenous mining dialogue group not a silver bullet. *The Independent Weekly.* Retrieved March 16, 2010 from www.independentweekly.com.au/news/local/news/general/indigenousminning-dialogue-group-not-a-silver-bullet-acf/1439732.aspx?storypage=0

Stolle-McAllister, J. (2005). *Mexican social movements and the transition to democracy.* Jefferson, NC: McFarland.

Storey, D., & Jacobson, T. (2004). Entertainment-education and participation: Applying Habermas to a population program in Nepal. In A. Singhal, M. Cody, E. Rogers, & M. Sabido (Eds.), *Entertainment education and social change* (pp. 377–397). Mahwah, NJ: Lawrence Erlbaum Associates.

Strati, A. (1999). *Organization and aesthetics.* London: Sage.

Strati, A. (2007). Sensible knowledge and practice-based learning. *Management Learning, 38,* 1, 61–77.

Swaminathan, M. S. (1983). *Science and the conquest of hunger.* Delhi: Concept.

Sweeney, G. (1993). Irish hunger strikes and the cult of self-sacrifice. *Journal of Contemporary History, 28,* 421–437.

Swiderska, K., Daño, E., & Dubois, O. (2001). *Developing the Philippines' Executive Order no. 247 on access to genetic resources.* London: International Institute for Environment and Development.

Swidler, A. (1986). Cultural power and social movements. In H. Johnston & B. Klandermans (Eds.), *Social movements and culture* (pp. 25–39). Minneapolis, MN: University of Minnesota Press.

Switzer, J. V. (2001). *Environmental politics: Domestic and global dimensions* (3rd ed.). Boston, MA: Bedford/St. Martins.

Tarrow, S. (1992). Mentalities, political cultures, and collective action frames: Constructing meanings through action. In A. D. Morris & C. M. Mueller (Eds.), *Frontiers in social movement theory* (pp. 174–202). New Haven, CT: Yale University Press.

Tarrow, S. (1993). Cycles of collective action: Between moments of madness and the repertoire of contention. *Social Science History, 17,* 281–307.

Tarrow, S. (1998). *Power in movement: Social movements and contentious politics.* Cambridge: Cambridge University Press.

Tarrow, S. (2005). *The new transnational activism.* Cambridge: Cambridge University Press.

Tarrow, S., & della Porta, D. (2005). Conclusion: Globalization, complex internationalism, and transnational contention. In D. della Porta & S. Tarrow (Eds.), *Transnational protest and global activism* (pp. 227–246). Lanham, MD: Rowman & Littlefield.

Teune, S. (2005). *Art and the re-invention of political protest.* Paper presented at the Third ECPR Conference, Budapest.

Thomas, H. (2003). *The body, dance, and cultural theory.* New York: Palgrave Macmillan.

Tiejun, W. (2001). Centenary reflections on the "three dimensional problem" of rural China. *Inter-Asia Cultural Studies, 2,* 2, 287–295.

Tihuwai Smith, L. (2006). *Decolonizing methodologies: Research and indigenous peoples.* New York: Zed.

Tilly, C. (1978). *From mobilization to revolution.* Reading, MA: Addison-Wesley.

Tomaselli, K., Dyll, L., & Francis, M. (2008). "Self" and "other": Auto-reflexive and indigenous ethnography. In N. Denzin, Y. Lincoln, & L. Tuhiwai Smith (Eds.), *Handbook of critical and indigenous methodologies* (pp. 347–372). Thousand Oaks, CA: Sage.

Tomlinson, J. (1991). *Cultural imperialism.* Baltimore, MD: Johns Hopkins University Press.

Tomlinson, M. R. (1999). From rejection to resignation: Beneficiaries' views on the South African government's new housing subsidy system. *Urban Studies, 36*, 8, 13–49.

Touraine, A. (1985). An introduction to the study of social movements. *Social Research, 52*, 749–787.

Trade and Environment Database (TED). (1998). *TED Case Studies: Basmati*. Last update 1998. Retrieved May 15, 2010 from www.american.edu/TED/Basmati.htm

Trade and Environment Database (TED). (2005). *Basmati: TED Case Study*. Retrieved August 10, 2010 from www.american.edu/TED/basmati.htm

UNDESA (2010). *The state of the world's indigenous peoples*. New York: Department of Economic and Social Affairs, Division for Social Policy and Development, Secretariat of the Permanent Forum on Indigenous Issues, United Nations.

United Nations (UN). (1947). *General Agreement on Tariffs and Trade*. Geneva: UN.

United Nations Development Programme (UNDP). (2004). *Human Development Report*. New York: Oxford University Press.

United States Agency for International Development (USAID). (1997). *New partnership initiative: A strategic approach in development*. Washington, DC: USAID.

United States Agency for International Development (USAID). (1998). Making a world of difference one family at a time. *Global Issues, 3*, 33–35.

United States Agency for International Development (USAID). (2002a). *Foreign Aid in the National Interest: Promoting Freedom, Security, and Opportunity*. Washington, DC: USAID.

United States Agency for International Development (USAID). (2002b). *Tools for alliance builders*. Washington, DC: USAID.

Valocchi, S. (2005). Collective action frames in the gay liberation movement, 1969–1973. In H. Johnston & J. A. Noakes (Eds.), *Frames of protest: Social movements and the framing perspective* (pp. 53–68). Lanham, MD: Rowman & Littlefield.

Verheul, E., & Cooper, G. (2001). *Poverty reduction strategy papers: What is at stake for health*. April 2001, 48RAP01001, Wemos. Retrieved December 3, 2002 from www.wemos.nl

Via Campesina Women's Working Group. (1996). *Report of the Via Campesina Women's Working Group Meeting*. San Salvador, El Salvador, August 6–8.

Via Campesina Women's Working Group. (1999). *Peasant women on the frontiers of food sovereignty: The Via Campesina Women's Working Group*. Final report to PROWID, June. Saskatoon, SK: NFU (National Farmers Union, Canada).

Vienet, R. (1967). Die Situationisten und die neuen Aktionsformen gegen Politik und Kunst. In *Der Beginn einer Epoche. Texte der Situationisten* (pp. 242–247). Hamburg: Edition Nautilus.

Volo, L. (2000). Global and local framing of maternal identity: Obligation and the mothers of Matagalpa, Nicaragua. In J. Guidry, M. Kennedy, & M. N. Zald (Eds.), *Globalizations and social movements: Culture, power, and the transnational public sphere* (pp. 127–146). Ann Arbor, MI: University of Michigan Press.

Wagner, D., & Cohen, M. B. (1991). The power of the people: Homeless protesters in the aftermath of social movement participation. *Social Problems, 38*, 543–561.

Waldman, R. J. (1992). Income distribution and infant mortality. *Quarterly Journal of Economics, 107*, 1283–1302.

Wallerstein, I. (1974). *The modern world system*. New York: Academic Press.

Wallerstein, I. (1997). Eurocentrism and its avatars. *New Left Review, 226*, 93–107.

Wallerstein, I. (2004). *World systems analysis: An introduction*. Durham, NC: Duke University Press.

Wallerstein, I. (2006). *European universalism: The rhetoric of power*. New York: New Press.

Walton, J., & Seddon, D. (1994). *Free markets and food riots*. New York: Academic Press.

Waltz, M. (2005). *Alternative and activist media.* Edinburgh: Edinburgh University Press.

Warkentin, C. (2001). *Reshaping world politics: NGOs, the internet and global civil society.* Lanham, MD: Rowman & Littlefield.

Warren, M. R. (1998). Community building and political power. *American Behavioral Scientist, 42,* 78–92.

Warren, M. R. (2001). *Dry bones rattling: Community building to revitalize American Democracy.* Princeton, NJ: Princeton University Press.

Weber, M. (1958). *The Protestant ethic and the spirit of capitalism.* New York: Charles Scribner's Sons.

Weber, M. (1964). *The sociology of religion.* Boston, MA: Beacon.

Weber, M. (1988). *The Protestant ethic and the spirit of capitalism.* New York: Charles Scribner and Sons.

Whitehead, K. (1996). *The feminist poetry movement.* Jackson, MS: University Press of Mississippi.

Wilkins, K. (Ed.) (2000). *Redeveloping communication for social change: Theory, practice, power.* Lanham, MD: Rowman & Littlefield.

Wilkinson, R. G. (1986a). Socio-economic differences in mortality: Interpreting the data on their size and trends. In R. G. Wilkinson (Ed.), *Class and health* (pp. 1–20). London: Tavistock.

Wilkinson, R. G. (1986b). Income and mortality. In R. G. Wilkinson (Ed.), *Class and health* (pp. 88–114). London: Tavistock.

Wilkinson, R. G. (1992a). Income distribution and life expectancy. *British Medical Journal, 304,* 165–168.

Wilkinson, R. G. (1992b). National mortality rates: The impact of inequality? *American Journal of Public Health, 82,* 1082–1084.

Wilkinson, R. G. (1996). *Unhealthy societies: The afflictions of inequality.* New York: Routledge.

Wilkinson, R. G. (2005). *The impact of inequality: How to make sick societies healthier.* New York: New Press.

Williams, D. R. (1999). Race, socioeconomic status, and health: The added effects of racism and discrimination. *Annals of the New York Academy of Sciences, 896,* 173–188.

Wong, K-F. (2003). Empowerment as a panacea for poverty: Old wine in new bottles? Reflections on the World Bank's conception of power. *Progress in Development Studies, 3,* 307–322.

Wood, R., Hall, D. M., & Hasian, M. A. (2008). The human genome diversity project: A case study in health activism. In H. M. Zoller & M. Dutta (Eds.), *Emerging perspectives in health communication* (pp. 431–446). New York: Routledge.

Woods, M. (2002). Food for thought: The biopiracy of jasmine and basmati rice. *Albany Law Journal of Science and Technology, 13,* 123–143.

World Bank. (2000a). *Transforming development: New approaches to developing country-owned poverty reduction strategies,* March 2000. Retrieved December 3, 2002 from www.world bank.org/poverty/

World Bank. (2000b). *Draft guidelines for participation in PRS and IPRS in the ECA region.* Retrieved December 3, 2002 from www.worldbank.org/participation/ECAPRSPs.htm

World Bank. (2000c). *Background on poverty reduction strategies.* Retrieved December 3, 2002 from www.worldbank.org/poverty/strategies/backgr.htm

World Bank. (2001). *Press release: Nicaragua to receive US$4.5 billion under the enhanced HIPC initiative, World Bank and IMF open way for debt relief.* News Release no. 2001/188/S. Washington, DC: World Bank.

World Bank. (2002). *Poverty reduction strategy source book*. Retrieved February 2, 2010 from http://siteresources.worldbank.org/INTPRS1/Resources/383606-1205334112622/13839_chap7.pdf

World Health Organization (WHO). (2003). *World Health Report 2003: Shaping the future*. Geneva: WHO.

World Health Organization (WHO). (2008). *World Health Report 2008: Social determinants of health*. Geneva: WHO.

World Trade Organization (WTO). (1994). *World Trade Agreement 1994*. Retrieved September 28, 2010 from www.jus.uio.no/lm/wta.1994/

World Trade Organization (WTO). (2005). *Understanding the WTO—Agriculture: Fairer markets for farmers*. Retrieved September 28, 2005 from www.wto.org

Yearley, S., & Forrester, J. (2000). Shell: A sure target for global environmental campaigning? In R. Cohen & S. M. Rai (Eds.), *Global social movements* (pp. 134–145). New Brunswick, NJ: Athlone.

Zoller, H. M. (2003). Health on the line: Identity and disciplinary control in employee occupational health and safety discourse. *Journal of Applied Communication Research, 31*, 2, 118–139.

Zoller, H. M. (2004). Dialogue as global issue management: Legitimizing corporate influence in the Transatlantic Business Dialogue. *Management Communication Quarterly, 18*, 2, 204–240.

Zoller, H. M. (2005). Health activism: Communication theory and action for social change. *Communication Theory, 15*, 341–364.

Zoller, H. M. (2006). Suitcases and swimsuits: On the future of organizational communication. *Management Communication Quarterly, 19*, 661–666.

Zoller, H. M., & Dutta, M. (2008a). Introduction: Communication and health policy. In H. M. Zoller & M. Dutta (Eds.), *Emerging perspectives in health communication: Interpretive, critical and cultural approaches* (pp. 358–364). Mahwah, NJ: Lawrence Erlbaum Associates.

Zoller, H. M., & Dutta, M. (2008b). Afterword: Emerging agendas in health communication and the challenge of multiple perspectives. In H. M. Zoller & M. Dutta (Eds.), *Emerging perspectives in health communication: Interpretive, critical and cultural approaches* (pp. 449–463). Mahwah, NJ: Lawrence Erlbaum Associates.

INDEX

Page numbers followed by 'n' refer to notes.

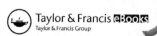